Alvaro Della Bona

Bonding to ceramics:

scientific evidences for clinical dentistry

2009

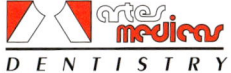

DENTISTRY

Bonding to ceramics:

scientific evidences for clinical dentistry

Alvaro Della Bona

2009

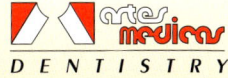

DENTISTRY

Bonding to ceramics: scientific evidences for clinical dentistry

ISBN 978-85-367-0091-5

Dados Internacionais de Catalogação na Publicação (CIP)
(Câmara Brasileira do Livro, SP, Brasil)

Edition

Editora Artes Médicas Ltda.

Publishing Director

Milton Hecht

Production Manager

Fernanda Matajs

Editorial Production / Cover

Júnior Bianchi

Illustrations

Cibele Santos

Printing

Gráfica RR Donnelley

Bona, Alvaro Della
    Bonding to ceramics : scientific evidences for
clinical dentistry / Alvaro Della Bona.
-- São Paulo : Artes Médicas, 2009.

    Bibliografia.
    ISBN 978-85-367-0091-5

    1. Cerâmica dentária   2. Odontologia clínica
3. Odontologia – Estética   4. Materiais dentários
5. Prótese dentária 6. Restaurações dentárias
I. Título.

08-11274   CDD-617.675
                                                  NLM-WU 360

Índices para catálogo sistemático:
1. Restaurações estéticas com cerâmicas :
        Odontologia   617.675

Editora Artes Médicas Ltda.

R. Dr. Cesário Motta Jr, 63 - Vila Buarque - 01221-020 - São Paulo - SP - Brasil

www.artesmedicas.com.br - artesmedicas@artesmedicas.com.br

Tel.: 55 11 3221-9033 - Fax: 55 11 3223-6635

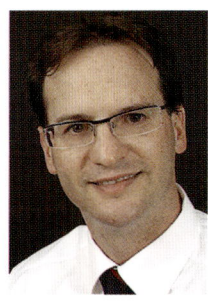

Alvaro Della Bona,
DDS, MMedSci, PhD, FADM

- Doctor of Dental Science at the University of Passo Fundo, RS, Brazil (1987).

- Preceptorship in Restorative Dentistry at the University of Texas Health Science Center at San Antonio, TX, USA (1992).

- Master of Medical Science in Restorative Dentistry at the University of Sheffield, UK (1994).

- Postgraduate Visiting Fellow in Dental Biomaterials at the University of Otago, New Zealand (1996).

- Doctor of Philosophy in Materials Science & Engineering at the University of Florida, USA (2001).

- Senior Professor at the Dental School, University of Passo Fundo, RS, Brazil.

- Vice-President of the Academy of Dental Materials (ADM).

- Chair of the IADR Ethics in Research Committee.

Preface

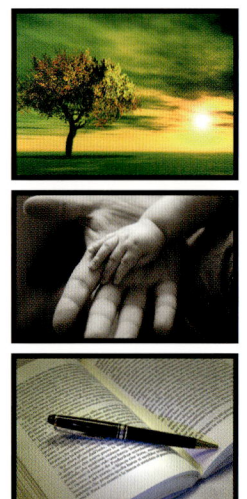

There is an adage I used to hear from my dad as a child: "There are three important things for a man in life: planting a tree, having a child and writing a book". Most people even say that this sequence of events is in the proper order, based on experience and responsibility. I was taught how to preserve the land and plant trees very early at school and enjoy passing that along to my children now. Writing a book is also a lengthy process closely associated with the desire for learning and teaching. As I am engaging in all the "important things", I feel the need to plant more "trees"…

Writing this book was a long, cumulative process involving learning, research laboratories, clinical experience and, most important, collaboration with outstanding people. So, part of this book is the result of international collaboration and the subsequent scientific research studies published in noted international journals, while the other part is evidence-based information illustrated by clinical procedures.

Interaction with many researchers in universities and industry around the world created the foundation for this project which endeavors to present the principles of matter, describing, from the atom to the structure, the basic properties of ceramics thereby providing a basis by which to understand the applications and failures of this material. Additionally, this book describes the importance between: (1) basic principles and properties as well as the development of experiments to obtain and/or test them; (2) ceramic microstructures, properties and failures; (3) in vitro experiments and clinical applications; and (4) properties and material selection according to the clinical application.

Therefore, this book is intended to enhance understanding for students, researchers and clinicians, to expand their knowledge in appropriate experimental design, in selecting an adequate ceramic material based on the clinical application, and in examining clinical failures, thereby improving materials, structures, designs, and clinical performance, which is, after all, the main evidence of a material's clinical success.

About the Author

James B Summitt, DDS, MS
Professor and Chairman
Department of Restorative Dentistry
University of Texas Health Science Center
at San Antonio
Author of the book "Fundamentals of
Operative Dentistry: a Contemporary
Approach".

Alvaro Della Bona is an amazingly energetic dentist, dental researcher, and dental educator, with a thirst for knowledge and understanding of his profession like no other individual I have ever known. I was fortunate to get to know and work with him shortly after he completed his dental school education. He came to San Antonio, Texas for a preceptorship in restorative dentistry at the University of Texas Health Science Center Dental School. I was amazed at his dedication and depth of understanding then, but he has continued his quest for more knowledge, and he has already contributed more in his relatively young life than most of us will in our entire professional lives.

Although his main areas of study and contribution have been in ceramics and the bonding of ceramic restorations, he has a vast knowledge of all of restorative dentistry, including endodontics, and of other areas of dentistry. His research contributions have been related to bonded direct restorations and endodontics as well as bonded ceramics. He is an outstanding mentor and friend to many. Everyone I know who has had the opportunity to work with him, including his mentors and his graduate school program director, has grown to have great admiration, respect, and fondness for him.

His passion for his profession, though tremendous, does not surpass his passion for God and for his family. He has a wonderful, beautiful wife and two terrific children, and his love for them and for God is apparent in each communication I have with him. He is one of those remarkable individuals who is able to maintain excellent balance in the important things in life.

Since I know him, his drive, and his depth of knowledge and understanding, and knowing his ability as a writer, I am confident that his book will be very beneficial for students, practitioners, and researchers, and I am looking forward with great anticipation to becoming familiar with it.

About the Author

Richard van Noort,

BSc, DPhil, DSc, FAD, FRSA
Professor in Dental
Materials Science
Department of Adult Dental Care
University of Sheffield
Author of the book
"Introduction to Dental Materials".

I first got to know Alvaro Della Bona back in 1992 when he joined our Masters Programme as a fresh young man, enthusiastic and thirsty for knowledge. He was a most exemplary student, and I would not be overstating the case by saying that he was one of the best students I have ever had the pleasure to work with. Unusually his research project was of such quality that we managed to get it published in the prestigious Journal of Dental Research. From the first day we met he impressed me with his enthusiasm, dedication, his hard work and his rapid grasp of new ideas and concepts in clinical dentistry. It was therefore no surprise to me that he should seek to carve out a career where research would have a high profile, which, I am pleased to say, he has done very successfully.

Alvaro Della Bona is a very engaging, likeable young man, who is well respected in the dental materials research community where he has worked with a number of well respected dental materials researchers.

This experience has allowed him to develop a worldwide reputation for research in dental ceramics and thus it comes as no surprise that he should at some point write a book on dental ceramics, something for which he is now eminently qualified. The process of writing a text book is a serious challenge as it requires a depth of knowledge and understanding well beyond what is being written about. I know Alvaro has the wherewithal to do exactly that and the time is right for him to meet this challenge head on and I am sure the reader will be in for a real treat. I know that I am looking forward to seeing the fruits of his labour.

About the Author

Dr. Simon E. Northeast
Specialist and Lecturer in
Restorative Dentistry
Department of Adult Dental Care
University of Sheffield
Sheffield, UK

Among the first students to study for the Master of Medical Science degree at Sheffield University was a confident and humorous young man from Brazil. Fresh from a Preceptorship in Texas, Dr Della Bona was keen to develop his clinical and research skills. Alvaro was an outstanding student, engendering respect and admiration from peers and tutors alike thanks to his breadth of knowledge, mature thinking, strong character and wit. Alvaro combined a sound academic background with exceptional clinical and practical skills which impressed all who worked with him. Sheffield University Dental School adopted resin bonded ceramic techniques from their outset and I can confidently say we provided one of the platforms from which Alvaro launched his clinical and academic career in ceramics and bonding. His later studies worldwide in New Zealand and Florida provided further foundations for carrying out independent research and skilled clinical practice focusing on adhesive ceramics. This provides an impetus to challenge and develop new materials and clinical techniques, something which benefits all dental practitioners.

As an experienced practitioner and internationally respected researcher in dental ceramics, the logical step for Alvaro was to collate and condense this vast experience into a book for the global benefit of the dental profession. I am sure Alvaro has risen to this challenge with the same dedication and enthusiasm which is his trademark. I am keen to read the finished product, providing an essential guide to recent research behind the ubiquitous all-ceramic dental restorations.

About the Author

Ken Anusavice, Ph.D.,
D.M.D., FADM, FACD
Distinguished Professor and Chair
Department of Dental Biomaterials
Associate Dean for Research
University of Florida
Author of the book "Phillips'
Science of Dental Materials".

I have known Alvaro Della Bona since 1998 when he became a Ph.D. student at the University of Florida (UF). During this time I co-chaired his Ph.D. committee with Dr. Jack Mecholsky of the Department of Materials Science and Engineering. Alvaro completed his Ph.D. in a remarkably short time period of 3.5 years. He received his PhD degree in 2001. This is amazing since most of our Ph.D. students require five or six years to complete their degrees at UF. What is even more remarkable is the fact that he published 10 peer-reviewed articles and translations of two of these articles, all of which were derived from his Ph.D. dissertation.

Alvaro received a Certificate of Award for Academic Achievement as an International Student in 1999 at University of Florida and he received the Paffenbarger Award from the Academy of Dental Materials in 2000. Dr. Della Bona has completed at least five years of leadership through research, training, service, and/or education beyond formal education. He has served on the Ethics in Research Committee of the International Association for Dental Research (IADR) from 2003 to the present and he will have served as Chair of this committee from 2007 to 2009. In addition, he has served on a similar committee in the Brazilian Division of the IADR. He is a scientist-educator of the highest ethical and moral character. He is an honest, conscientious, caring, and empathic team player who can be counted on to assist in research and to support professional organizations with the high energy and passion for which he is well known.

Alvaro places his highest priority on his family but this love of family is difficult to differentiate from his love of friends and their families. It is my belief that he sees us as part of his family. He keeps track of the progress of our families and shares in our celebrations as well as rare periods of sadness. He is one of the most empathic individuals I have ever met. He always reaches out to those that are disadvantaged but at the same time he celebrates the achievements of others who are blessed with good fortune and health.

I am positive that Alvaro's pursuit of excellence that is exhibited in his professional career will extend into the same high quality and excellence reflected in this book. His unique insights into what is important in scientific research and the dental profession will undoubtedly be transferred to a book of high value to dental educators, oral health scientists, and practicing dentists.

Acknowledgements

This book is based on knowledge gathered during the Preceptorship program in Restorative Dentistry at the University of Texas Health Science Center at San Antonio (UTHSCSA), U.S.A. with Dr. James B. Summitt and Dr. Nasser Barghi and sponsored by the Rotary Foundation; followed by the Master of Medical Science (MMedSci) program in Restorative Dentistry at the University of Sheffield, UK, with Dr. Richard van Noort and Dr. Simon E. Northeast; the postgraduate visiting fellowship at the University of Otago, New Zealand, with Dr. James A. A. Hood (*in memoriam*); and, mainly, during the PhD program in Materials Science and Engineering at the University of Florida (UF), USA, with Dr. Kenneth J. Anusavice and Dr. John J. Mecholsky Jr. I am very grateful to each of my mentors for providing me numerous hours of guidance, sage advice, and thought-provoking discussion. They have my continued admiration, respect, and friendship.

I also extend my gratitude to others that have helped me appreciably along this journey: Dr. Tom Berry, Dr. José dos Santos Jr. and Dr. John O Burgess, at UTHSCSA; Dr. Chiayi Shen, Dr. Tomas J. Hill, Allyson A. Barrett and Mr. Robert "Ben" Lee, at UF; Dr. Luisa Amelia Dempere and Mr. Wayne Acree at MAIC-UF; Dr. Paul H. DeHoff at UNCC; Dr. J Robert Kelly at UCHC, and Dr. Jason Griggs at UMMC.

My thanks for the support and understanding of my colleagues at the University of Passo Fundo, particularly to Mr. Carlos A. Kochenborger, Mr. Tadeu da Rocha Pereira and Mr. Armando J. Antonio.

Most of the ceramic restorations shown in this book were made by the author and/or Mr. Ireno T. Britto at Coral Dental Laboratory. Thanks Britto for the excellent work and for the long lasting work relation.

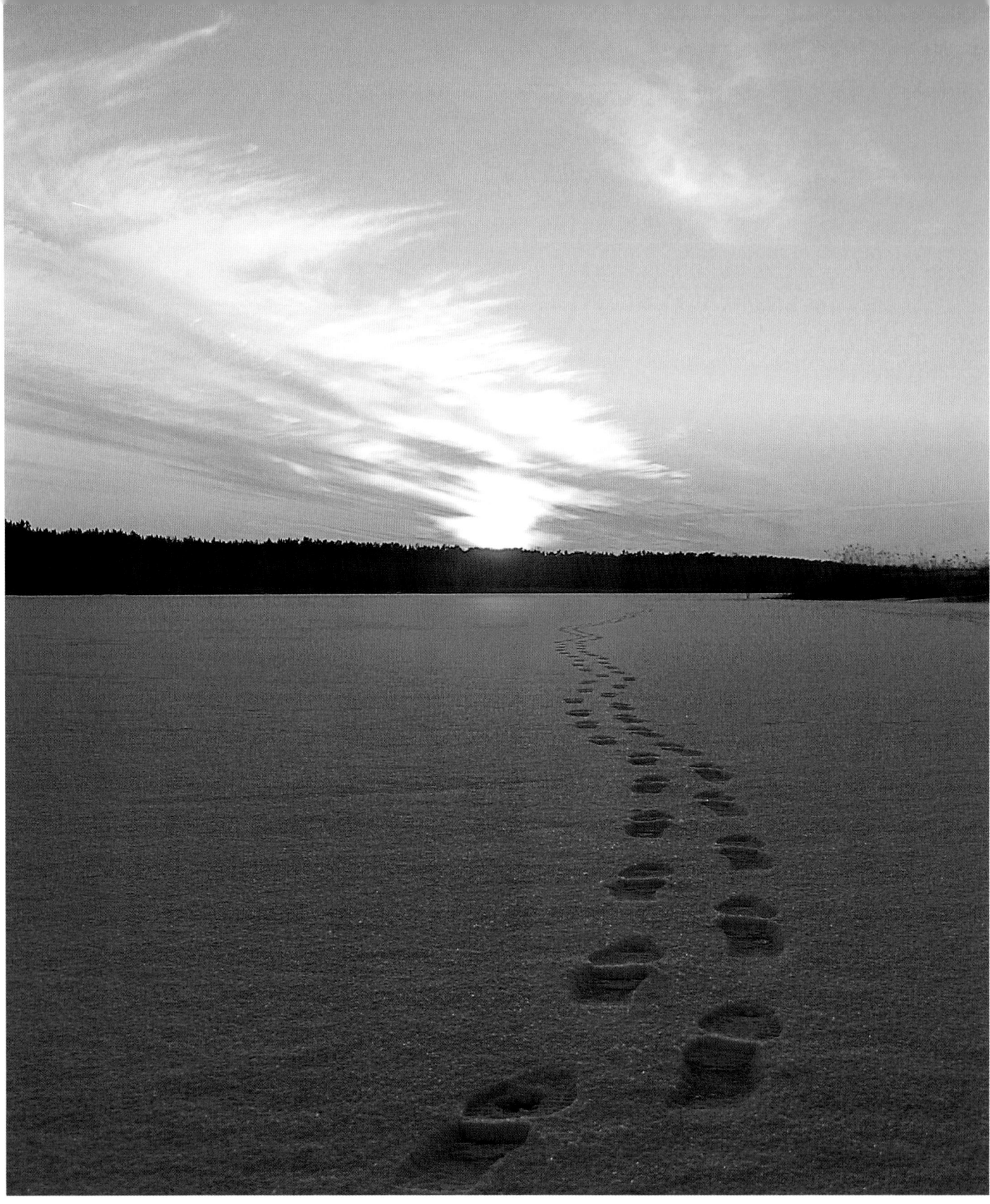

To my parents, **Carlos** and **Zelima**, and sister, **Carla**,

for teaching me to appreciate love, joy and kindness.

And to my wife, **Carla**, and our children, **Izadora** and **Diogo**,

for giving me the gift to continue sharing these feelings.

Contents

Chapter *1*

History and development of dental ceramics

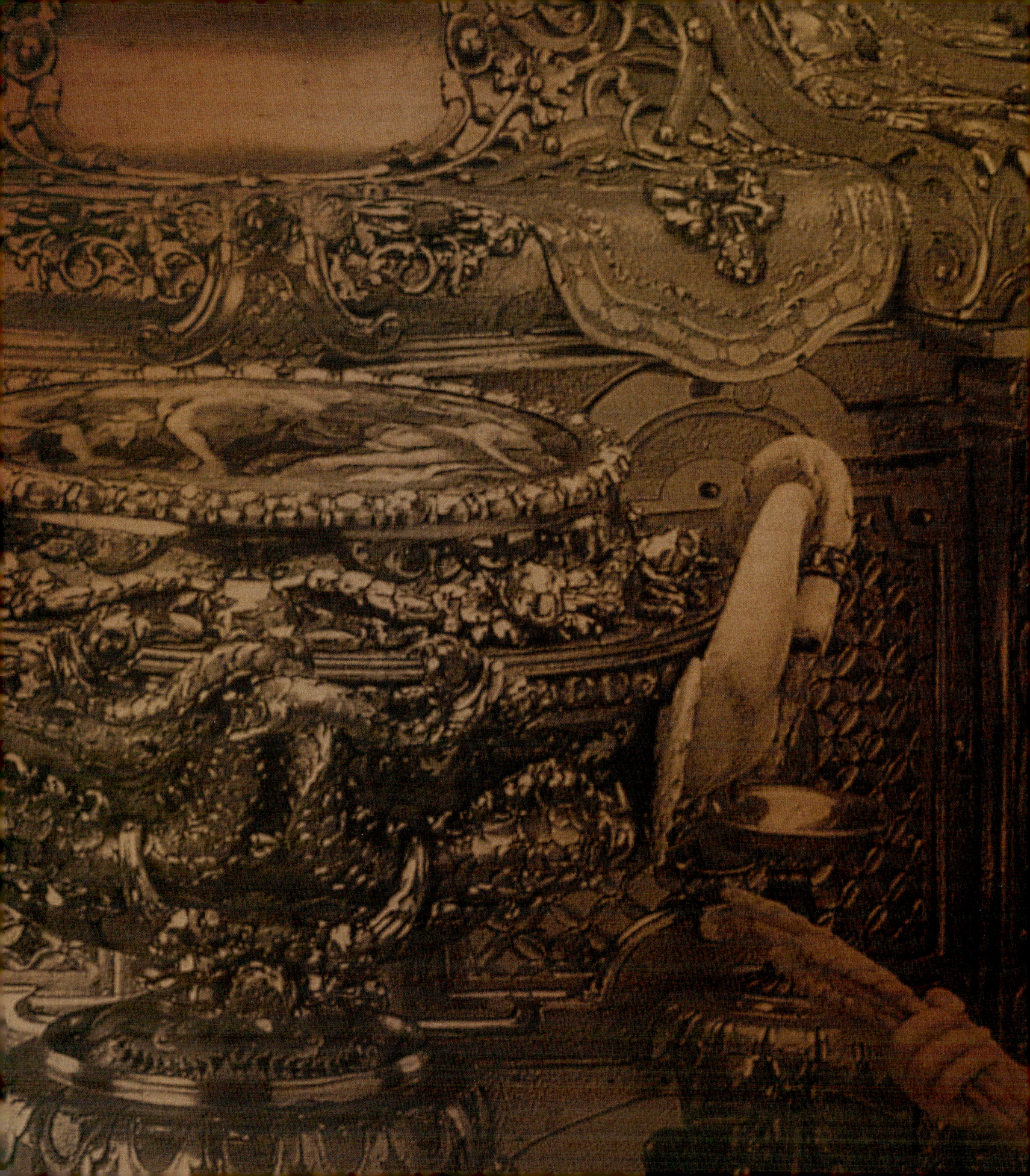

Introduction

The adhesion phenomenon is a molecular attraction between two substrates. Evidence-based dentistry has showed that adhesive bonding is basically dependent upon (1) the properties and behavior of the adhesive and (2) the structure and surface treatment of the adherend. Thus, it is important to learn about the microstructure, composition, properties and behavior of the ceramics to understand and improve the adhesion to these materials.

Therefore, this first chapter presents a brief history on the development of ceramics, since its origin as a domestic utensil up to its use in dentistry. The historical aspects of the first teeth replacements and the progress of dental ceramics are also considered.

Ceramic: An inorganic compound with nonmetallic properties typically composed of metallic (or semimetallic) and nonmetallic elements.

Dental ceramic: Inorganic, non-metallic material which is specifically formulated for use, when processed according to manufacturers instructions, to form the whole or part of a dental restoration or prosthesis.

Dentine ceramic: Dental ceramic material used to form the overall shape and basic color of a dental restoration or prosthesis, simulating the natural tooth dentine.

Enamel (veneering) ceramic: Dental ceramic material used to overlay either partially or wholly the dentine ceramic and also to form the more translucent incisal third of a dental restoration or prosthesis, simulating the natural tooth enamel

Dental porcelain: Predominantly glassy, dental ceramic material used mainly for esthetics in a dental restoration or prosthesis.

Originating from the Greek word *Keramos*, the oldest known human-made **ceramics** date back 26 thousand years. These ceramics were found in Czechoslovakia (Czech Republic since 1993) and were in the form of animal and human figurines, slabs, and balls (Fig. 1.1). They were made of animal fat and bone mixed with bone ash and a fine claylike material. After forming, the ceramics were fired at temperatures between 500-800°C in domed and horseshoe shaped kilns partially dug into the ground with loess walls. While it is not clear what these ceramics were used for, it is not thought to have been a utilitarian one. The first use of functional pottery vessels is thought to be in 9000 BC. These vessels were most likely used to hold and store grain and other foods.

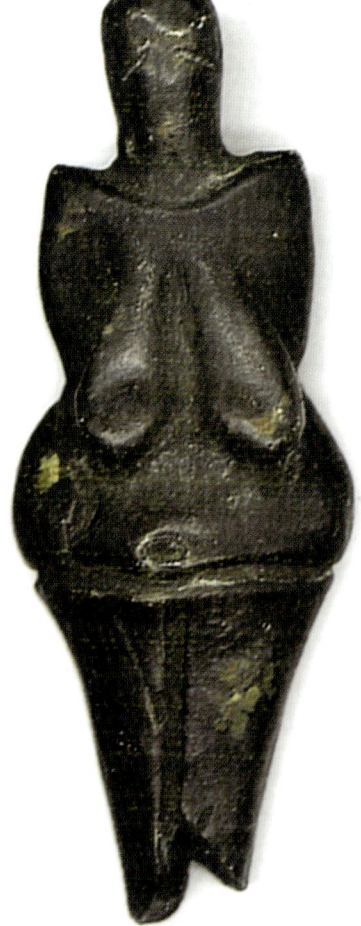

Figure 1.1 - The Venus of Dolní Věstonice (*Věstonická Venuše* in Czech) is a ceramic statuette of a nude female figure dated to, approximately, 24000 BC. The palaeolithic settlement of Dolní Věstonice in Moravia, Czech Republic has been under systematic archaeological research since 1924, led by Karel Absolon. This Venus statuette, together with figures of animals and more than 2000 balls of burnt clay found at Dolní Věstonice, is the oldest known ceramic in the world. The statuette has a height of 111 mm (4.4 inches), and a width of 43 mm (1.7 inches) at its widest point and is made of a clay body fired at a relatively low temperature. The figurine was discovered on July 13, 1925 in a layer of ash, broken into two pieces. Once on display at the Moravian Museum in Brno, it is now protected and only rarely accessible to the public.

It is thought that ancient **glass** manufacture is closely related to pottery making, which flourished in upper Egypt about 8000 BC. While firing pottery, the presence of calcium oxide (CaO) containing sand combined with soda (Na_2O) and the overheating of the pottery kiln may have resulted in a colored **glaze** on the ceramic pot. Experts believe that it was not until 1500 BC that glass was produced independently of ceramics and fashioned into separate items.

Since these ancient times, the technology and applications of ceramics (including glass) has steadily increased. We often take for granted the major role that ceramics have played in the progress of humankind.

Dental ceramic, also known as **dental porcelain**, or simply porcelain, is one of the most fascinating and fast developing material within the science and technology of dental materials.

Vanity rather than a wish to improve mastication almost certainly instigated the first false teeth. The Greeks and the Phoenicians used gold wire to attach false teeth to the natural teeth in the mouth. The Etruscans, however, excelled all at **dental bridge** work. They lived about 700 BC, where is now Tuscany, northern Italy, and could solder together wide bands of pure gold that would fit over natural teeth and hold the false ones with the addition of gold pins. These removable or "fixed" bridges were often made out of human or animal teeth (Fig. 1.2).

Glass: An inorganic nonmetallic compound that lacks a crystalline structure.

Glaze: Layer or coating of a vitreous substance fired to fuse to a ceramic object to color, decorate, strengthen or waterproof it. Glazing is functionally important for earthenware vessels, which would otherwise be unsuitable for holding liquids due to porosity. Glaze is also used on functional and decorative stoneware and porcelain. Glazes may also enhance an underlying design or texture of either the natural aspect of the material or an inscribed, carved or painted design.
Glazed dental ceramic: Dental ceramic material which is overlayed and fired at a reduced temperature compared to dentine or enamel ceramic, to produce a thin coherent sealed surface, the level of gloss being determined by the firing conditions.
Dental glaze (medium): Surface appearance obtained when the gloss is clinically and esthetically acceptable.

Dental prosthesis (dental bridge): An artificial replacement (prosthesis) of one or more teeth (up to the entire dentition in either arch) and associated dental/alveolar structures. Dental prostheses usually are subcategorized as either fixed dental prostheses or removable dental prostheses.

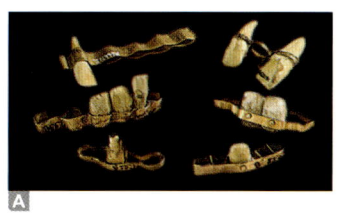
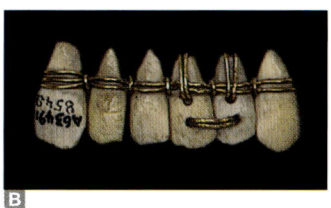
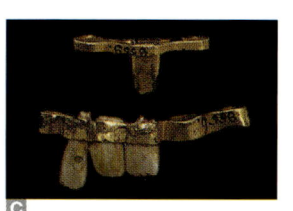

Figure 1.2 - **A**- Etruscan bridges (about 700 BC) using human and animal teeth hold together with gold bands and pins. **B**- A Phoenician bridge (1000-210 BC) using gold wire to hold artificial teeth together. **C**- Romans (about 400 BC) also used gold bands to make bridges. You can find these dental bridges at the Science Museum, London, UK.

Although the desire and history of replacing missing teeth started almost three thousand years ago, the ceramics were used in dentistry just after 1770s.

The art of making ceramic pieces demanded a great deal of technique, skill and persistence. In the beginning there were some problems with manipulating the raw material. As the clay-water mixture is very sticky, the addition of sand or ground shells improved its handling. Nevertheless, the problems of shrinkage and gases (CO_2) released during the uncontrolled firings could offer a great risk to the integrity and resistance of the final product. Such gases could remain as internal air bubbles or explode in the direction of the surface, causing a great deal of porosity and many cracks.

Controlled and gradual increase in temperature attenuated this problem, since the gases and vapors diffused slowly toward the surface of the piece, without causing major ruptures; this process is still used in manufacturing conventional ceramic pieces.

The need to reach high and uniform temperatures led to the invention of ceramic furnaces. The first furnaces were capable of attaining temperatures of 900°C producing earthenware pieces or burnt clay crockery. These products were still porous, and therefore unsuitable for containing liquids. This porosity was minimized by fusing a thin glassy layer onto the surface, called glazing. This technology was used in places such as Turkey in the years 5500 BC.

The art and development of ceramics had a very slow and late start in Europe and adequate furnaces only appeared at the end of the 15th century. In contrast, stoneware had already been known in China since 100 BC and the ceramic art technology had been dominated since the 10th century. "The ceramic was as white as snow and the wall thickness of the vases was so thin (from 2 to 3 mm) that it was possible to see light through them. Their internal structure was so firm that when one tapped a plate, it sounded like a bell".

The selection of materials and the correct method of manufacture were always of greatest importance in the faithful reproduction of legitimate Chinese porcelain. Many affirmed having discovered the secret of Chinese porcelain. In 1671, Charles II, went as far as authorizing the registration of a patent in the name of John Dwight of Fulham, but the product was no more than white stoneware.

As commercial trade improved in the 17th century, the fine Chinese porcelain arrived in Europe. Until then there was a complete lack of interest in "table dishes". The majority of the population used wooden plates and the nobles used metal dishes. Gold plates were used just on special occasions. Nevertheless, the appearance of Chinese porcelain stimulated the European market to qualify its product as it was practically impossible to meet the entire demand importing from the East.

At that time, good "imitations" were produced. The white appearance was imitated with the application of a stannic oxide glaze, but the translucence of legitimate Chinese porcelain could not be reproduced. In 1708, in Dresden, Germany, the first pieces of what it was called "white porcelain" were produced (Fig. 1.3). Some other manufacturers, now famous (Majolica - Italy, Wedgewood – England, and Delfts Blue - Holland), were incapable of producing genuine porcelain, but they made their names with high quality stoneware.

Figure 1.3 - The covered beaker (1713), modeled by Johann J. Irminger (1635-1724) and produced at Meissen porcelain factory, at Albrechtsberg Castle, Meissen, Germany. The factory was established, in 1710, by Augustus the Strong, elector of Saxony, who was also an avid collector of Chinese and Japanese porcelains. This beaker, was reserved for Augustus' private collection, and in 1725, he presented it to the king of Sardinia as a rare and fine gift. The first white porcelain pieces for show were successfully produced by Johann Friedrich Böttger, in Dresden, and they were manufactured for sale at Meissen beginning in 1713. This beaker is at the Carnegie Museum of Art, Pittsburgh, PA, USA. Courtesy of Dr. J. Robert Kelly.

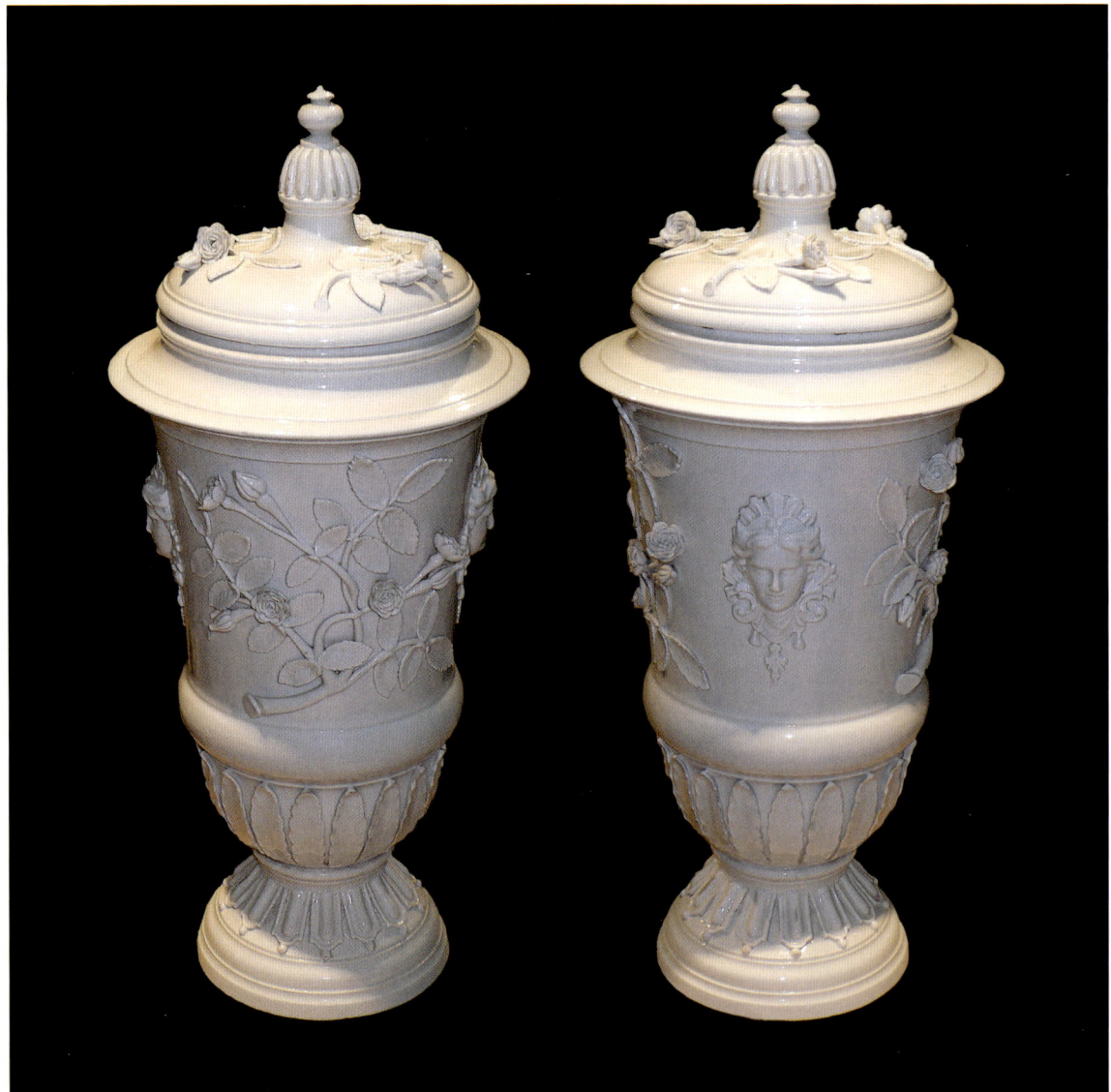

The secret of the Chinese porcelain was kept until 1712, when a Jesuit missionary by the name of Père François Xavier d'Entrecolles sent the first of two letters with samples and detailed instructions of the porcelain manufacturing process to France. d'Entrecolles did his missionary work in Ching-tê-chên (today referred to as Jingdezhen), the Chinese porcelain center at the time, becoming involved with the local artisans and learning about the porcelain process. In Europe, the samples were analyzed and the components were identified as kaolin, silica and feldspath (feldspar). Kaolin (kaolinite), or China clay, is a hydrated aluminum silicate ($Al_2Si_2O_5(OH)_4$). Silica, in the form of quartz, remains as a thin dispersion after sinterization. Feldspath (petuntse, also called Chinese porcelain stone) is a mixture of aluminum, potassium and sodium silicates (Fig. 1.4).

Unknown to d'Entrecolles, Böttger had already unraveled the secret of porcelain manufacture, leading to the establishment of the Meissen Porcelain Manufactory in 1710 (Fig. 1.3).

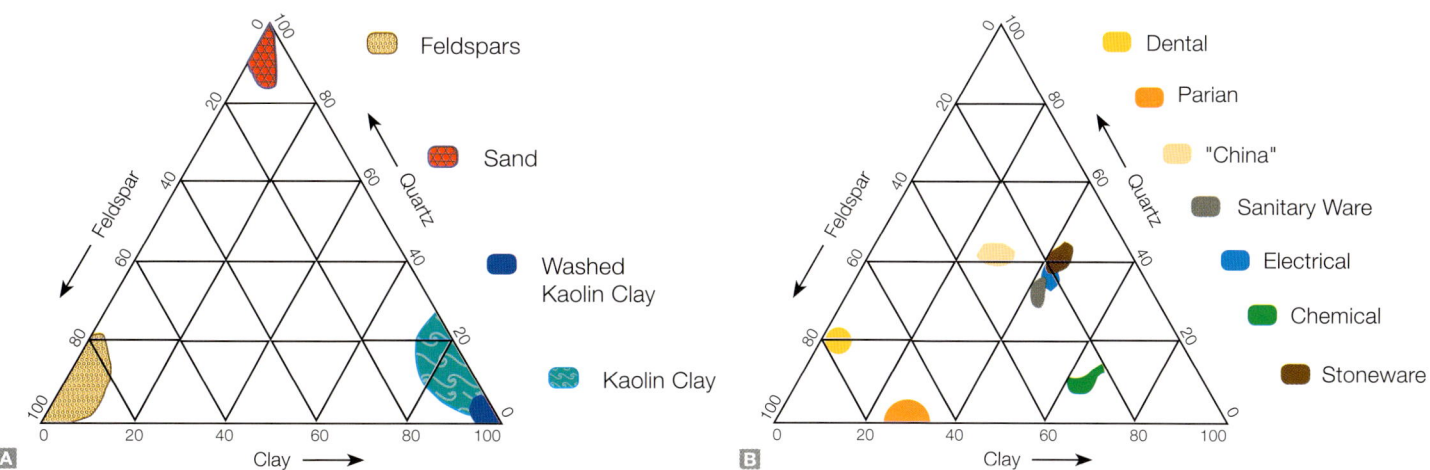

Figure 1.4 - A- Diagram showing the raw materials (feldspar, sand and kaolin clay) in relation to the main ceramic components (feldspar, quartz and clay). B- Diagram showing some types of ceramics in relation to the main ceramic components (feldspar, quartz and clay). Determining the amount and type of feldspar (albite: sodium feldspar; orthoclase: potassium feldspar; and anorthite: calcium feldspar) is important for dental ceramics. However, as the feldspar is white, inorganic shade pigments have to be incorporated into the glass matrix to produce the different tooth shades. Courtesy of Dr. J. Robert Kelly.

Once the mystery had been revealed, it did not take long for porcelain pieces to be manufactured in Europe in any shape, color and translucence, which immediately revealed its potential for dentistry.

The principles of metal-ceramic work were actually demonstrated by some European jewelers almost four centuries ago. They use glass or porcelain to enamel metals, such as gold and silver, to produce wonderful art products. The "golden coffee set" (1697-1701) and the "Fabergé imperial Easter eggs" (1885-1917) are very good examples of how jewelers (Johann and Georg Dinglinger; and Peter Carl Fabergé) mastered the enameling of metals (Fig. 1.5), ...and took another century to the dental profession to use it...

Figure 1.5 - A) The "Moscow Kremlin egg" (or the Uspenski Cathedral egg) is part of the "Fabergé imperial Easter eggs" (1885-1917). This egg was made under the supervision of the Russian jeweler Peter Carl Fabergé in 1906, for the last Tsar of Russia, Nicholas II who presented it to his wife, the Tsaritsa Alexandra Fyodorovna. This is by far the largest of the 69 known Fabergé eggs and was inspired by the architecture of the Cathedral of the Assumption (Uspenski) in Moscow, where all the Russian Tsars were crowned, including Nicholas. The Cathedral dome (in white opalescent enamel) is removable, and the remarkably crafted interior of the church can be seen. Its carpets, tiny enameled icons and High Altar on an oval glass plate are made visible through four triple windows, surmounted by a gold cupola and flanked by two square, two circular stylized turrets, the former based on the Spassky Tower. The tower bears the coat-of-arms of the Russian Empire and Moscow, inset with 'chiming clocks'. It stands on a crenelated gold base and octagonal white onyx plinth designed as a pyramid, and built of smaller pyramids. The surprise in this egg is music. The base of the egg contains a gold 'music box' that plays traditional Easter hymns when a clockwork mechanism is wound up by a gold key. It is currently held in the Kremlin Armoury Museum in Moscow.
B) Images of the "golden coffee set" by Johann M. Dinglinger (draft and goldsmith work), Georg F. Dinglinger (porcelain enamel) and Paul Heermann (ivory sculptures). It was created from 1697 to 1701. All drinking vessels have a solid gold body enameled with porcelain. This set is part of the Green Vault (Grünes Gewölbe) museum in Dresden, Germany. It contains the largest collection of treasures in Europe, and it is often referred to as a walk-in treasure chest. The building is part of the Dresden castle and it was founded by Augustus II the Strong in 1723.

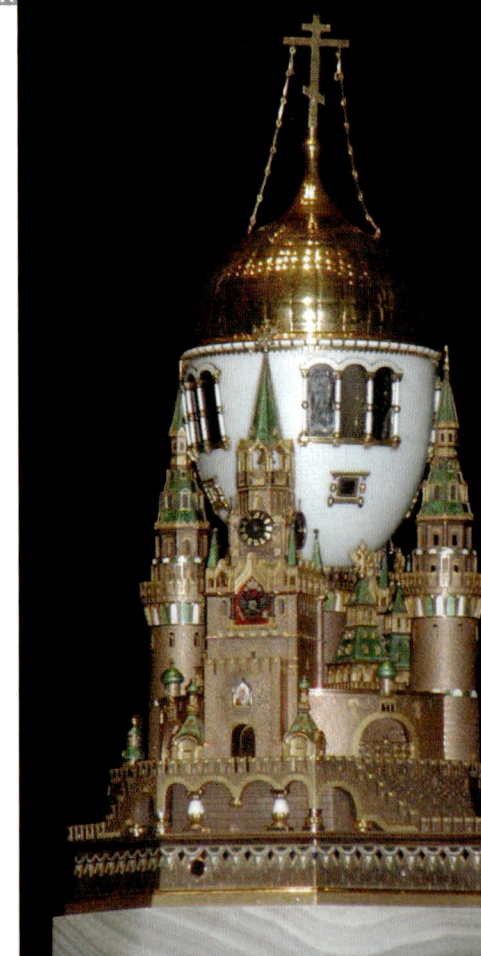

Introduction

The objective of this chapter is to present the atomic structure and the principles of matter, which are important to understand the behavior of ceramics. Thus, it is essential to gain some knowledge on physical-chemical reactions at atomic level because they influence on: the material properties (chapter 3), the ceramic surface treatments (chapter 4), and the adhesion longevity of ceramic restorations and repairs (chapter 5).

Atom: The name atom comes from the Greek and means "uncuttable" or "the smallest indivisible particle of matter", i.e., something that cannot be divided. The atom is the smallest unit of an element that retains its chemical properties. An atom has an **electron cloud** consisting of negatively charged **electrons** surrounding a dense **nucleus**. The nucleus contains positively charged **protons** and electrically neutral **neutrons**. When the number of protons in the nucleus equals the number of electrons, the atom is electrically neutral; otherwise it is an **ion** and has a net positive or negative charge. **Anion** is a negatively charged ion that has more electrons than protons. A positively-charged ion, which has fewer electrons than protons, is known as a **cation**.

An atom is classified according to its number of protons and neutrons: the number of protons determines the **chemical element** (atomic number – Z) and the number of neutrons determines the **isotope** of that element. Common examples of a chemical element or pure chemical substance are oxygen (O), hydrogen (H), silicon (Si), iron (Fe), gold (Au), and carbon (C). As of 2008, 117 elements have been observed, 92 of them occur naturally on Earth and 80 have stable isotopes (namely all elements with Z from 1 to 82, except elements 43 (Tc) and 61 (Pm)). Elements with atomic numbers 83 (Bi) or higher are inherently unstable, and undergo radioactive decay. The elements from atomic number 83 (Bi) to 94 (Pu) have no stable nuclei but are found in nature.

All chemical matter consists of these elements. New elements of higher atomic number are discovered from time to time, as products of artificial nuclear reactions.

All materials are built up from atoms and molecules that are held together by atomic interactions. The nature of the **atoms** and their arrangements determine the microstructure and composition of the solid, consequently, the properties of the material.

Whenever two atoms are brought together they may link to form a molecule via one of the three possible primary bonds: covalent, ionic, and metallic. The strength of the bonds and their ability to reform after breakage have a significant influence on the physical properties of a material.

The covalent bond can be very strong, as in diamond, or weak, as with bismuth, which melts at about 270^0C. Bond energies and melting temperatures (T_m) are directly related (Table 2.1). The covalent bond occurs when atoms share their electrons so that each electron shell reaches an inert configuration. As the two atoms approach one another and the orbitals of the electrons begin to overlap, a molecular orbital is formed where the two electrons are shared between the two nuclei (Fig. 2.1A). Since the electrons will spend most of their time in the region where the orbitals overlap, the bond is highly directional. This type of bond occurs in dental resins and ceramics, in which the carbon or the silicon atoms have four valence electrons forming sp3 hybrid configurations that can be stabilized by combining with hydrogen or oxygen, respectively (Fig. 2.1).

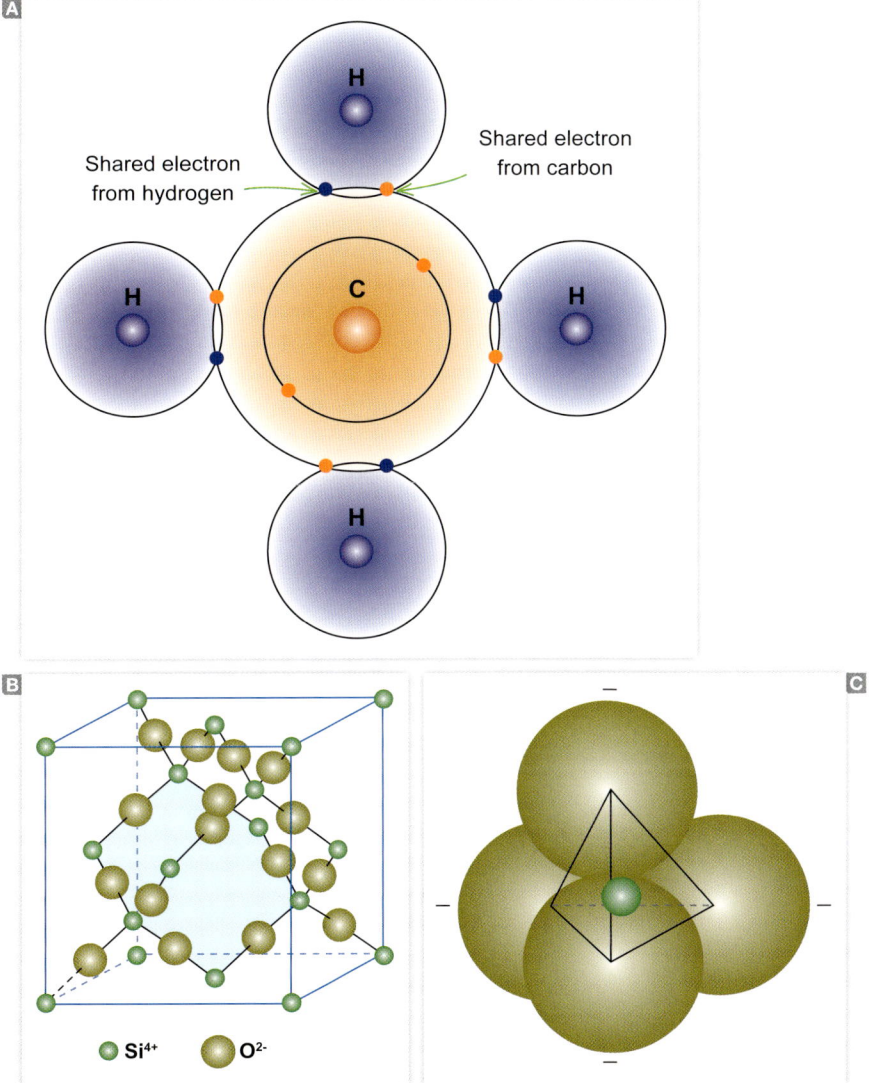

Figure 2.1 - Schematic representation of covalent bond. (**A**) Covalent bonding in a molecule of methane (CH$_4$); characterized by electron sharing and precise bond orientations. (**B**) Three-dimensional representation of silicon (Si) and oxygen (O) atoms in a reduced-sphere unit cell of cristobalite (a polymorph of SiO$_2$). The tetrahedral symmetry for the Si atoms can be clearly seen (**Fig. 2.10 A**); the third and fourth oxygen atoms, in some cases, are contained in the adjacent unit cell (not in the image). Note that a hexagon with Si atoms on the corners and O atoms on the edges has been shaded; a two-dimensional representation of such hexagons is shown in **Fig. 2.10 C**. The charge distribution between the atoms is not uniform but cone-shaped (**C**), and the angle between the bond axes (valence angle) is 109°28'. This arrangement also applies for carbon, in the diamond cubic structure.

⤷⤶

Bonding energy: energy required to separate two atoms that are chemically bonded to each other (Fig. 2.4 and Table 2.1).

Melting temperature (*melting point*, T_m): Equilibrium temperature at which heating of a pure compound or substance produces a change from solid to liquid state. The T_m of a glass is the temperature at which the viscosity is 10 Pa·s (100 P); the glass is fluid enough to be considered a liquid (Fig. 2.11 and Table 2.1).

⤷⤶

Ionic bonds (Fig. 2.2) result from the mutual attraction of positive (cations) and negative (anions) charges with a reduction in the total energy of the pair as they approach, such as the case of sodium and chlorine (Na^+ and Cl^-). As sodium has a single valence electron and the chlorine has seven electrons in its outer shell, an interaction between these two atoms results in the stable (inert) compound sodium chloride (NaCl). The resulting configuration is based on a charge and size balance, depending on the electrostatic fields that surround the ions, which can interact with any other ions in the vicinity, and therefore forming a not directional bond, meaning the magnitude of the bond is equal in all directions around the ion. The **bond energies** are relatively large, as reflected in high **melting temperature** (T_m) (Table 2.1). Ionic materials are characteristically hard and brittle, and electrically and thermally insulators. This is the predominant atomic bond in ceramic materials.

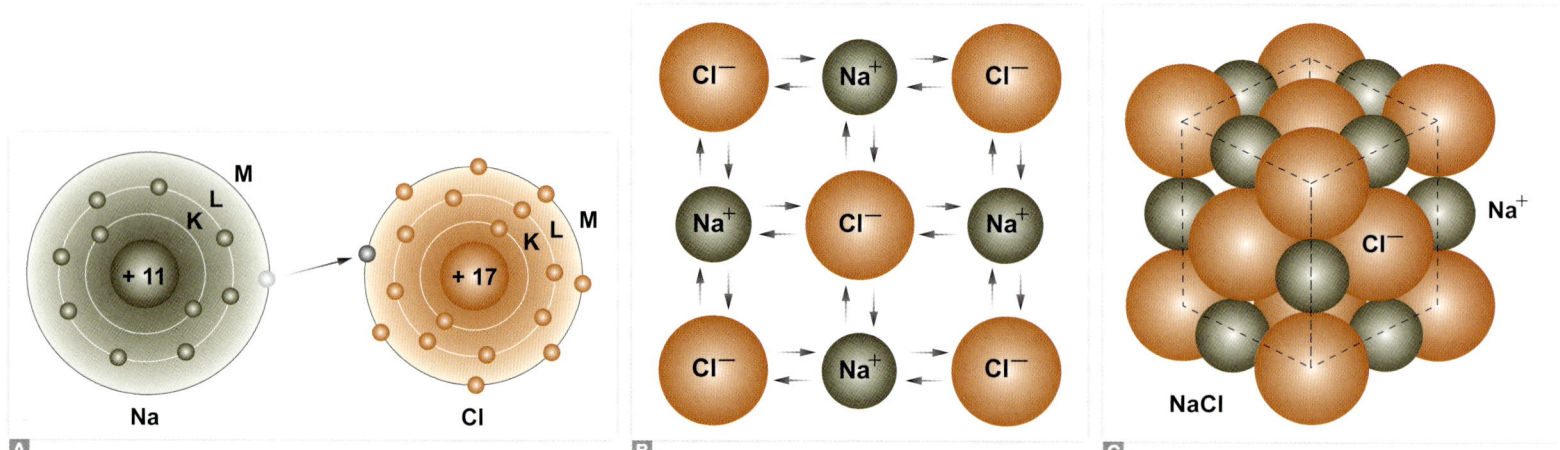

Figure 2.2 - Schematic representation of ionic bond. **A**) Formation of Na^+Cl^- by transferring one electron from Na to Cl yielding Na^+ and Cl^- ions. **B**) Illustration of ionic bonding in sodium chloride (NaCl). **C**) The face-centered cubic (FCC) structure of NaCl (**Fig 2.9**).

The metallic bond is also non-directional. It occurs when an aggregate of metal atoms is brought close together forming a "sea" or "cloud" of free electrons surrounding the atoms (Fig. 2.3). So, these cluster structures, which have lower energy electron orbitals than the ones of individual atoms, are responsible for the excellent electrical and thermal conductivity of metals and also for their ability to deform plastically, differing much from ceramics. The electrical and thermal conductivities of metals are controlled by the degree of freedom of the electrons through the crystal, whereas their deformability is associated with the **slip** of atoms along crystal planes.

Slip: Process by which plastic deformation is produced by a dislocation motion. By an external force, parts of the crystal lattice glide along each other, resulting in a changed geometry of the material. Depending on the type of lattice, different slip systems are present in the material. More specifically, slip occurs between planes containing the smallest Burgers vector.

Dislocation: It is a crystallographic defect, or irregularity, within a crystal structure. The presence of dislocations strongly influences many of the material properties.

Vacancy: Unoccupied atom lattice site in a crystalline solid.

Crystal lattice: The regular geometrical arrangement of points in crystal space (structure).

Burgers vector (b): Represents the magnitude and direction of the lattice distortion of dislocation in a crystal lattice.

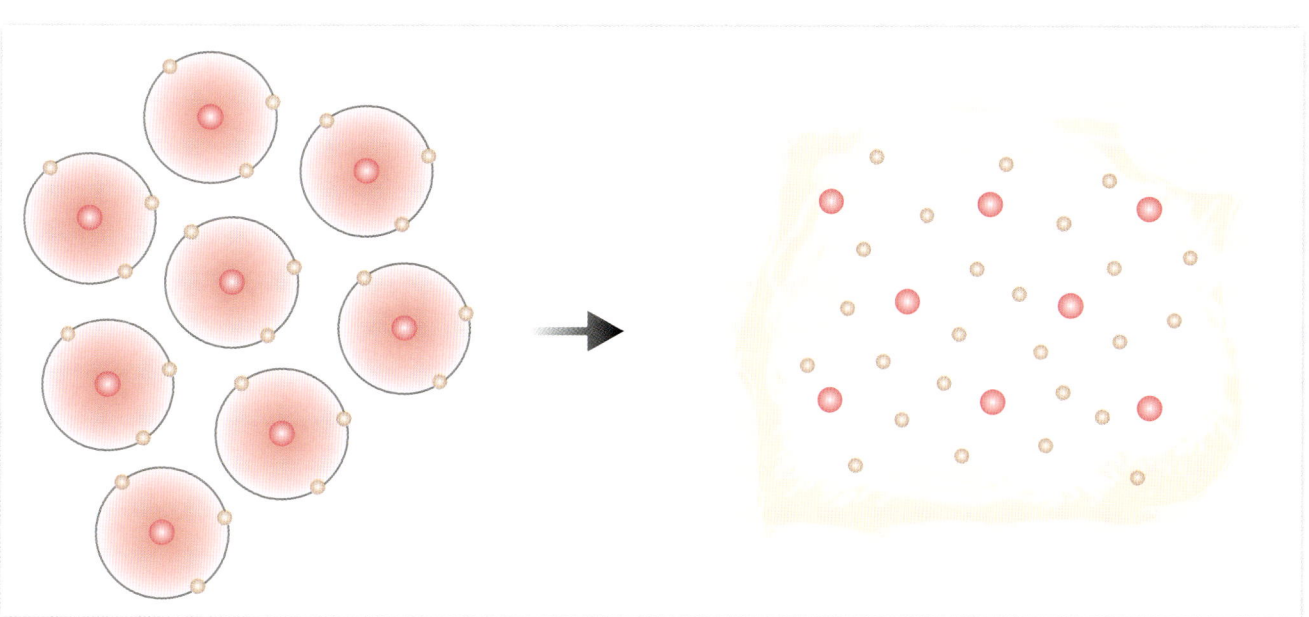

Figure 2.3 - Schematic representation of metallic bond. It is characterized by electron sharing and formation of a "sea" of electrons surrounding the nuclei.

As one can imagine, the controlling factor in any interatomic bond formation is energy and a bond only forms if it results in a lower energy molecule than the sum of the energies of the separate atoms (E_a). As the atoms are brought closer together, the total energy from both atoms ($2E_a$) begins to fall, until it reaches a minimum (E_m) at a distance a_0. As the atoms are brought more closely together, the energy increases due to repulsion between their clouds of electrons and nuclei (Fig. 2.4). The amount of energy necessary to separate the atoms, is the bond energy, which varies from the strongest covalent to the weakest metallic bonds (Table 2.1). It is all about energy!

Conversely to primary bonds, the secondary bonds occur with no sharing of electrons. In this type of bond, charge variations among molecules or atomic groups induce polar forces that attract the molecules. The secondary bonds are responsible for some processes where no primary bonds are present, such as the adhesion phenomenon of ice to glass windows.

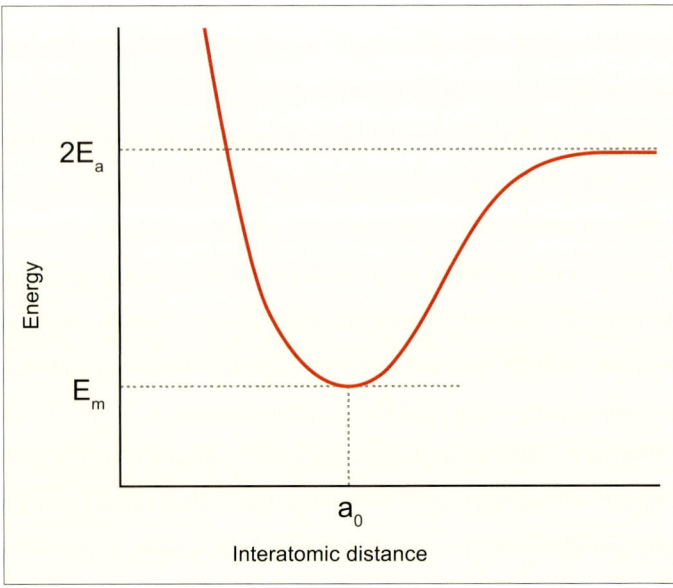

Figure 2.4 - A typical energy-separation curve for two atoms, each of energy E_a. The bond energy is $2E_a - E_m$.

Table 2.1 - Typical bond energies and melting temperatures (T_m) for various substances according to their type of bond.

Bonding Type	Substance	Bond energy (eV/atom, ion, molecule)	T_m (°C)
Covalent	C (diamante)	7.4	>3550
	Si	4.7	1.410
Ionic	MgO	5.2	2.800
	NaCl	3.3	801
Metallic	Al	3.4	660
	Hg	0.7	-39
Hydrogen bond	H_2O	0.52	0
	NH_3	0.36	-78
van der Waals	Cl_2	0.32	-101
	Ar	0.08	-189

The hydrogen bond, which is associated with the positive charge of hydrogen caused by polarization, is a special case of dipole-dipole interaction. The typical example is the asymmetric water (ice) molecule where the covalent bonds between the oxygen (O) and hydrogen (H) atoms (4.4 eV) leave, at one side, positive charge hydrogen protons (H^+) that are not shielded by surrounding electrons, and on the other side the electrons that fill the outer orbit of the oxygen atom provide a negative charge (Fig. 2.5). A necessary condition for the formation of a hydrogen bond is that an electronegative atom (O^-, in the case of ice, water) should be in the neighborhood of the hydrogen atom that is bonded to an electronegative atom (again O^-, for ice). In the case of ice, this secondary bond energy is only about 0.5eV, and is readily overcome by heating above 0°C (Table 2.1). The hydrogen bond is important because it accounts for the extensive adsorption possible by organic

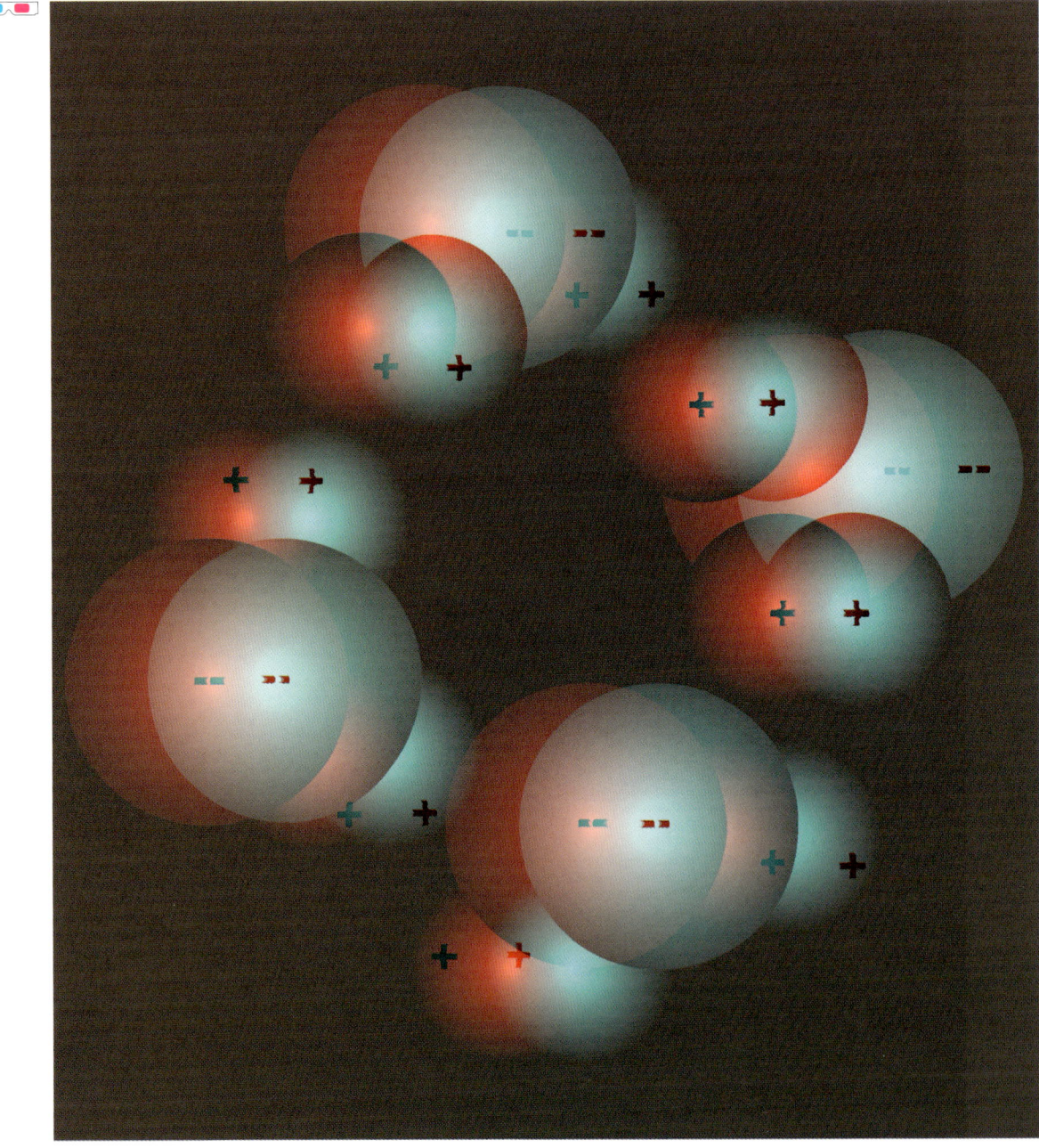

Figure 2.5 - Schematic representation of hydrogen bond formation between water molecules. The polar water molecule binds adjacent water molecules via an H●●●O interaction between these molecules.

molecules, including proteins, and is therefore considered essential to the life processes. It is also important for the intermolecular reactions in many organic compounds, such as the sorption of water by synthetic dental resins. Yet, secondary bonding forms the basis of the molecular attraction in molecular solids.

Another example of secondary bonds is the van der Waals forces, which are a short range of force of physical attraction that promotes adhesion between molecules of liquids or molecular crystals. This occurs because the electrostatic field around the atom may fluctuate and its charge becomes momentarily positive and negative, attracting other similar dipoles.

The energy or the degree of interaction between the atoms is also associated with the state (main phase) of the matter: gas, liquid or solid. A phase is defined as a structurally homogeneous part of the system having its own distinct structure and associated properties. Much of the information about the control of microstructure or phase structure of a system is conveniently shown in a **phase diagram** (Fig. 2.6). Many of microstructures develop from **phase transformations**, which are changes that occur between phases when the temperature is altered (typically upon cooling). Therefore, phase diagrams are used to predict phase transformations and resulting microstructures.

Important zirconia-based ceramic systems are shown in figure 2.6. Upon heating, the monoclinic phase in pure zirconia (zirconium oxide – ZrO_2) starts transforming to the tetragonal phase at 1187 °C (1461 K), peaks at 1197 °C (1471 K), and finishes at 1206 °C (1480 K). On cooling, the transformation from the tetragonal to the monoclinic phase starts at

Phase diagram: A graphical representation of the relationships between environmental constraints (*e.g.*, temperature and pressure), composition, and regions of phase stability, ordinarily under equilibrium conditions.
Phase transformation: A change in the number and/or character of the phases that constitute the microstructure of a material, meaning, it is the transformation of a thermodynamic system from one phase to another. It is also named phase transition.

27

1052 °C (1326 K), peaks at 1048 °C (1322 K), and finishes at 1020 °C (1294 K), exhibiting a hysteresis behavior that is well known for this material. As this transformation has many characteristics of martensitic transformation in metals, the zirconia tetragonal-to-monoclinic phase transformation is also known as martensitic transformation.

A relatively large volume change accompanies this zirconia phase transformation, with a unit cell of monoclinic occupying about 4% more volume than when tetragonal, which could result in the formation of ceramic cracks if no stabilizing oxides were used. Ceria (CeO_2), yttria (Y_2O_3), alumina (Al_2O_3), magnesia (MgO) and calcia (CaO) have been used as stabilizing oxides. So, as the monoclinic and $CaZr_4O_9$ phases do not form under normal cooling conditions (as predicted from the phase diagram, Fig 2.6 A), consequently, the cubic and tetragonal phases are retained, and crack formation due to phase transformation is circumvented.

It is also important to consider that the stabilization of the tetragonal and cubic structures requires different amounts of dopants (stabilizers). The tetragonal phase is stabilized at lower dopant concentrations than the cubic phase, as shown in the room temperature region of the ZrO_2–Y_2O_3 phase diagram (Fig. 2.6 B). Yet, another way of stabilizing the tetragonal phase at room temperature is to decrease the crystal size (the critical average grain size is < 0.3 μm). This effect has been attributed to a surface energy difference.

Consequently, zirconia-based ceramics used for biomedical purposes, typically exist as a metastable tetragonal partially stabilized zirconia (PSZ) at room temperature (Table 2.2). Metastable means that trapped energy still exists within the material to drive it back to the monoclinic state. It turned out that the highly localized stress ahead of a propagating crack is sufficient to trigger zirconia grains to transform in the vicinity of the crack tip. In this case the 4% volume increase becomes beneficial, essentially squeezing the crack to close and increasing toughness (Fig. 3.11).

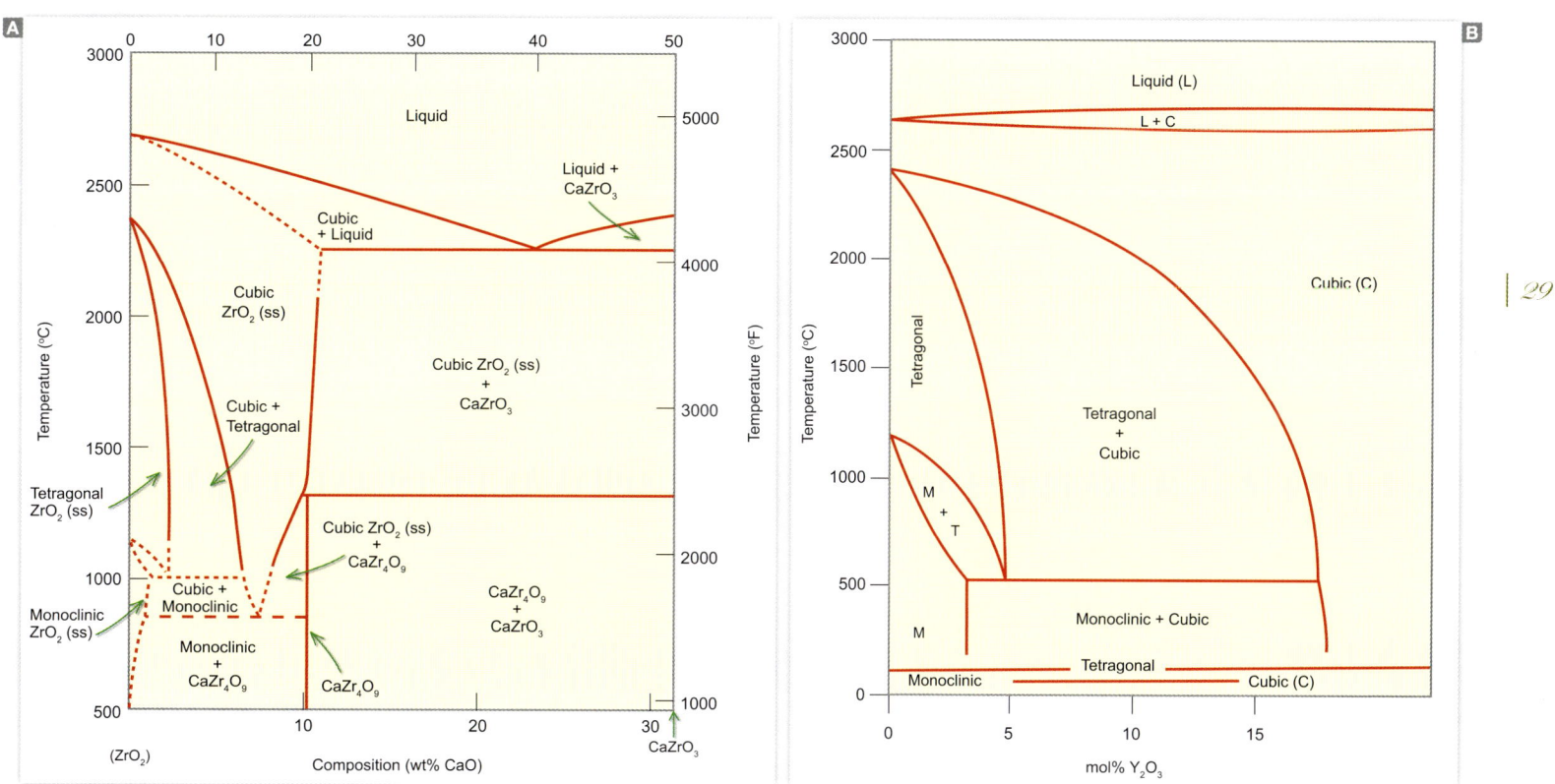

Figure 2.6 - (**A**) A portion of the zirconia-calcia phase diagram (binary system). The ZrO_2 phases have three different crystal structures: cubic (C), tetragonal (T), and monoclinic (M) (**Fig 2.8**). The horizontal axis extends to only about 31 wt% CaO (50 mol% CaO), at which $CaZrO_3$ forms. (**B**) Zirconia-rich end of the yttria-zirconia phase equilibrium diagram. Although pressure is also a parameter that influences the phase structure, it remains virtually constant in most applications; thus these phase diagrams are for a constant pressure of 1 atm. ss= solid solution.

Zirconia is a very interesting biomaterial because of the following properties: high strength (σ), fracture toughness (K_{IC}), and hardness (H); wear resistance and good frictional behavior; electrical insulation; low thermal conductivity (k); corrosion resistance in acids and alkalis; modulus of elasticity (*E*) similar to steel; and coefficient of thermal expansion (α) similar to iron. Additionally, its fine grain size enables excellent surface finishes and the ability to hold a sharp edge (Tables 1.1, 2.2 and 3.3). However, as with most ceramic, materials properties are dependent on many factors such as starting powders and fabrication techniques. Many ceramic fabrication techniques have been applied to zirconias, including: dry pressing, isostatic pressing, injection moulding, extrusion and tape casting. Addition of impurities during processing may also introduce flaws and degrade properties.

There are, however, many different types of zirconias: partially stabilized zirconia (PSZ), tetragonal zirconia polycrystals (TZP), fully stabilized zirconia (FSZ), transformation toughened ceramics (TTC), zirconia toughened alumina (ZTA), transformation toughened zirconia (TTZ). The stabilizers will also be noted as a prefix to the mentioned abbreviations. They will sometimes be used in conjunction with numbers which indicate the amount of the stabilizing agent added. Typical examples include Y, Ce, Mg and A, which correspond, respectively, to yttria, ceria, magnesia and alumina. So a material denoted as 3Y-TZP is a tetragonal zirconia polycrystal with an addition of 3mol% of yttria as a stabilizer. These zirconias have evolved as researchers and manufacturers sought to exploit the different properties of the various phases. Some of the phases are stable at high temperatures and need to be "frozen" in such that they can be used at room temperatures, while others exploit toughening mechanisms that are only found in these and few other materials.

Table 2.2 - Typical properties of some types of zirconia.

Property	Y-TZP	Ce-TZP	ZTA	Mg-PSZ
Density (g/cm³)	6.0	6.1	4.2	5.7
H (GPa)	11	9	12	10
Flexural σ (MPa)	800-1400	350-500	450-650	700-900
Compressive σ (MPa)	2000	-	-	2000
E (GPa)	205	215	380	205
Poisson's ratio	0.3	-	-	0.23
K_{IC} (MPa•m$^{1/2}$)	5-9	15-20	4-5	8-15
α (ppm/°C)	10	8	8	10
k (W/m•°K)	2	2	23	1.8

H= hardness (Vickers); σ= strength; E= elastic modulus; K_{IC}= fracture toughness; α= coefficient of thermal expansion; k= thermal conductivity.

Examples of commercially available ceramics:
Y-TZP- DC Zirkon (DCS Precident, Schreuder & Co.), Cercon (Dentsply Prosthetics), Lava (3M ESPE), In-Ceram YZ (Vita Zahnfabrik);
Ce-TZP- Nanozir (Matsushita Electrical Works, Ltd.);
ZTA- In-Ceram Zirconia (Vita Zahnfabrik);
Mg-PSZ- Denzir-M (Dentronic AB).

Atomic vibration: The vibration of an atom about its normal position in a substance.

Diffusion coefficient: Proportionality constant representing the amount of a substance diffusing through a unit area and a unit thickness under the influence of a unit concentration gradient at a given temperature.

Diffusion: Mass transport by atomic motion.

The three main phases of matter can be distinguished based on the interatomic and intermolecular movement. In the gaseous state there is little or no resistance to the relative movement of atoms or molecules, while in the liquid state the resistance to movement is considerably greater, but molecules can still flow past each other with great ease. In solids the movement of atoms and molecules is restricted to a local **vibration**, although some interatomic movement is possible through **diffusion**. Considering this information, coupled with the knowledge that anions and cations in ceramic materials are often significantly different in size, one can explain the relative success of the ion exchange process used for strengthening dental ceramics (Fig. 2.7). This method introduces residual compressive stresses into the surface of a ceramic, challenging the crack propagation. Such effect, however, is no deeper than 100 μm and, therefore, the strengthening effect can be lost if the ceramic surface is ground or worn.

Energy is also required for a solid-to-liquid transformation. The attraction between atoms in the solid state must be greater than that in either the liquid or the gaseous state. If this was not true, atoms would separate easily in metals, deforming readily and they could also exist in the vapor phase at low temperatures. Temperature, however, also has an effect on the materials' behavior. A metal typically fails from a ductile failure process, however it can experience a brittle fracture at low temperatures. Any similarity to the Titanic failure?

Ceramics are compounds of metallic elements, and non-metallic substances such as oxides, nitrides and silicates. These materials are very

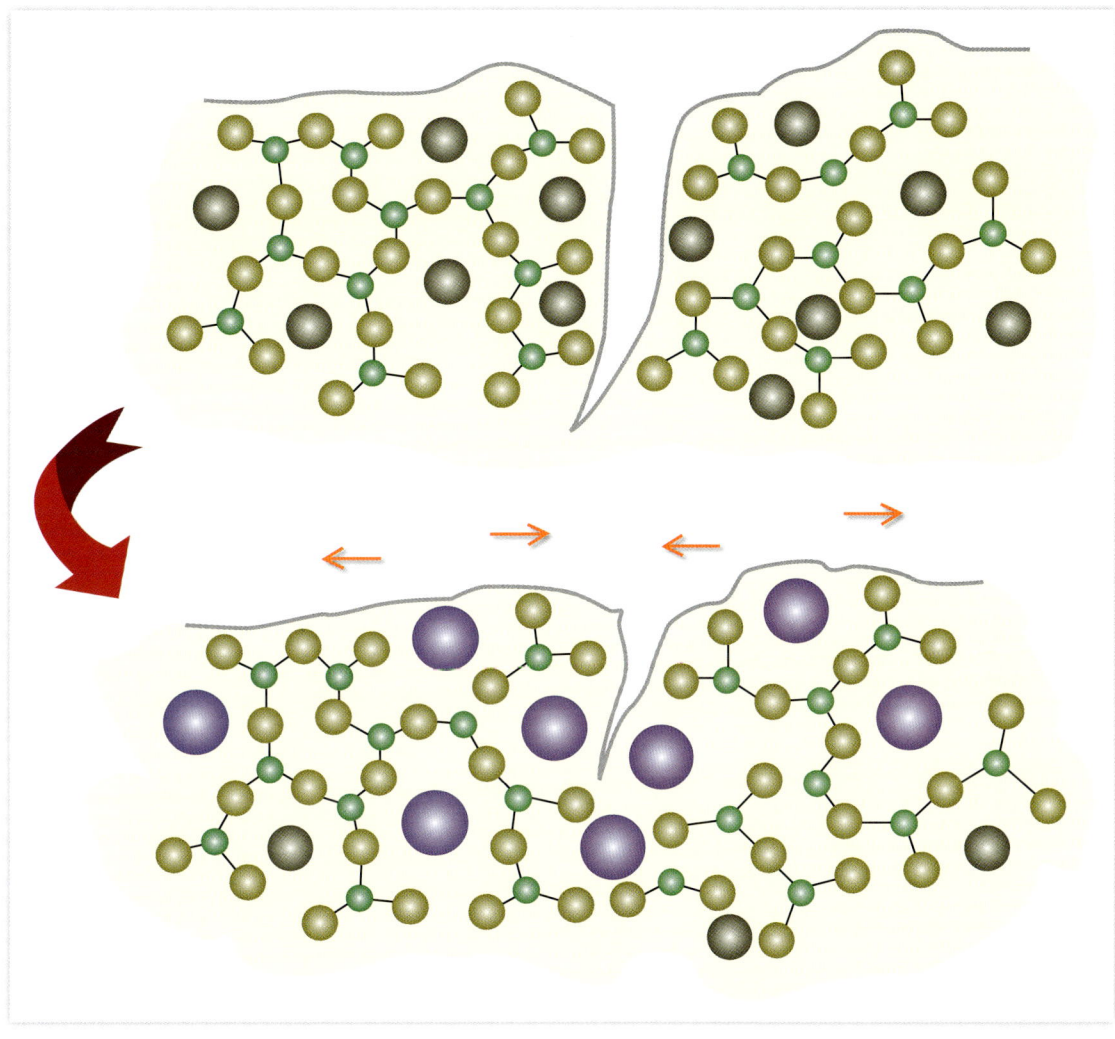

- Silicon
- Oxygen
- Sodium
- Potassium

Figure 2.7 - Schematic representation of the ion exchange process. It often involves the exchange of sodium (Na), a relatively small diameter ion and a common constituent of glasses, for potassium (K) that is about 35% larger than the Na ion. This process is usually accomplished by applying a potassium-rich slurry to the ceramic surface that is heated for some time (*e.g.*, 450ºC for 30 min).

❦❧

Packing fraction (atomic packing factor - APF): The fraction of volume in a unit cell or crystal structure that is occupied by atoms or ions. It is dimensionless and always less than unity. For practical purposes, the APF of a crystal structure is determined by assuming that atoms are rigid spheres.

❦❧
---

stable because of their high interatomic primary (ionic and covalent) bond strengths and high **packing efficiency**. Ceramics can appear as either crystalline or amorphous (glass) solids (Fig. 2.10C and D).

The atoms in crystalline materials are positioned in a periodic (repetitive) pattern forming a three-dimensional grid known as lattice (Fig. 2.8). The arrangement of atoms into a repeatable lattice is called crystal structure. As explained in Fig. 2.4, an external force is needed to move the atoms closer together or further apart. This interatomic spacing is the configuration of minimum energy (E_m), and in order to achieve it there is a tendency for the atoms to adopt a regular close-packed arrangement. The densest packing of atoms is obtained when they are arranged in a regular symmetrical manner, forming a crystalline structure (Fig. 2.9). An important feature of such structure is that from any atom, the arrangement of its neighbouring atoms is identical. Metals and ionic solids, such as most ceramics, are usually crystalline at room temperature. Any solid in which there is no symmetry of the atoms is said to be amorphous (Fig. 2.10).

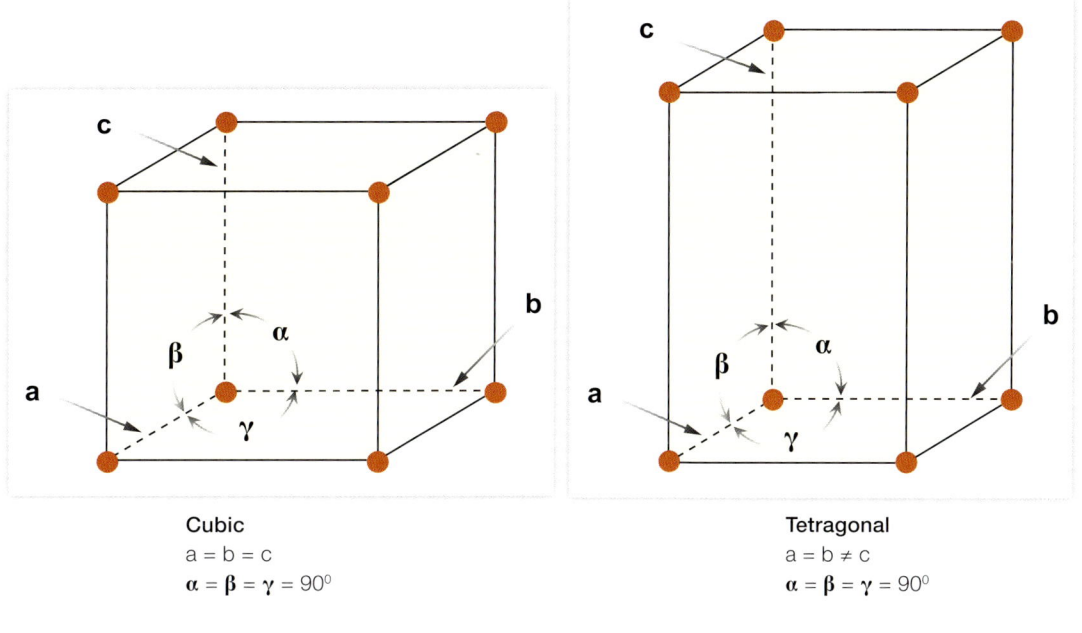

Cubic
a = b = c
α = β = γ = 90⁰

Tetragonal
a = b ≠ c
α = β = γ = 90⁰

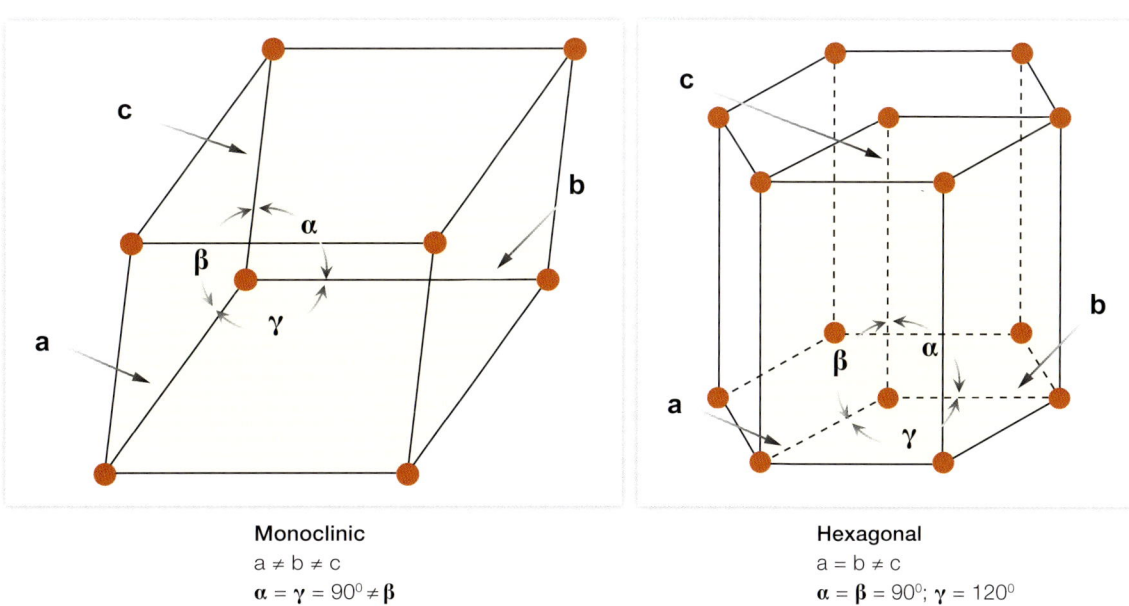

Monoclinic
a ≠ b ≠ c
α = γ = 90⁰ ≠ β

Hexagonal
a = b ≠ c
α = β = 90⁰; γ = 120⁰

Figure 2.8 - There are 14 possible Bravais lattices grouped into 7 lattice types (unit cell geometry) according to the different lattice parameters of the crystal structure. These parameters are: the edge or axial lengths (a, b, c) and the interaxial angles (α, β, γ). These 7 crystal systems are cubic, tetragonal, hexagonal, monoclinic, triclinic, orthorhombic, and rhombohedral. The first four types are the most important for ceramics and are schematically shown in this Figure, along with their axial relationships and interaxial angles.

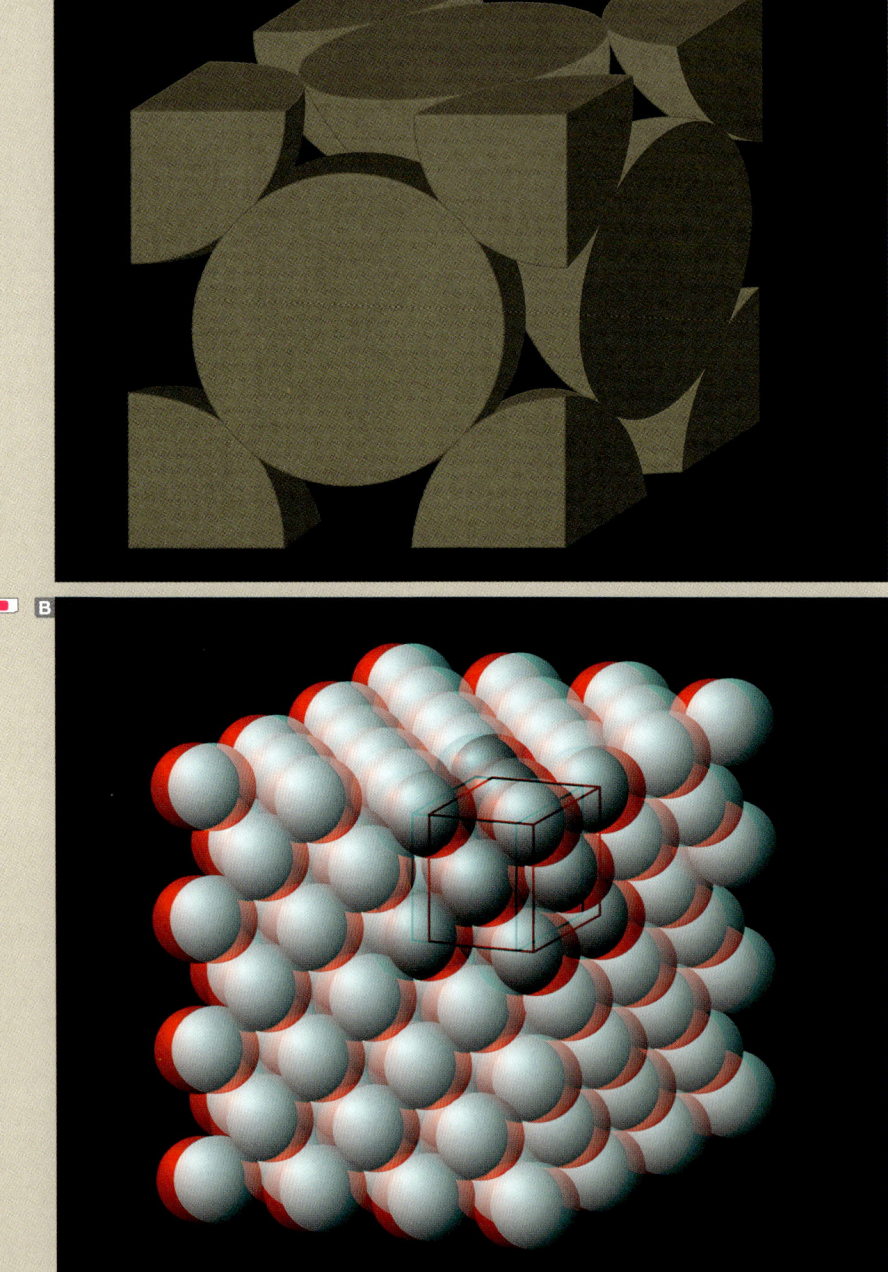

Figure 2.9 - **A**) Schematic representation of a unit cell for the face-centered cubic (FCC) crystal structure. There are 8 atoms in the corners that are shared among 8 unit cells (8 x 1/8 = 1 atom) and 6 face-centered atoms that are shared between 2 unit cells (6 x 1/2 = 3 atoms). Therefore, a FCC cell can hold 4 whole atoms. Aluminum (Al), gold (Au), silver (Ag), and platinum (Pt) are just few examples of this crystal structure, which is also shown in **Figure 2.2C** for NaCl compound. **B**) A structure of many atoms arranged as a repeating FCC unit cell.

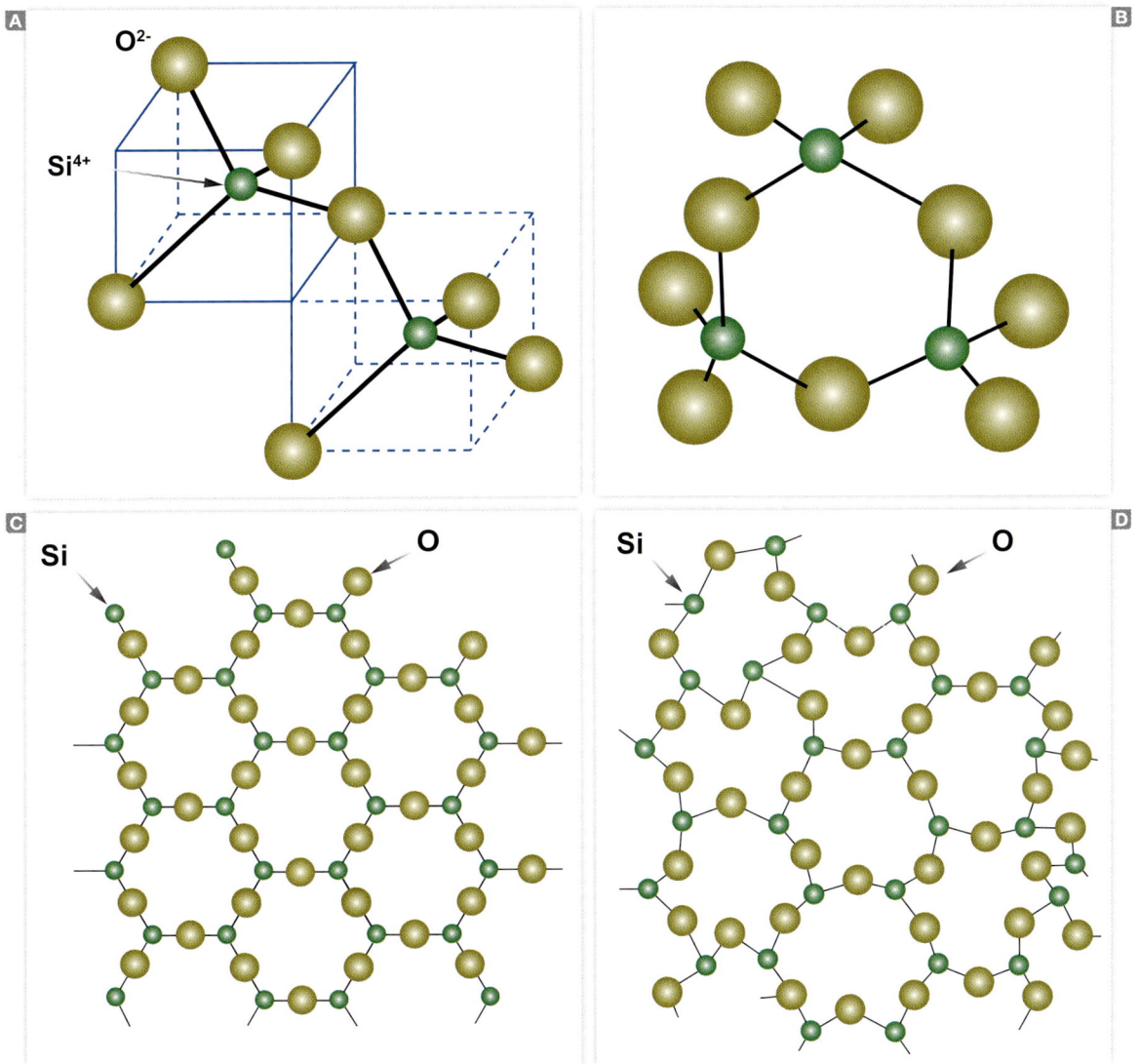

Figure 2.10 - Schematic representations of silica. **A**) Spacial arrangement of the oxygen atoms with respect to silicon. **B**) A silica ring $(Si_3O_9)^{6-}$. **C**) Two-dimensional representation of crystalline silica structure (see also **Fig. 2.1 B** for the three-dimensional structure), and **D**) amorphous glass. The fourth bond of Si is not seen because it points into the paper plane.

Glass transition temperature (T_g):
Temperature at which a sharp increase in
the thermal expansion coefficient occurs,
indicating increased molecular mobility.
Temperature at which, upon cooling,
a noncrystalline ceramic or polymer
transforms from a supercooled liquid to a
rigid glass (red line (b) in Fig. 2.11 A).
Supercooled liquid: A liquid that has
been cooled at a sufficiently rapid rate to
a point below the temperature at which an
equilibrium phase change can occur.

A representative example of ceramic structure is the silica (SiO_2). Despite of its simple chemical formula, it can exist in many different forms (polymorphism) and it is the basis of many ceramic formulations, such as alumino-silicate glasses used in glass ionomer cements, or combined with potassium, sodium or calcium in feldspathic ceramics. Crystalline silica (quartz, tridymite, and β-cristobalite – Fig. 2.11 B) is partly ionic and partly covalently bound in tetrahedral form (Fig. 2.1 B and C). In amorphous noncrystalline silica (glass, fused silica, or vitreous silica), the Si-O bond is mostly covalent, meaning that each bond is strong and directional (Fig. 2.10). Additions of modifying elements, such as sodium, loosen up the strong bonds and make the material pliable at lower temperatures (695^0C for soda-lime-silica glass compared to 1580^0C for fused silica). Soda (Na_2O) and lime (CaO) considerably lower the viscosity, and thus the **glass transition temperature** (T_g), by causing extensive disruption of the network. Oxides of titanium, zinc, lead and aluminium can all take part in the formation of the glassy network, and produce stiff network structures.

As mentioned, the temperature can produce phase changes and also a change of the state (main phase) of the material. A solid crystalline ceramic structure can melt when heated to its crystal melting transition temperature (T_m), therefore changing from solid to liquid state, which is accompanied by a change in the volume of the material. A plot (volume vs temperature) can show a distinct increase in the specific volume at a specific temperature (the melting point - T_m) (blue line (a) in Fig. 2.11 A). As the specific volume is effectively the inverse of the density, the increase in volume at T_m is not surprising since the material changed from an ordered crystalline structure to a disordered liquid, and the packing density of the atoms in the liquid is considerably less than in the crystalline solids. In the case of heating an amorphous solid, it does not show a discrete solid-liquid transition, but a gradual increase in the volume. The temperature at which this change in the slope of the specific volume occurs is the glass transition temperature (T_g) (red line (b) in Fig. 2.11 A). This expansion upon heating and contraction on cooling produces changes in the volume and, consequently, in the length of a solid. Thus, the fractional change in length divided by the change in temperature is named as (linear) coefficient of thermal expansion (CET or α_l). Therefore, the T_g can be defined as the temperature at which a sharp increase in the CET occurs, indicating increased molecular mobility.

Conversely, the liquid-solid transformations are also dependent on temperature changes, and the resulting solid depends on the cooling rate. Therefore, liquid silica on cooling can form either glasses or crystalline solids. When crystallization occurs on cooling (Fig. 2.11 A, curve a), there is a sharp, distinct reduction in the volume because of configurational contraction, as there is a large increase in the packing fraction when changing from a disordered liquid to an ordered crystalline solid. Once this sharp contraction has been completed, the material continues to contract by normal thermal contraction. If crystallization does not occur (Fig. 2.11 A, curve b), the liquid undergoes both normal thermal contraction and configurational contraction, forming an unstable **supercooled liquid** between T_m and T_g, whereupon the rate of contraction slows down significantly, the liquid becomes so

Vitrification: During firing of a ceramic body, the formation of a liquid phase that upon cooling becomes a glass-bonding matrix.

Devitrification: Process in which a glass (noncrystalline or vitreous solid) transforms to a crystalline solid.

Glass-ceramics: A fine-grained crystalline ceramic material that was formed as a glass and subsequently devitrified (or crystallized), that is, a ceramic consisting of a glass matrix phase and at least one crystal phase produced by controlled crystallization of the glass.

Annealing: Process of slowly cooling glass to relieve internal stresses after it was formed. Glass which has not been annealed is liable to crack or shatter when subjected to a relatively small temperature change or mechanical shock. Annealing glass is critical to its durability. If glass is not annealed, it will retain many of the thermal stresses caused by quenching and significantly decrease the overall strength of the glass.

The glass is heated until the temperature reaches a stress-relief point, that is, the *annealing temperature* (also called *annealing point*) at a viscosity, η, of 10^{13} Poise (or 10^{12} Pa-s), at which the glass is still too hard to deform, but is soft enough for the stresses to relax. The piece is then allowed to heat-soak until its temperature is even throughout. The time necessary for this step varies depending on the type of glass and its maximum thickness. The glass is then slowly cooled at a predetermined rate until its temperature is below the *strain point* ($\eta = 10^{14.5}$ Poise). Following this, the temperature can safely be dropped to room temperature at a rate limited by the heat capacity, thickness, thermal conductivity (k), and CET of the glass.

viscous that configurational changes can no longer take place, and the liquid structure has been frozen in as a glass. So, if the liquid is cooled quickly, the solid formed is likely to be a glass, and the process is known as **vitrification**. Yet, it is possible that a small amount of crystallization occurs in the production of a glass, although the rate of the crystals' growth is very low. This process is known as **devitrification** and it may happen when the glass is kept at an elevated temperature for a long time, allowing some reorganization of the molecules. The glass will tend to take on a translucent appearance, due to the scattering of light from the surfaces of the small crystals. This is the basis of the formation of **glass-ceramics**.

As for devitrification, glasses and ceramics containing a glass phase can be annealed to allow molecular or atomic rearrangement. The annealing point is the temperature at which residual stresses in a glass are eliminated within about 15 min, and it corresponds to a glass viscosity of about 10^{12} Pa-s. This **annealing** process should be used after grinding or polishing ceramic containing a glass phase or glasses in preparation to any research protocol involving sample indentation, such as hardness measurements and fracture toughness techniques as indentation fracture (IF) and indentation strength (IS). For this purpose, the glass or ceramic containing glass can be annealed at a temperature 50^0C above its T_g.

Solid-solid transitions also occur with changing temperature. Silica, for example, is in the form of quartz at room temperature; it changes into tridymite at 870°C; and at 1471°C changes into cristobalite that finally melts at 1713°C (Fig. 2.11 B).

A dilatometer is often used to detect these temperature-volume transformations. Two other common thermal analysis techniques are the thermogravimetric analysis (TGA), in which weight loss is monitored during heating, and the differential thermal analysis (DTA), in which the changes in sample temperature relative to a standard are monitored during heating. DTA is often used to determine the location of phase boundaries (Fig. 2.11 C).

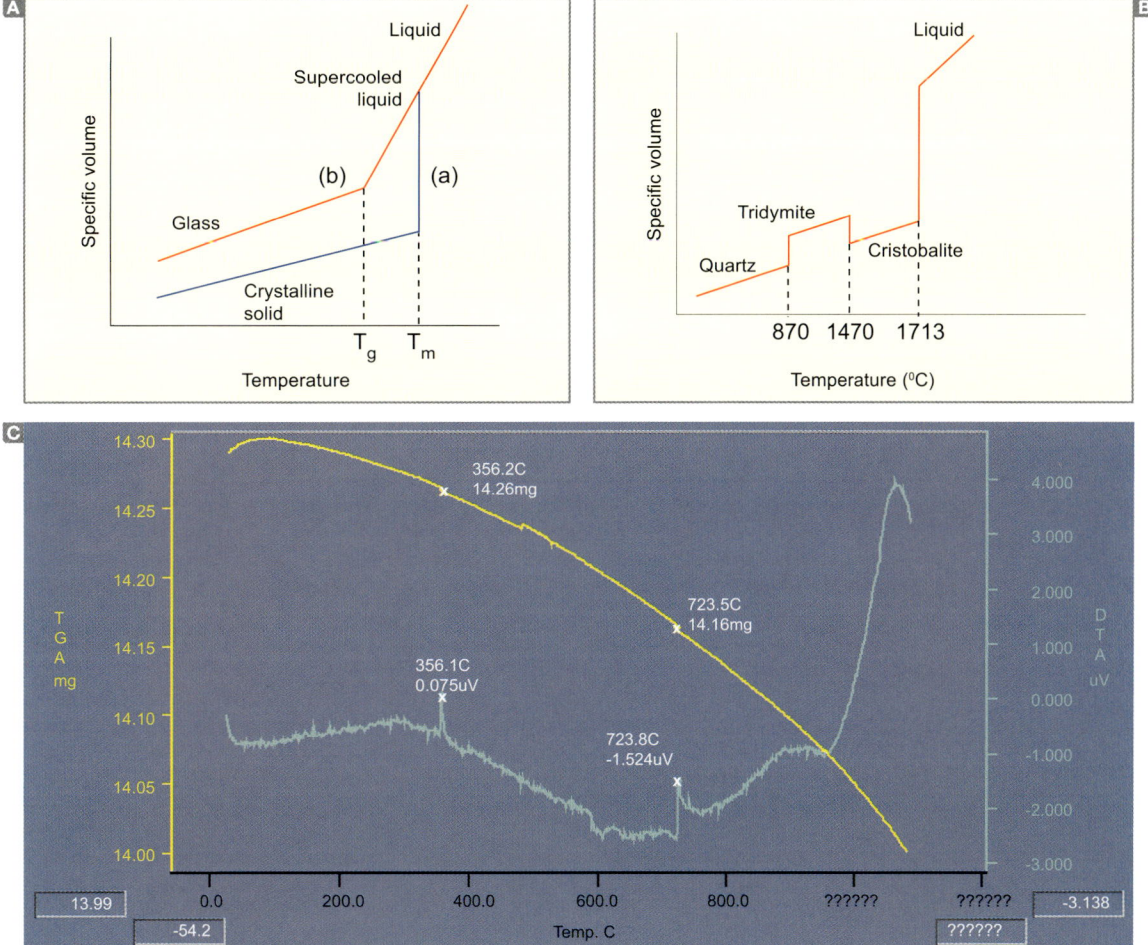

Figure 2.11 - (**A**) Solid-liquid transitions shown by the volume vs temperature curves for a material that can form a crystalline solid (a) or a glass (b). (**B**) Solid-solid transitions for silica at different temperatures. (**C**) A plot of TGA (yellow) and DTA (blue) curves for a ceramic showing two peaks at 356⁰C and 723⁰C due to phase changes.

Selected readings

- Anusavice KJ. *Phillips' science of dental materials*. 11th ed. Philadelphia: W.B. Saunders, 2003.
- Callister Jr WD. *Materials Science and Engineering: an Introduction*. 7th ed. New York: John Wiley & Sons, Inc. 2007.
- Kingery WD, Bowen HK, Uhlmann DR. *Introduction to ceramics*. 2nd ed. New York: John Wiley & Sons, Inc. 1975.
- Schaffer JP, Saxena A, Antolovich SD, Sanders Jr TH, Warner SB. *The science and design of engineering materials*. Chicago: Richard D Irwin, Inc., 1995.
- van Noort R. *Introduction to dental materials*. 3rd ed. London: Mosby, 2007.

Chapter *3*

Characterizing the microstructure, composition, and basic properties of ceramics

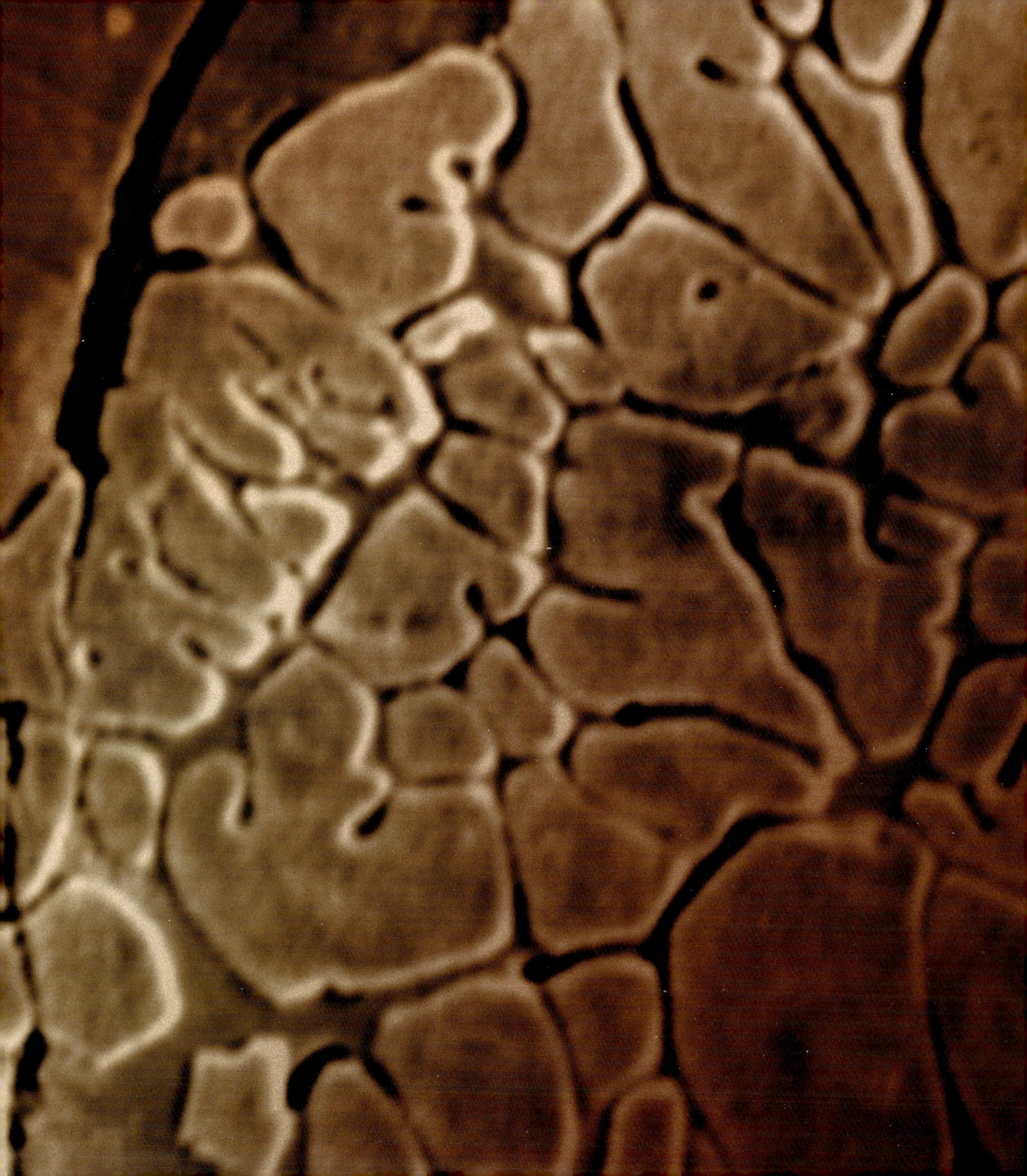

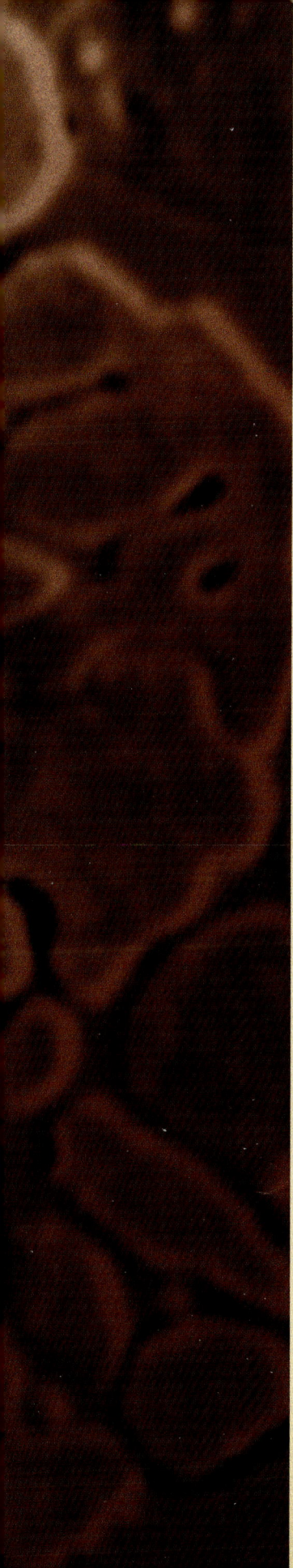

Introduction

This chapter presents and discusses the most important and useful properties, methods and procedures to characterize ceramic materials. Such knowledge is essential to plan and execute any research project involving dental ceramics and to understand the microstructure, composition and properties in relation to the structural design, performance and survival of all-ceramic restorations. This information should be coupled with clinical evidences aiming to support clinical procedures, which will be presented in chapters 4 and 5.

The appeal of ceramics as structural dental materials is based on their light weight, remarkable **optical properties** (Fig. 3.1), high hardness values, chemical inertness, and anticipated unique **tribological** characteristics. A major goal of current ceramic research and development is to produce tough, strong ceramics that can provide adequate esthetic appearance and reliable performance in dental applications.

Materials characterization and manufacturing are part of the technology innovation process. Microscopic examination is an useful and important part of the study and characterization of materials (Fig. 3.2). Examination of microstructures is often related to material properties and the information is used to predict structural properties and improve the design of new materials. Therefore, quantitative microstructural analyses provide an association among the constitution, physical properties, and structural characteristics of materials.

Tribology: It is the science and technology of interacting surfaces in relative motion. It includes the study and application of the principles of friction, lubrication and wear. The tribological interactions of a solid surface's exposed face with interfacing materials and environment may result in loss of material from the surface. The process leading to loss of material is known as "wear". Major types of wear include abrasion, adhesion (friction), erosion, and corrosion.

Optical property: It is a material's response to exposure to electromagnetic radiation and, in particular, to visible light. Materials that are capable of transmitting light with relatively little absorption and reflection are **transparent**. Light that is transmitted into the interior of transparent materials experiences a decrease in velocity, and , as a result, is bent at the interface; this phenomenon is named **refraction**. **Translucent** materials are those through which light is transmitted diffusely, that is, light is scattered within the interior. **Opaque** materials are impervious to the transmission of visible light. Some materials are capable of absorbing energy and then reemitting visible light in a phenomenon called **luminescence**, which is classified according to the magnitude of the delay time between absorption and reemission events. If reemission occurs for times much less than one second, it is named **fluorescence**; for longer times, it is called **phosphorescence**.

Figure 3.1 - When using ceramics (*e.g.* VM system), it is possible to mimic the light transmission, therefore the appearance, of a natural dentition structure. With permission of Mr. Claude Sieber.

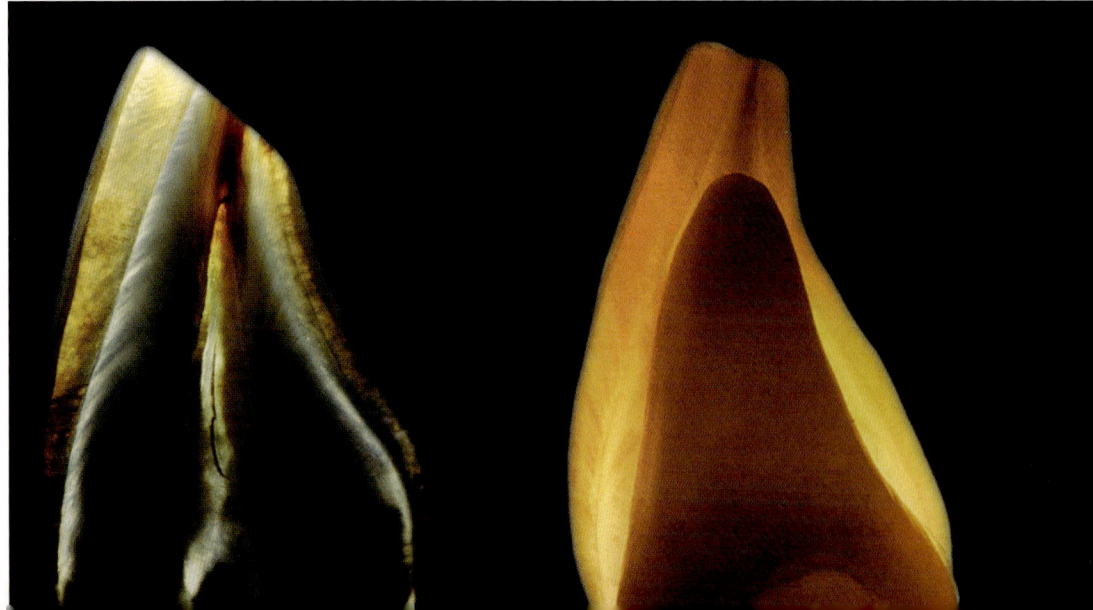

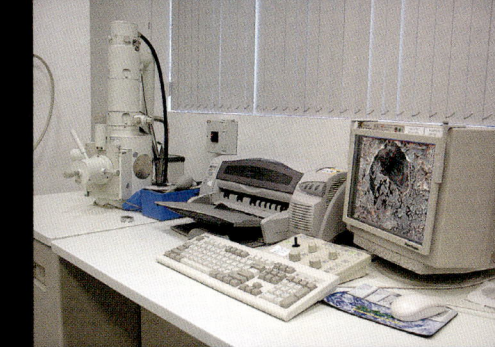

Figure 3.2 - The microstructure, critical defects and surface topography should be examined using a scanning electron microscope (SEM).

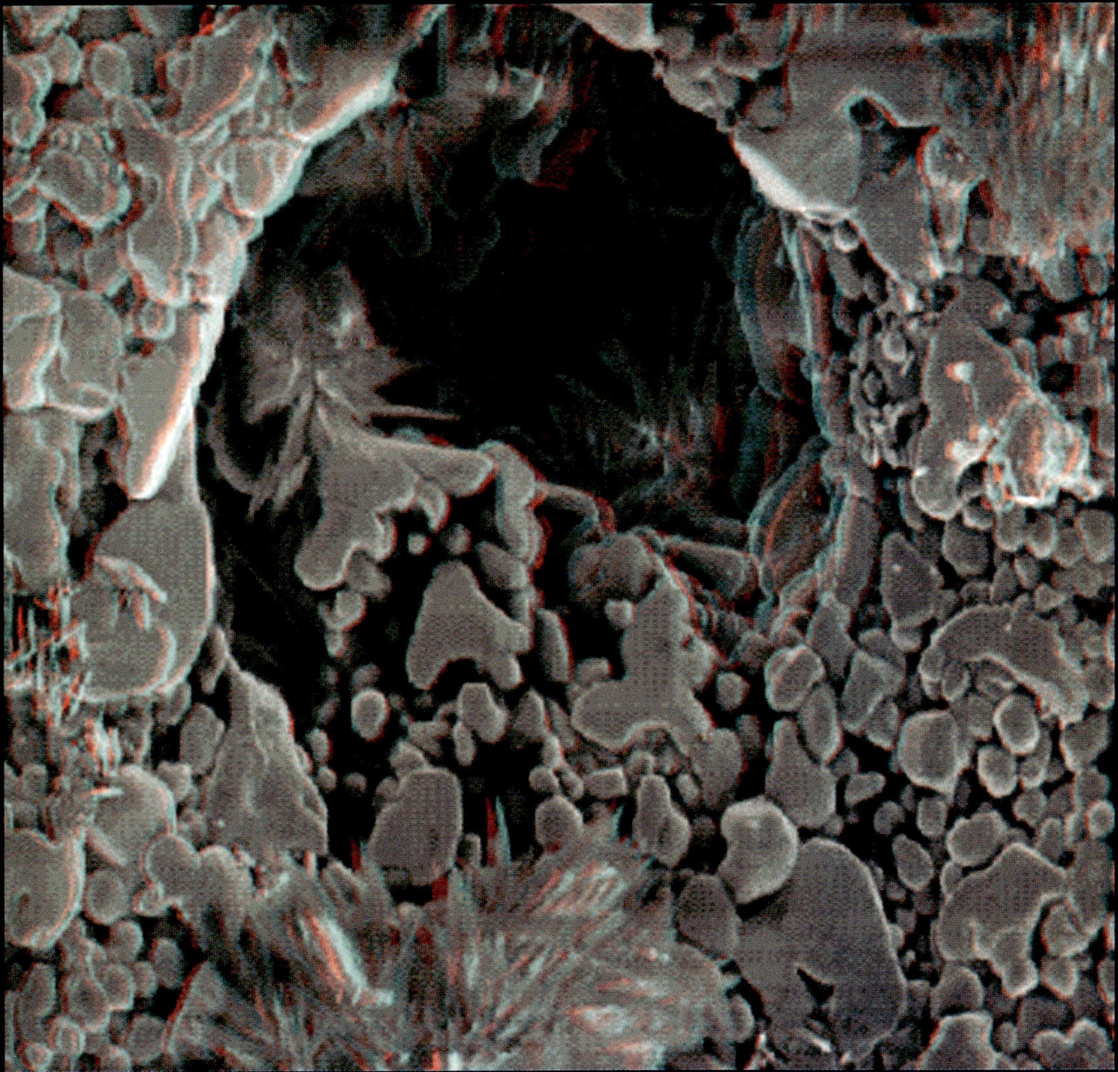

Grain boundary: The interface separating two adjoining grains (crystals) having different crystallographic orientations.

Surface energy quantifies the disruption of intermolecular bonds that occurs when a surface is created. In the physics of solids, surfaces must be intrinsically less energetically favorable than the bulk of a material; otherwise there would be a driving force for surfaces to be created, and surface is all there would be. Therefore, the surface energy is the excess energy at the surface of a material compared to the bulk.

Structurally, ceramics fall into three main categories as follows: (1) crystalline or polycrystalline (no glass content), (2) particle-filled glasses or partially crystalline (with either low or high glass content), and (3) amorphous glasses (Fig. 3.3). Examples of structurally different dental ceramics are shown in the following pages. Most of crystalline ceramics, except for single crystals, are actually polycrystalline because they are made up of a large number of small crystals, or grains, separated from one another by **grain boundaries** (Fig. 3.3 A). The atoms are bonded less regularly along a grain boundary, and consequently, there is an interfacial or grain boundary energy similar to the **surface energy**. Therefore, grain boundaries are more chemically reactive than the grains themselves and this concept has been used to enhance the observation of different material phases by lightly etch the ceramic surface before microscopy analysis (Fig. 3.4 B). This rationale is also applied to create micromechanically retentive ceramic surfaces by acid etching, improving the bond to resin (Fig. 3.4 C).

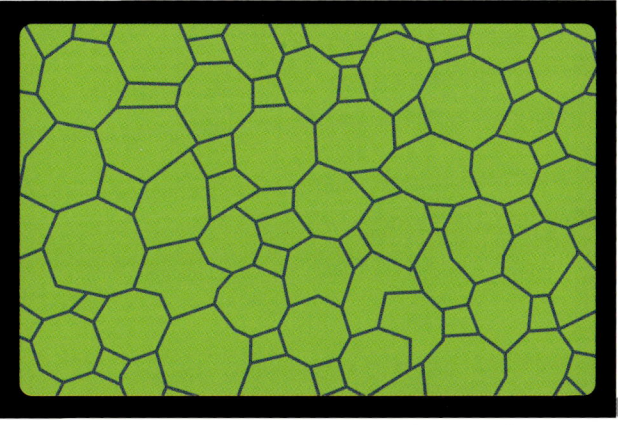

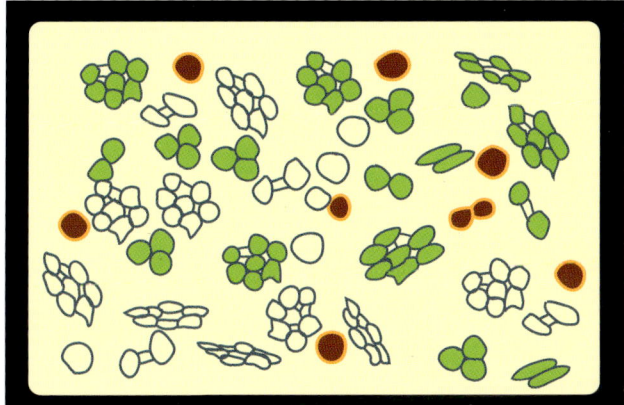

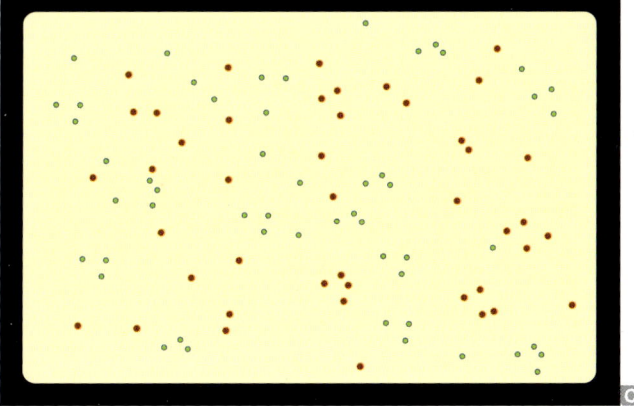

Figure 3.3 - Schematic representations of ceramic structures.
A- A crystalline ceramic material, also named as polycrystalline ceramic (no glass content ceramic material). As there is no glass, the crystals are link to each other through their boundaries (Fig. 3.10).
B- A particle-filled glass, also called partially crystalline ceramic. The glass content surrounding the crystalline phase(s) can vary (Figs. 3.4 B, 3.5 A, 3.7 A).
C- The amorphous glass may have few inclusions or defects within the predominantly glassy phase (Figs. 3.19 D, 4.7 A).

Figure 3.4 - SEM photomicrographs of a leucite reinforced glass-ceramic (IPS Empress, Ivoclar). **A**- Back scattered image (BSI) of the microstructure showing the leucite grains, the glass matrix and some cracks associated with the leucite grains (x3000). **B**- Secondary electron images (SEI) of a lightly etched ceramic surface. It was used a 2% hydrofluoric acid (HF) for 15 s. Note the structure of the leucite grains (x5000). **C**- SEI of etched ceramic surface using 9.8% HF for 90 s to produce a clinically acceptable retentive surface for resin bonding (x1000).

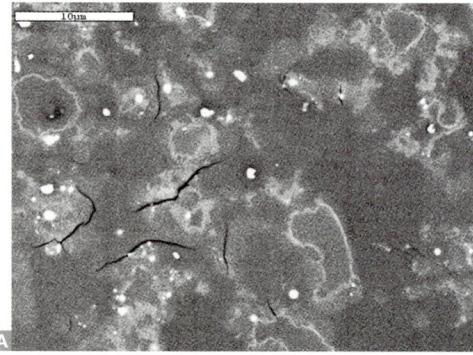

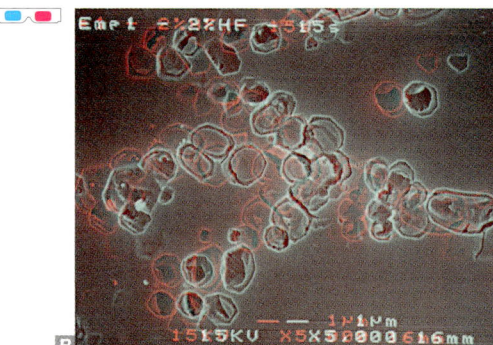

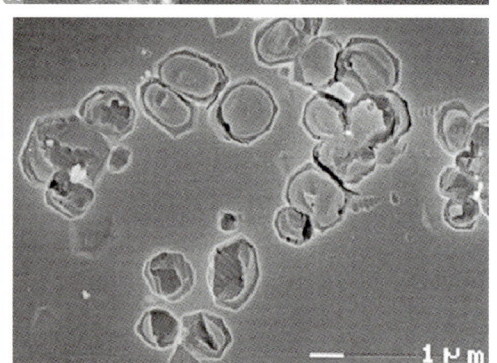

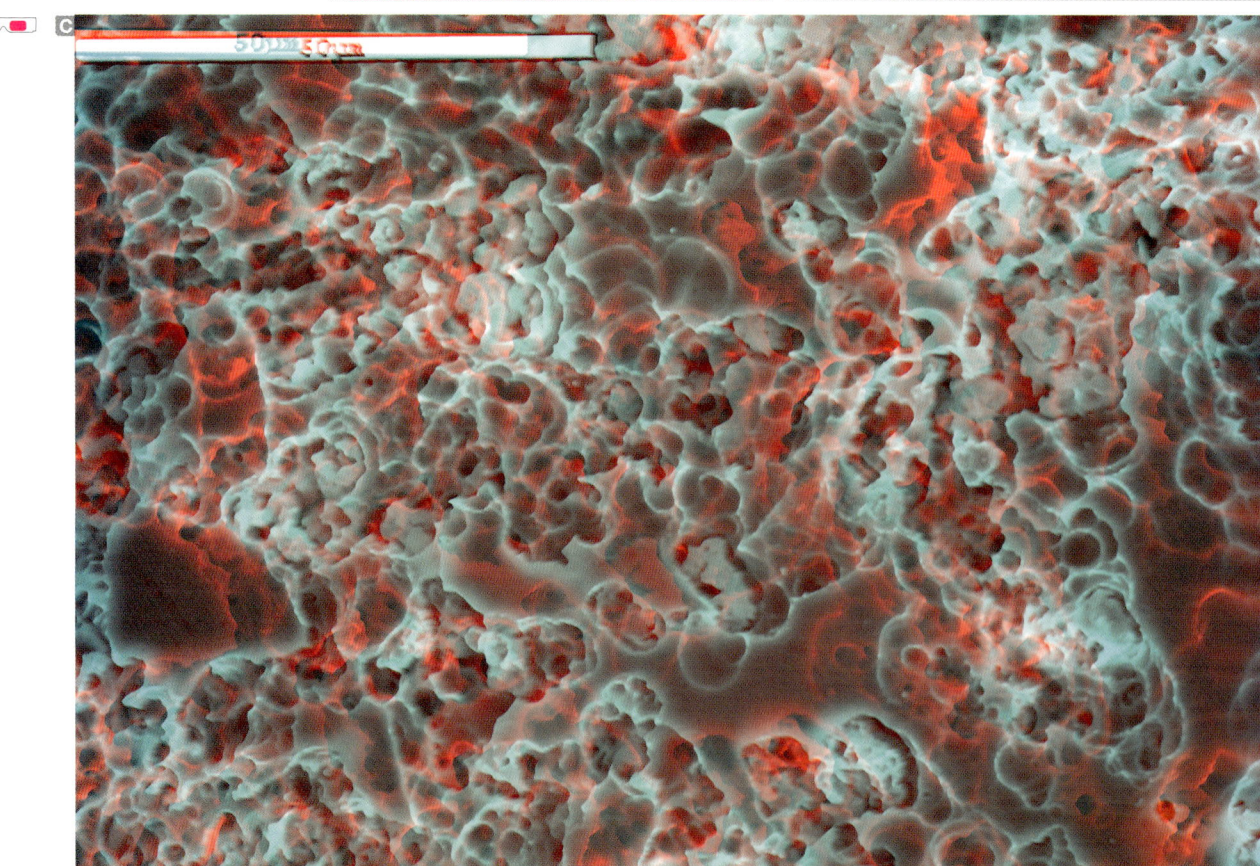

There are important relationships between chemical composition, atomic structure, fabrication process, microstructure, and properties of polycrystalline ceramics. The role of the fabrication process, for example, is to produce microstructures with desired chemical characteristics and properties. Each processing step has the potential for producing undesirable microstructural flaws in the ceramic body that can limit its properties and reliability. Thus, the microstructure, which refers to the nature, size, shape, quantity, and distribution of the structural elements or phases in the ceramics, has a profound effect on physical properties. In addition, recent ceramic research has concentrated on developing a fundamental understanding of ceramic damage/failure modes as influenced by microstructure, which is discussed later in this chapter.

The structure of each phase in dental ceramics depends greatly upon the firing conditions such as pre-heating temperature, heating rate, final firing temperature, hold-time at final temperature, atmosphere in firing oven, and the cooling rate. The coefficient of thermal expansion (CET), strength (σ) values, chemical **solubility**, transparency, and appearance are some of the properties that show some dependency on the degree and manner to which the structure is fired.

Researchers usually examine the properties introduced above by preparing ceramic samples according to the manufacturer´s instructions and following an appropriate international standard, such as the ISO standard 6872. After fabricating the ceramic samples, it is necessary to have them at same surface polishing level, which can be achieved using a sequence of SiC metallographic papers and alumina or diamond abrasive paste.

Solubility: It is a physical property referring to the ability of a given substance, the solute, to dissolve in a solvent. Chemical interaction between the ceramic and the environment at the crack tip can have a profound effect on the rate of crack growth (**static fatigue**).

51

Scanning electron microscope (SEM) images the sample surface by scanning it with a high-energy beam of electrons in a raster scan pattern. The electrons interact with the atoms at or near the surface of the sample producing signals that contain information about the sample's surface topography, composition and other properties such as electrical conductivity. The types of signals produced by an SEM include secondary electrons, **back scattered electrons** (BSE), characteristic X-rays, and transmitted electrons. These types of signal all require specialized detectors for their detection that are not usually all present on a single machine. Using the most common or standard detection mode, **secondary electron imaging** (SEI), the SEM can produce very high-resolution images of a sample surface, revealing details about 1 to 5 nm in size. Back-scattered electrons (BSE) are beam electrons that are reflected from the sample by elastic scattering. BSE are often used in analytical SEM along with the spectra made from the characteristic x-rays. Because the intensity of the BSE signal is strongly related to the atomic number (Z), BSE images can provide information about the distribution of different elements in the sample. **Characteristic X-rays** are emitted when the electron beam removes an inner shell electron from the sample, causing a higher energy electron to fill the shell and release energy. These characteristic X-rays are used to identify the composition and measure the abundance of elements in the sample.

Specific X-ray wavelengths are selected and counted, either by **wavelength dispersive spectroscopy** (WDS) or **energy dispersive spectroscopy** (EDS). WDS utilizes Bragg diffraction from crystals to select X-ray wavelengths of interest and direct them to gas-flow or sealed proportional detectors. In contrast, EDS uses a solid state semiconductor detector to accumulate X-rays of all wavelengths produced from the sample. Chemical composition is determined by comparing the intensities of characteristic X-rays from the sample material with intensities from known composition (standards). Count from the sample must be corrected (*e.g.*, PRZ or ZAF methods) for matrix effects to yield chemical compositions. The resulting chemical information is gathered in textural context (Fig. 3.5). Variations in chemical composition within a material (zoning), such as a mineral grain or metal, can be readily determined.

Fourier-transform spectroscopy is a measurement technique whereby spectra are collected based on measurements of the temporal coherence of a radiative source, using time-domain measurements of the electromagnetic radiation or other type of radiation. It can be applied to a variety of types of spectroscopy including optical and infrared (IR).

In addition, the samples have to be sonically cleaned in distilled water to complete the baseline preparation process.

A **scanning electron microscope** (SEM), with back scattered imaging (BSI) and secondary electron imaging (SEI) capability, followed by energy dispersive spectroscopy (EDS) or wavelength dispersive spectroscopy (WDS), X-ray photoelectron spectroscopy (XPS), X-ray diffraction (XRD), and Fourier-transform infrared reflection spectroscopy (FTIR) are the usual analytical instruments and methods to perform quantitative and qualitative analyses of the microstructure and composition of ceramics. Few studies examined and compared the surface and bulk composition of commercially available feldspathic ceramics. The authors reported a small increase of Si in the surface layer and a reduction of K and Na in the bulk composition, which were considered to be virtually indistinguishable. These results suggest that the compositional analysis protocol can use methods, such as WDS and EDS that collect data up to 1 μm from the ceramic surface, to estimate the composition of the material.

Whenever compositional analyses (SEM-EDS) are part of the research protocol (Fig. 3.5), the ceramic specimens should be mounted on aluminum stubs using carbon coating paste or tape for better conductivity. Then, the polished and/or lightly etched ceramic surface should be carbon coated to avoid any signal interference and/or masking of element peaks by the gold and palladium present in gold coating procedures. As mentioned, to enhance the observation of microstructural features (*e.g.*, grains and grains boundaries), acid-sensitive ceramic specimens can be lightly etched with 2% hydrofluoric acid (HF) for few seconds (10-15 s), followed by rinsing in running water for 30 s, and air dried (Fig. 3.4 B). The BSE mode is often preferred for the SEM analysis (Figs. 3.5 A; and 3.7 A). The overall surface composition and/or each ceramic phase composition can be determined by either EDS or WDS using an electron microprobe X-ray analyzer connected to the SEM (Fig. 3.5). Compositional correction methods, such as ZAF and PRZ, are normally used (Fig. 3.5 B, C, D; Fig. 3.7 D, E). PRZ is a type of matrix correction scheme that uses a set of equations to correct for X-ray absorption, atomic number effect, and fluorescence from different elements in the sample.

For topographical analysis (SEM), mounted ceramic samples should be sputter-coated with gold-palladium and examined using the SEI mode.

The XRD is often used to determine or confirm the presence of a crystalline phase. Most of the XRD equipments use powder samples. Therefore, ceramic specimens have to be ground down to powder, mixed with an adhesive (*i.e.*, 1:7 collodian – amyl acetate), and placed on a glass slide sample area. Therefore, this method would show no crystalline phase in amorphous glasses. The FTIR can also be used to identify any ceramic crystalline phase.

The microstructural features of crystalline materials such as volume fraction (V_V) and average area of crystals ($\bar{A}$) are important parameters in the materials characterization and can be estimated using **stereologic** principles and a method known as point counting, as recommended by the ASTM E562 (Fig. 3.6). The method uses clear plastic grids with a number of systematically spaced points. The grid is placed on a photomicrograph and the number of points lying on the crystals ($P\alpha$) is counted and divided by the total number of grid points (P_T).

Stereology describes the relationship between measurements made on the two-dimensional plane of polished surfaces and the three-dimensional microstructural features to be sampled.

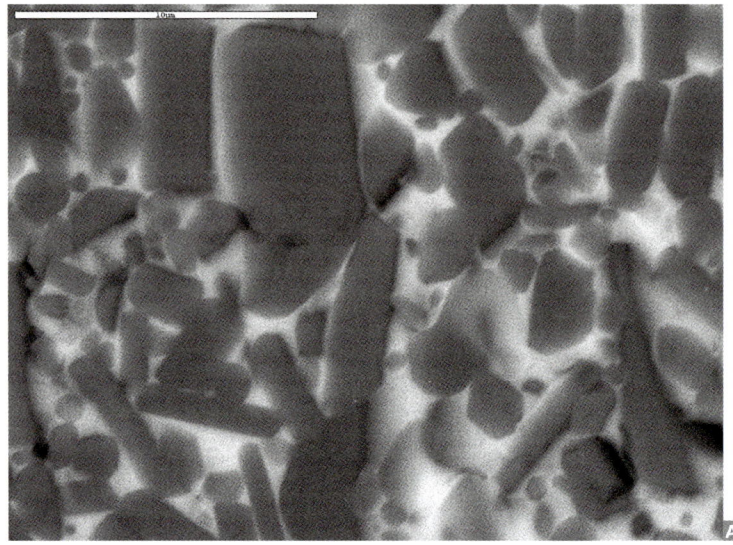

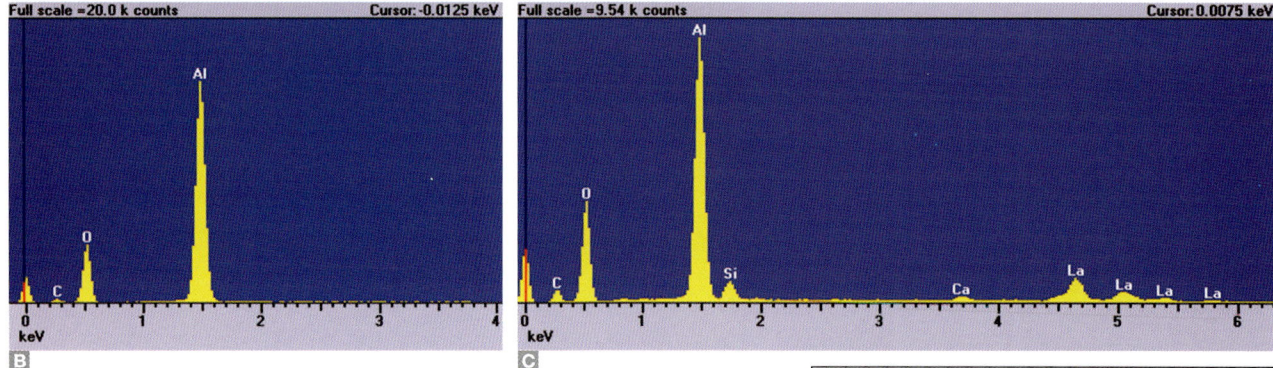

Figure 3.5 - Ceramic surfaces can be examined using SEM-EDS to obtain representative images of the microstructure and a semi-quantitative analysis of the composition. **A**- A BSI photomicrograph of a glass-infiltrated alumina-based ceramic (In-Ceram Alumina, Vita). The dark phase is alumina infiltrated by a lanthanum oxide-based glass (light phase); the top white bar is 10 μm. The semi-quantitative compositional analyses using EDS and ZAF correction show alumina crystals (**B**) and alumina and La_2O_3-based glass for the overall ceramic composition (**C**). **D**- A report on the semi-quantitative results quantifying the element intensity peaks from images **B** and **C**; without carbon and oxygen for the overall composition (**C**) and without carbon for the aluminium oxide crystals (**B**).

B- In-Ceram Alumina: Alumina crystal without C

SEMQuant results. Listed at 2:57:30 PM on 3/17/05
System resolution = 65 eV
Quantitative method: ZAF (4 iterations).
Analyzed all elements and normalized results.

Elmt Spect. Type Element % Atomic %
O K ED 49.93 62.71
Al K ED 50.07 37.29
Total 100.00 100.00
****

C- In-Ceram Alumina: overall without C and O

SEMQuant results. Listed at 3:06:47 PM on 3/17/05
System resolution = 66 eV
Quantitative method: ZAF (4 iterations).
Analyzed all elements and normalized results.

Elmt Spect. Type Element %
Al K ED 79.27
Si K ED 3.58
Ca K ED 1.02
La L ED 16.13
Total 100.00

A point lying on a crystal boundary is counted as half. This procedure is repeated on several fields from different sections selected without bias. The point fraction (P_P) is given by: $P_P = P\alpha/P_T$. Studies have shown that P_P is equal to the area fraction (A_A) and to the volume fraction ($P_P = A_A = V_V$). In addition, the average area of the crystals ($\bar{A}$) can be calculated by dividing the crystalline V_V by the number of crystals within a given measurement area (N_A) [$\bar{A} = V_V/N_A$]. As for any dental composite, the size of the particles (crystals) is greatly related to the wear. The larger the crystals, the greater the wear. Recently, the V_V has being estimated using an auto beam-area measurement function based on intensity histograms generated by a computer program (*e.g.*, Link ISIS program) that is attached to the SEM operating in BSI mode (Fig. 3.7 B, C).

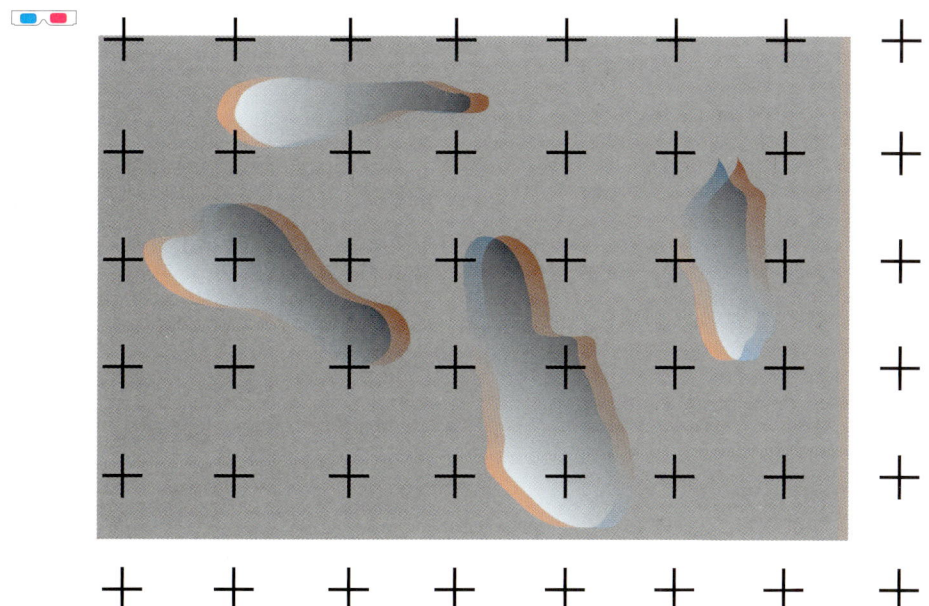

Figure 3.6 - Schematic representation of a clear plastic grid with a number of systematically spaced points (grid points, P_T) placed on a photomicrograph to count the number of points lying on the crystals ($P\alpha$). Once the point fraction (P_P) is determined ($P_P = P\alpha/P_T$), the V_V can be estimated ($P_P = V_V$).

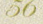

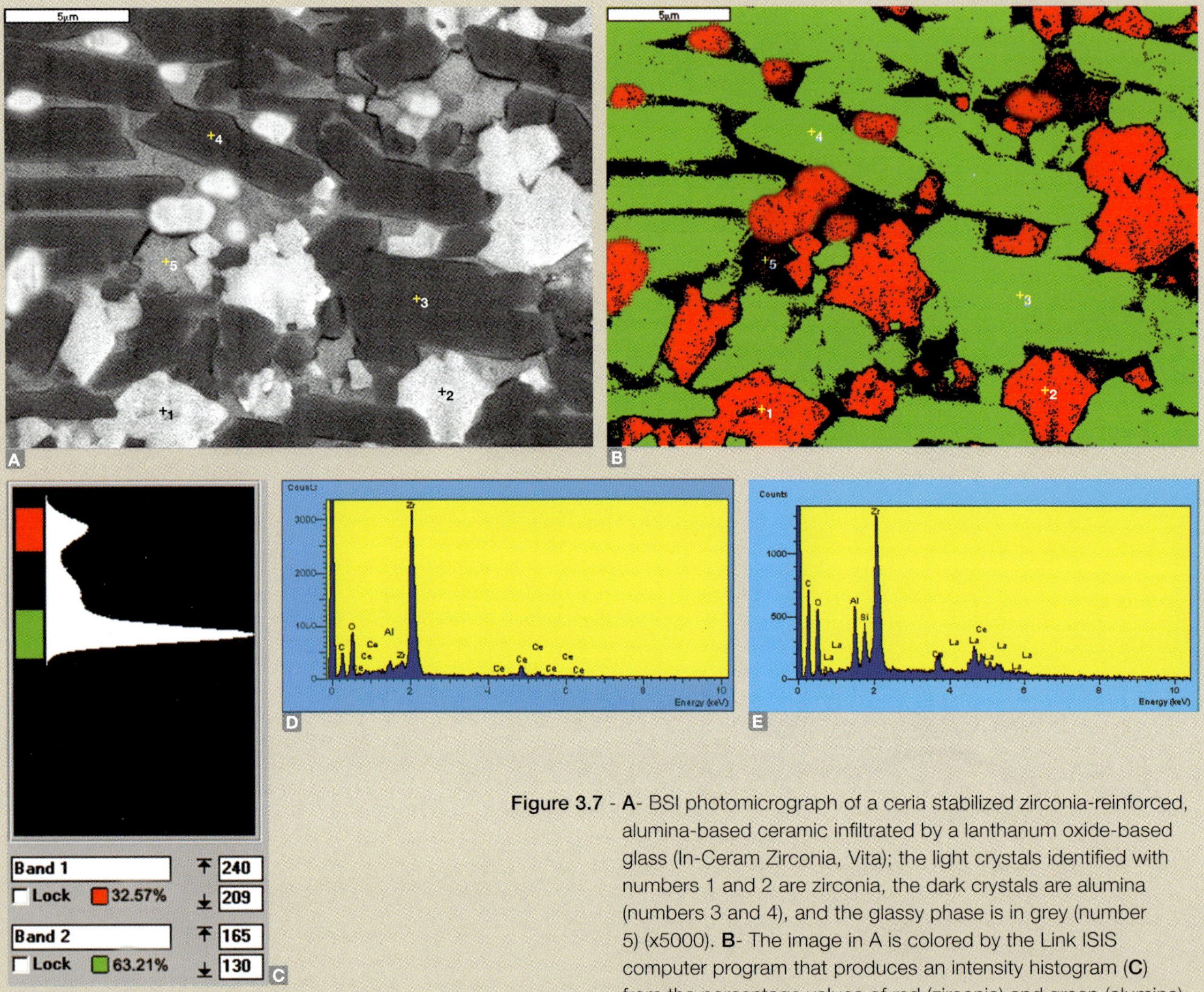

Figure 3.7 - **A**- BSI photomicrograph of a ceria stabilized zirconia-reinforced, alumina-based ceramic infiltrated by a lanthanum oxide-based glass (In-Ceram Zirconia, Vita); the light crystals identified with numbers 1 and 2 are zirconia, the dark crystals are alumina (numbers 3 and 4), and the glassy phase is in grey (number 5) (x5000). **B**- The image in A is colored by the Link ISIS computer program that produces an intensity histogram (**C**) from the percentage values of red (zirconia) and green (alumina), calculating the Vv. Semi-quantitative EDS analyses with ZAF correction show the composition of zirconia crystals (**D**) and the overall ceramic area (**E**). Note the presence of cerium (Ce) to stabilize the zirconia.

In addition, learning about the crystal structure of materials is important to understand the volume (V) and the density (ρ) of materials. The volume of crystalline materials and their volume changes with temperature are closely related to the crystal structures, as explained in chapter 2. The volume of a glass is largely determined by the nature of the vitreous network. The density is directly determined by the crystal structure, that is, the efficiency of atomic packing, which depends on the number of atoms per cubic centimeter and on the atomic weight of the constituents. So, the density (g/cm^3) of a sample can be effectively determined using a helium pycnometer after calculating the sample volume. For ceramics, the density is a minimum value for the pure network former and increases as modifier ions are added.

The microstructure of some dental ceramics has been studied and related to physical properties. The high-expanding mineral, leucite ($K_2O \bullet Al_2O_3 \bullet 4SiO_2$), is often associated with spontaneous microcracks that result from a thermal expansion mismatch between leucite and the surrounding glass matrix (Fig. 3.4 A; Fig. 3.8 A). This type of microcracking can be minimized by reducing the leucite particle size and by obtaining a homogeneous distribution of these particles throughout the ceramic (Fig. 3.8 B), as it was done for the ceramic Fortress (Chameleon Dental Products) in the 1990´s. These inherent microcracks are rarely observed in high crystalline content ceramics and in glass-infiltrated or hot-pressed ceramics (Figs. 3.5 A; 3.7 A; 3.9; 3.10; 3.12).

It was shown (chapter 2) that atomic organization influences the properties of materials, such as ceramics. The greater the crystal organization at atomic

Quasi-plasticity: A type of deformation below the contact (diffuse micro-damage) driven by shear stress.

level, the harder for the crack to propagate. Microstructural parameters, such as V_V and crystal size, are also important for the interpretation of fracture processes. Grain size and crystal structure are correlated with crack propagation resistance, regardless of processing or composition. When the grain size of the material becomes large with respect to flaw size, the crack does not encompass enough grains to be considered polycrystalline, resulting in a reduction in both fracture toughness and fracture strength. Yet, the dominant damage mode in any given material is dictated by the microstructure: (1) fine microstructures with minimal internal weakness tend to exhibit macroscopic cracks; and (2) coarse microstructures with enhanced internal weakness tend to exhibit micro-cracked or quasi-plastic zones. Both cracks and **quasi-plasticity** can lead to degradation of properties, and ultimately compromise the useful lifetimes of restorative structures, in different ways. The two modes may be interactive: the quasi-plasticity can enhance or inhibit fracture by redistributing tensile stresses (Peterson *et al.*, 1998; Rhee *et al.*, 2001).

The effect of crystallization as a toughening mechanism for glass-ceramics has been adopted by some manufacturers (*e.g.*, Ivoclar and Dentsply - Figs. 3.9 and 5.25). It is known that a morphology that makes crack propagation more difficult, requiring more energy, increases toughness. Therefore, a combination of toughening techniques can be microstructurally designed to optimize the toughness and strength of glass-ceramics (Fig. 3.9) and high crystalline content ceramics, such as alumina-base (Fig. 3.5), zirconia-base (Fig. 3.10) and zirconia-reinforced (Fig. 3.7) ceramics.

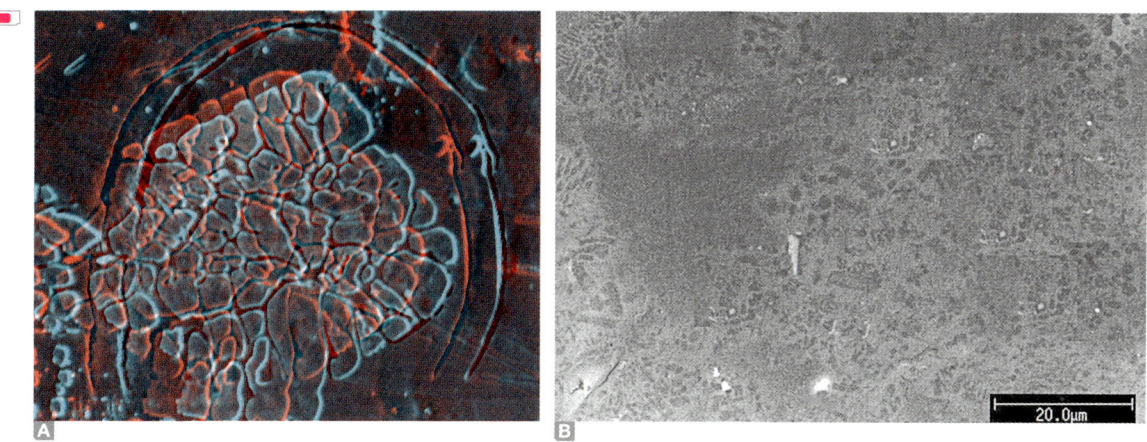

Figure 3.8 - **A**- SEI photomicrograph of a leucite cluster associated with a crack in a feldspathic ceramic (VMK95, Vita). **B**- BSI photomicrograph of a leucite reinforced feldspathic ceramic (Fortress, Chameleon Dental Products). No intrinsic cracks can be observed, which are often associated with leucite clusters. The leucite grains are homogeneously distributed throughout the material, improving the strength of this ceramic material (x1000).

59

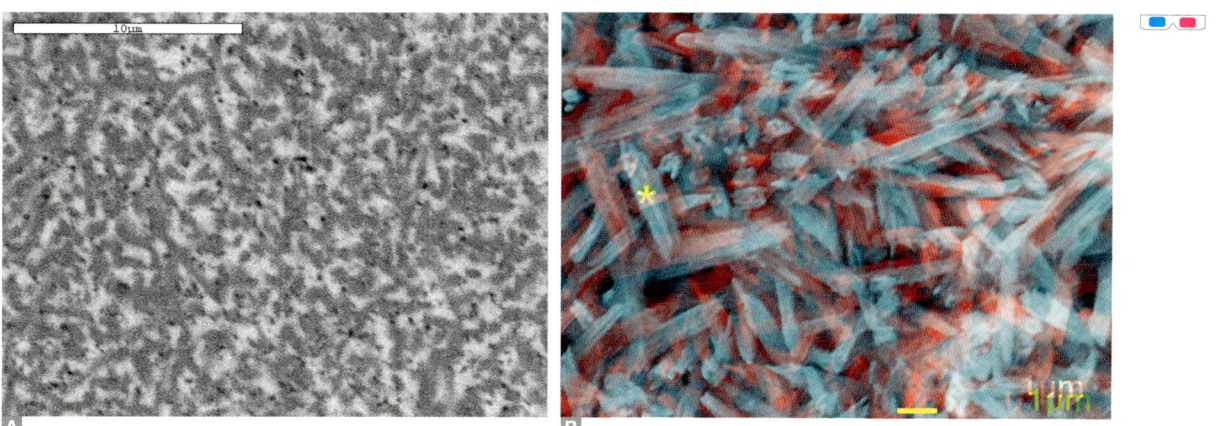

Figure 3.9 - Photomicrographs of a hot-pressed lithium disilicate-based ceramic (IPS Empress 2, Ivoclar). **A**- BSE image of a polished surface; the top white bar is 10 μm. **B**- The ceramic surface was acid etched (10% HF for 90 s) to reveal the lithium disilicate crystals (*), which were confirmed by XRD (yellow bar is 1 μm).

✦

Toughness (K): A measure of the amount of energy absorbed by a material as it fractures. It is indicated by the total area under the material's tensile stress-strain curve (Fig. 3.14).

✦

One of the most interesting polycrystalline ceramic available for dentistry is the transformation toughened zirconia. The impressive mechanical properties of zirconia are mainly due to the tetragonal to monoclinic phase transformation (chapter 2). This transformation that can be induced by cooling (Fig. 2.6) and-or external stresses, such as impact, grinding, and polishing, resulting in about 4% increase of volume, producing compressive stresses in the vicinity of a crack tip and arresting crack propagation (Fig. 3.11). Therefore, the crack must overcome this constraint to propagate, increasing the fracture **toughness** of zirconia compared to other ceramics. Thus, this transformation decreases the local stress intensity.

The transformation toughening depends on (1) the composition, size, and shape of the zirconia particles, (2) the type and amount of the stabilizing oxides (chapter 2), (3) the interaction of zirconia with other phases, and (4) the fabrication processing. Moreover, transformation toughening is not the only mechanism acting in zirconia-based ceramics. Microcrack toughening, contact shielding and crack deflection, can also contribute, to a different degree, to the toughening of the ceramic. In general, the toughness contribution from transformation (about 15 MPa•m$^{1/2}$) exceeds that for microcracking (2 - 6 MPa•m$^{1/2}$) or deflection (2 - 4 MPa•m$^{1/2}$) mechanisms. Yet, at a given temperature, the transformation-toughening contribution for 2mol% Y-TZP decreased from approximately 12 - 2.5 MPa•m$^{1/2}$ as grain size decreased from 2 to 0.5 μm, and for a 12mol% Ce-TZP this same range occurred over a much broader grain size range (8 - 0.25 μm).

Changing of the structure due to sintering

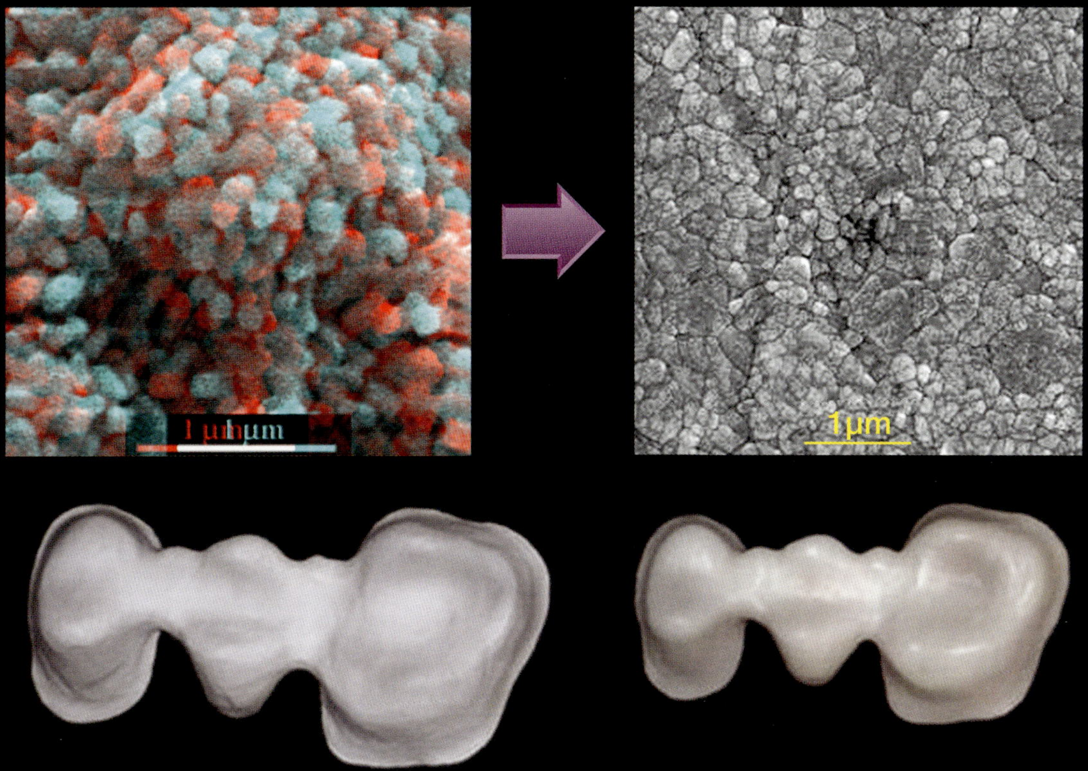

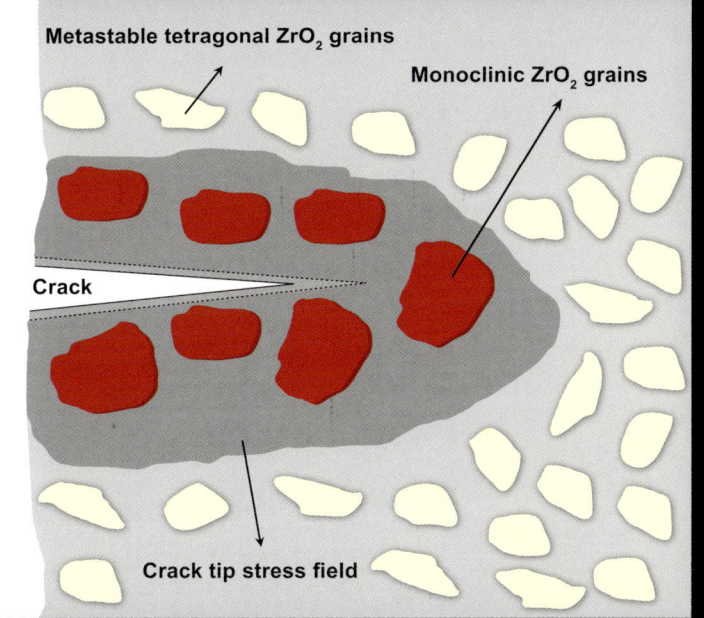

Figure 3.10 - The ZrO$_2$ crystals in the yttria stabilized zirconia-based ceramic (Cercon, Dentsply Prosthetics) contract (shrink) during sintering, resulting in a compact structure.

Metastable tetragonal ZrO$_2$ grains

Monoclinic ZrO$_2$ grains

Crack

Crack tip stress field

Figure 3.11 - Schematic representation of the transformation toughening mechanism that increases fracture toughness of zirconia-based ceramics. At the crack tip stress field the zirconia crystals transform from tetragonal to monoclinic, resulting in a volume increase that constrains crack propagation.

Low temperature degradation (LTD)
- It is a slow transformation from the metastable tetragonal zirconia phase to the more stable monoclinic phase that occurs in surface grains in a humid environment at relatively low temperatures (150–400°C). Classically, LTD initiates at the surface of polycrystalline zirconia and later progresses toward the bulk of the material. The transformation of one grain is accompanied by an increase in volume that causes stresses on the surrounding grains and microcracking. Water penetration exacerbates the process of surface degradation and the transformation progresses from neighbor to neighbor. The growth of the transformation zone results in severe microcracking, grain pullout and finally surface roughening, which ultimately leads to strength degradation. Some of the factors that promote LTD are the grain size, the amount of stabilizer, and the presence of residual stresses. As a consequence, the FDA (Food and Drug Administration), in 1997, cautioned against steam sterilization of zirconia femoral heads for total hip prostheses and specifying that it could cause phase transformation and roughening of the material, later leading to increased wear on the acetabular component.

With strength and fracture toughness greater than that of alumina ceramics (Table 3.3 and Fig. 3.22), transformation toughened zirconia represents an exciting potential material for ceramic substructure. Possible problems with these zirconia ceramics may involve long-term instability in the presence of water (**low temperature degradation**- LTD), porcelain compatibility issues, and some limitations in case selection due to opacity. It is prudent to keep in mind that some forms of zirconia are susceptible to aging and that processing conditions can play a critical role in the LTD of zirconia. However, the clinical data (presented in chapter 5) show no major problems related to the zirconia-based ceramic restorations.

As mentioned, most of today's high-strength ceramic materials are based on alumina and/or zirconia. Zirconia-based ceramics have been used for a great number of applications in the bioengineering field, including dentistry, because of their superior mechanical properties (Table 2.2). One of the first and most popular of such systems is the In-Ceram (Vita). It was patented in 1987, and it was developed using an alumina slip casting technique to build the framework that is fired to form an open-pore microstructure, which is infiltrated with lanthanum oxide (La_2O_3)-based glass. Therefore, the values indicating the high mechanical properties of this system depend upon the complete wetting of the porous microstructure by glass infiltration. The addition of about 30% of zirconia (In-Ceram Zirconia, Vita) resulted in an increase in flexural strength values from 500 MPa to about 750 MPa (Fig. 3.22).

Therefore, the In-Ceram Zirconia (Fig. 3.7) was developed by adding zirconia to In-Ceram Alumina (Fig. 3.5), combining the toughening mechanisms of zirconia with the established technology used for the partially-sintered glass-infiltrated alumina to produce stronger, tougher all-ceramic restorations that can be successfully used as posterior three-unit fixed bridges.

The success of the glass-infiltrated ceramics and the patent expiration (April, 2007) instigated the release of similar ceramics from other manufacturers. These new ceramic products were carefully examined and characterized (Della Bona *et al.*, 2008). In addition, Vita also introduced new methods to apply the ceramic slip of the In-Ceram system, such as the electrophoretic deposition (EPD) and the vacuum driven methods (Figs. 3.5, 3.7, 3.12, 3.13, and Table 3.1).

SEM-BSI, EDS, XRD analyses resulted in very similar microstructure and composition for all ceramics, except for Ceramcap (CC) that showed a lead (Pb) oxide-based glass matrix instead of a La_2O_3-based glass matrix. The Pb is a heavy and toxic metal that should decrease the ceramic glass transition temperature (T_g), increase the glass expansion, and reduce the glass viscosity that is beneficial for glass infiltration. The CC ceramic also showed lower values for E, ν and Vv. In addition, the ceramics Alglass (AG), Turkom-Cera (TC) and CC showed significantly lower strength than the other ceramics (Table 3.1). Based on these results, Anvisa (Brazilian Regulatory Agency) took CC out of the Brazilian market.

The Vitro-Ceram (VC) ceramic showed a third phase of about 3% of yttria stabilized zirconia crystals.

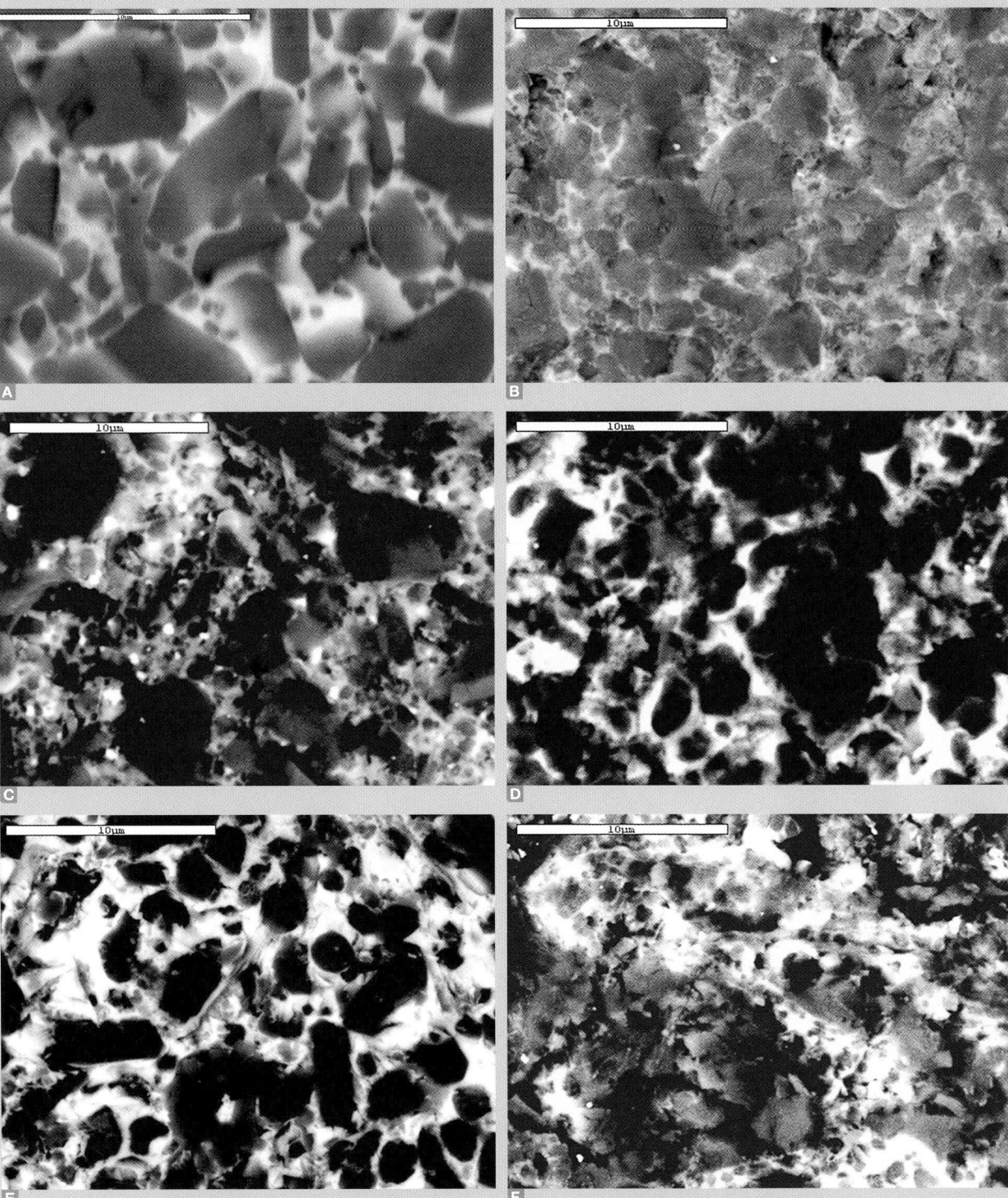

Figure 3.12 - BSE photomicrographs of glass infiltrated alumina-based ceramics. **A**- In-Ceram Alumina electrophoretically deposited (Vita); as should be expected the microstructure is very similar to the original In-Ceram Alumina (Fig. 3.5 A). **B**- In-Ceram Alumina fabricated using the vacuum driven method (Vita); the alumina crystals are closed pack compared to the original material (Fig. 3.5 B). **C**- Vitro-Ceram/Alumina (Angelus, Londrina, PR, Brazil) revealed a yttria stabilized zirconia phase (small white particles) in addition to the alumina and lanthanum oxide-based glass. **D**- Turkom-Cera (Turkom-Ceramic, Kuala Lumpur, Malaysia). **E**- Ceramcap (Foto Ceram, Catalão, GO, Brazil) showed a lead-based glassy phase. **F**- Alglass (EDG, São Carlos, SP, Brazil) a disorganized microstructure with about 20% of porosity. (x5,000 for all images; white bar is 10 μm).

Table 3.1 - Mean and standard deviation values for some properties of slip casting glass infiltrated alumina-based ceramic materials shown in figure 3.12.

	σ_{3P} (MPa)*	m*	K_{IC} (MPa•√m)*	E (GPa)	ν	H (GPa)*	ϱ (g/cm³)	Vv (%Al₂O₃)
IZ	638±64a	14±3 a	4.7±0.1 a	246±5	0.26	10.8±0.5bc	4.4±0.01	62±4
IA	489±62b	9±4 b	4.0±0.1 b	280±4	0.25	12.1±1.1ab	3.8±0.01	74±3
IAE	485±63b	9±2 b	4.0±0.1 b	277±3	0.26	12.9±1.1a	3.8±0.01	75±3
AEM	517±37b	16±5 a	4.2±0.1 b	300±4	0.25	11.3±0.5b	4.0±0.01	72±3
VC	529±67b	9±3 b	3.9±0.2 bc	284±5	0.24	12.4±0.4ab	3.8±0.01	62±3
TC	332±44c	8±2 b	3.7±0.1 c	245±3	0.25	9.3±0.7c	4.2±0.02	63±3
AG	233±26d	9±3 b	3.0±0.2 d	239±2	0.25	8.5±0.8c	3.6±0.02	57±2
CC	258±28d	9±2 b	3.1±0.1 d	166±1	0.23	7.4±0.5d	4.2±0.02	42±2

* Similar letters show no statistical difference (p>0.05). IZ- In-Ceram Zirconia (Vita); IA- In-Ceram Alumina (Vita); IAE- In-Ceram Alumina electrophoretically deposited (Vita); AEM- In-Ceram Alumina fabricated using the vacuum driven method (Vita); VC- Vitro-Ceram (Angelus, Brazil); TC- Turkom-Cera (Turkom-Ceramic, Malaysia); AG- Alglass (EDG, Brazil); and CC- Ceramcap (Foto-Ceram, Brazil). σ_{3P}- 3-point flexural strength; m- Weibull modulus; K_{IC}- fracture toughness using SEVNB method; E- elastic modulus; ν- Poisson's ratio; H- hardness; ϱ- density; Vv- volume fraction of Al₂O₃. (Della Bona et al., 2008).

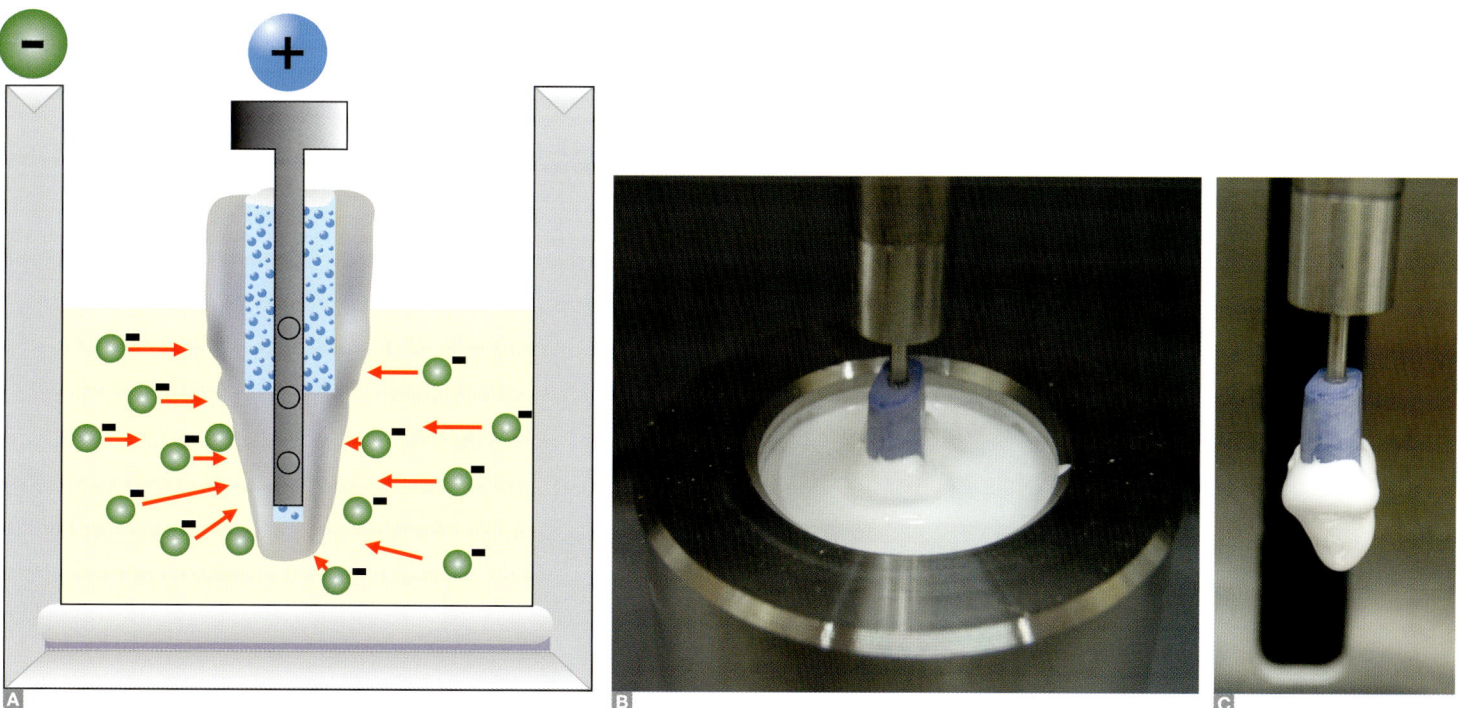

Figure 3.13 - **A**- Schematic representation of the electrophoretic deposition (EPD) of the In-Ceram slip (Vita). When an electric field is applied to a colloidal suspension, the particles move with a velocity that is proportional to the applied field strength. The motion is called electrophoresis. **B**- In the EPD an electrical polarity is applied to the mold (+) that is opposite to the polarity at the surface of the ceramic particles (-), which are electrically attracted to the mold surface and deposit as a uniform compact. **C**- When desired thickness of deposit is achieved the mold is removed from the container of slip (CeHa WHITE ECS, C. Hafner GmbH Co.). Figure 5.30 shows a clinical case using this method.

Strength: Maximum stress that a structure can withstand without sustaining a specific amount of plastic strain (**yield strength**) or stress at the point of fracture (**ultimate strength**). In fact, **the ultimate tensile strength** or simply **tensile strength** is the tensile stress (in a tensile test specimen) at the point of fracture.

Stress: Force per unit area within a structure subjected to an external force or pressure. **Compressive stress** is the ratio of compressive force to cross-sectional area perpendicular to the axis of applied force. **Tensile stress** is the ratio of tensile force to the original cross-sectional area perpendicular to the direction of applied force. **Shear stress** is the ratio of force to the original cross-sectional area parallel to the direction of the force applied to a test specimen.

Strain (ε): Change in length per unit initial length. **Elastic strain** is the deformation that is recovered upon removal of an externally applied force or pressure. **Strain rate** is the change in strain per unit time during loading of a structure.

Additionally, microstructure and composition are also controlling factors in the development of micromechanical retention produced by ceramic surface primers, such as acids, airborne-particle abrasion methods and electrodeposition technology and, therefore, affecting the bonding mechanisms to resin. This subject will be thoroughly discussed in the next chapter.

Therefore, quantitative and qualitative microstructural analyses provide an association among the constitution, physical properties, and structural characteristics of materials. In addition, the microstructure characterization is necessary to calculate relevant mechanical properties and to support further arguments on fracture and bonding phenomena. It is difficult to discuss materials behavior without proper material characterization, which should be the first step of any research proposal involving materials. Even though materials science and engineering knowledge is important to perform research, it always should be clinically oriented.

In addition to the microstructural features and properties described above, there are other physical and mechanical properties used to characterize the behavior of ceramics, such as: elastic modulus (E), Poisson's ratio (ν), hardness (H), fracture **strength**, toughness (K), and fatigue parameters.

The elastic or Young's modulus (E) is a measure of the relative stiffness, or the material's resistance to elastic deformation. The greater the modulus, the stiffer the material, or the smaller the elastic **strain** (ε) that results from the application of a given **stress** (σ) [$E = \sigma/\varepsilon$] (Fig. 3.14). The elastic modulus of a material can be directly related to the interatomic bonding forces and it is an important design parameter used for computing elastic deflections.

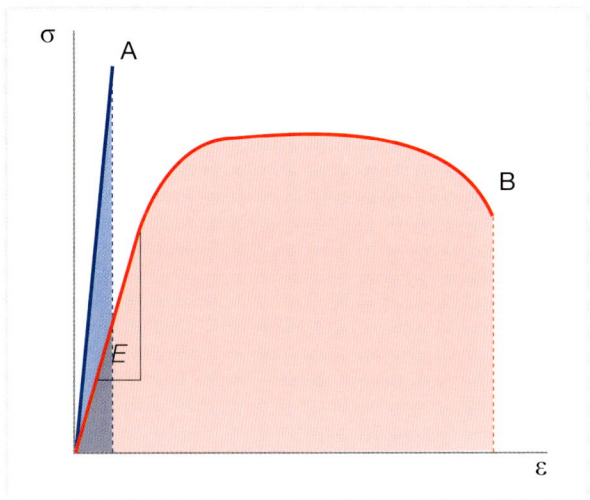

Figure 3.14 - Typical graph of σ-ε curves for different materials (A-ceramic; B-metal). *E* is measured by the slope of the elastic region (straight line) of the stress-strain graph. Although the stiffness of a dental restoration can increase by increasing its thickness, the *E* does not change. The total area (blue- and red-shaded) under each σ-ε curve indicates the material's toughness.

Poisson's ratio (ν) is the ratio of the lateral to axial strain. Theoretically, a typical ν value for isotropic materials is 0.25, but the maximum may be as high as 0.50. It is related to the shear modulus (G) and elastic modulus [$E = 2G(1 + ν)$].

The dynamic elastic modulus (*E*) and Poisson's ratio (ν) can be determined by means of ultrasonic waves and a computer program based on a set of equations (1 and 2) that uses the time of flight (TOF), density (ρ), and the thickness (t) of the sample.

$$(1) \quad v = \frac{TOF_s^2 - 2TOF_L^2}{2\left(TOF_s^2 - TOF_L^2\right)}$$

$$(2) \quad E = \frac{\rho t}{TOF_L^2}\left(1+v\right)\left(1-2v\right)\left(1-v\right)$$

The subscripted letters are longitudinal (L) and shear (s).

The procedure involves piezoelectric transducers and an ultrasonic pulse apparatus to determine the TOF through the ceramic specimens. Longitudinal and shear (transverse) TOF values are obtained and used to calculate the ν and E of the materials, which are also necessary for any finite element analysis (FEA). FEA is often used to simulate and evaluate structures under stress, determining the type and direction of stresses and displacements in mechanical objects and systems (Fig. 3.18 C and D).

Hardness (H) is a measure of material's resistance to plastic deformation. In a hardness test a load is placed on an indenter that is driven into the surface of the specimen. The degree to which the indenter penetrates the sample is a measure of the material's ability to resist plastic deformation. The Vickers indenter, a squared-based pyramidal-shaped diamond indenter with face angles of 136^0, is frequently used to measure the H of ceramic materials (ASTM C1327-03). The H values can be presented as Vickers hardness number (HV) that is a dimensionless number, or in Kg/mm^2 and MPa units (Fig. 3.15). The latter (MPa) seemed to be preferred because it can be easily related to other properties. Material's properties such as tensile strength, wear resistance due to friction, and fatigue resistance have been predicted from hardness data.

A pilot study can be performed to calculate the appropriate indentation load (P) to be applied. For this purpose, indent a sample of the material applying progressive loads, measure the crack length (c, in m), and graph $P/c^{3/2}$ versus P (the applied load, in N) for each indentation. The region for which the indentation load is constant is the appropriate load level for indentation (Fig. 3.15).

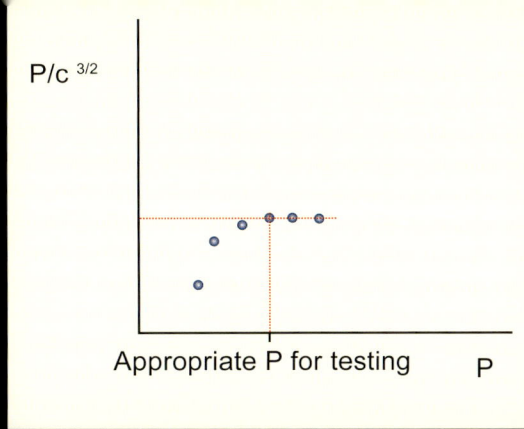
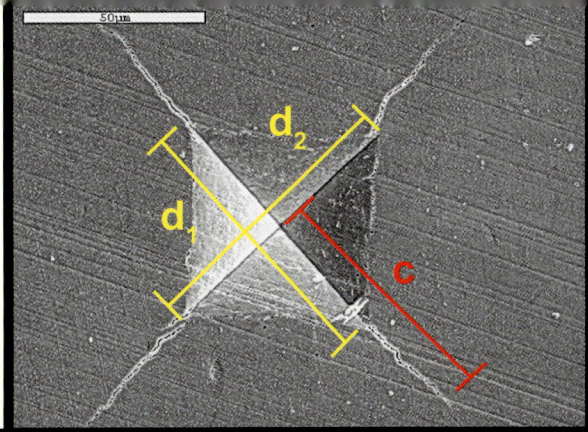

$$H = 0.0018544 \ (P/d^2)$$

P= load (in N); d= average length of the two diagonals (d1+d2/2) of the indentation (in mm); N/mm2= MPa
C= Crack length (in m)

Figure 3.15 - To find out the appropriate load (P) to indent a material, run a pilot study applying progressive loads, then graph $P/c^{3/2}$ versus P (the applied load) for each indentation. Once the appropriate P is selected, the hardness (H) can be calculated following the instructions of the ASTM C1327-03.

As ceramics are unable of plastically deform, the most prevalent cause of clinical failure is the catastrophic fracture. A mechanical failure occurs when the applied stress becomes greater than the strength of the material, which is dependent on the size of the initiating crack present in a particular sample or component. In other words, when a crack is loaded or stressed in mode I (Fig. 3.20) building up enough energy, it propagates catastrophically producing two new surfaces: the fracture surfaces. The large number of pre-existing ceramic cracks, coupled with a low **fracture toughness**, limit the strength of ceramics and cause a large variability in strength and time-dependency. Variability in strength is a consequence of the distribution in crack sizes, and the time dependency of strength results from the slow growth of these flaws to dimensions critical for catastrophic failure.

Fracture toughness: Conventional fracture mechanics parameter indicating the resistance of a material to crack extension (propagation). The critical stress intensity factor (K_c) at the beginning of a rapid crack propagation in a solid containing a crack of known shape and size. **Stress intensity factor** is a measure of the relative amount of increased stress at the tip of a crack of a given shape and size when the crack surfaces are displaced in the opening mode.

As structural reliability of dental ceramics is a major factor in the clinical success of ceramic restorations and complex stress distributions are present in most practical conditions, it has been reported that the strength data alone cannot be directly extrapolated to predict structural performance. Therefore, failure predictions for ceramics depend on the experimental parameters that measure the strength distribution and time dependency of strength. These parameters can be determined by measuring strength as a function of stressing rate in a test environment that simulates the service environment (Fig. 3.16). Thus, well designed experiments coupled with a reliability analysis can optimize rational design decisions that ensure the successful use of ceramics in demanding structural applications.

As previously defined, strength is the stress necessary to cause either fracture (ultimate strength) or a specific amount of plastic deformation (yield strength). As ceramics are unable to plastically deform, the strength refers to the ultimate stress that is required to cause fracture, most often associated with the presence of flaws within the tensile stress region. Thus, the strength of ceramics is often measured using flexural tests.

The flexural strength is generally considered as a meaningful mechanical property for brittle materials that are much weaker in tension than in compression. Several flexure test methods have been used to assess this property, including biaxial flexural, three-point and four-point bending tests (ISO 6872:2008) (Fig. 3.16). These test methods have been used for strength evaluation of single-component brittle materials and multilayered structures such as glass veneer on core ceramic specimens and metal-ceramic structures.

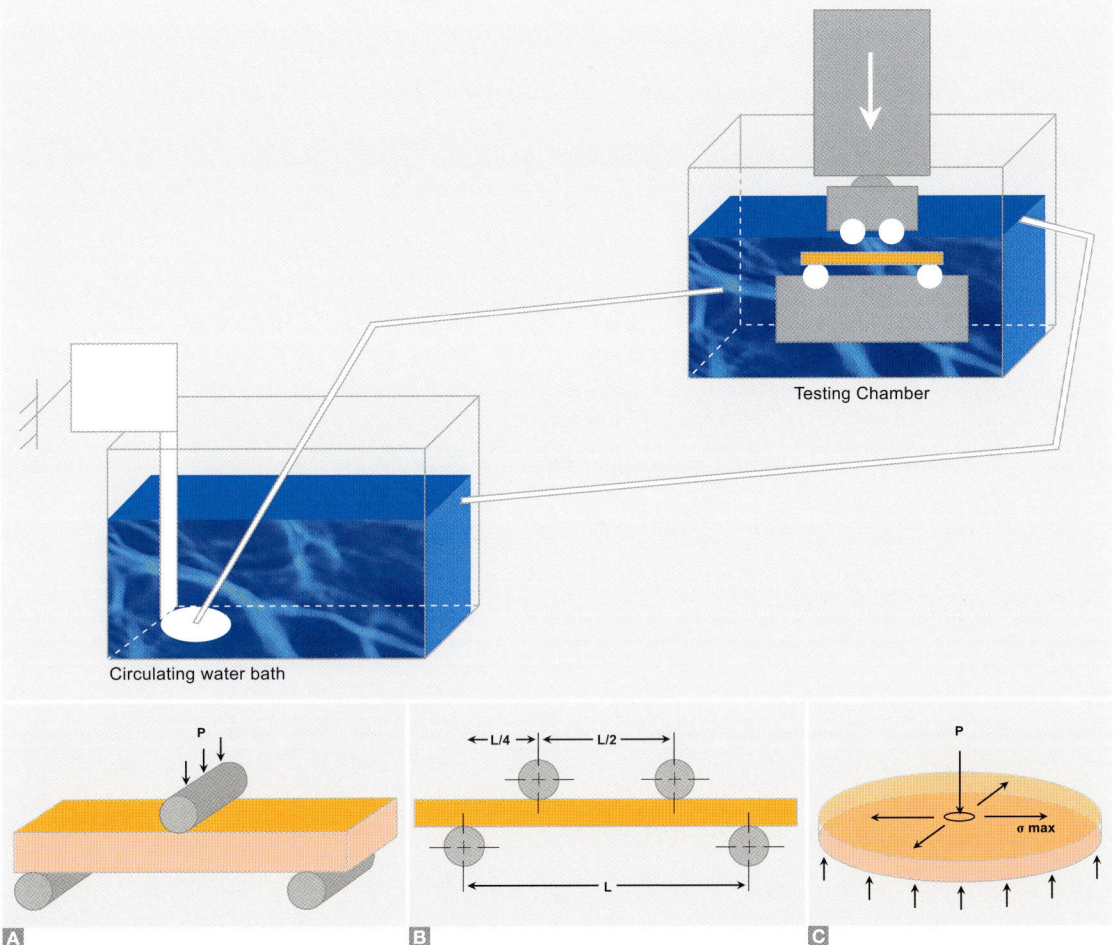

Figure 3.16 - Schematic representation of the most popular flexure test methods supported by the ISO standard 6872. **A**- three-point bending; **B**- four-point bending; and **C**- biaxial flexural test. A test environment that simulates the service environment (37°C distilled water) is also shown at the top. The water is maintained at 37°C (Isotemp Immersion Circulator, Fisher Scientific) and circulates to the testing chamber placed in the universal testing machine where any test method can be performed (the image is showing a four-point flexure test).

As explained above, it is expected that mean flexural strength values vary according to the test method and test environment. Same ceramic material can show up to 30% higher values if tested in three-point bending at room atmosphere than in four-point bending under water. In fact, a change in test method alone can result in significantly different mean flexural strength values. As an example, testing the slip casting In-Ceram Zirconia (Vita) in 3-point bending and 4-point bending, according to the ISO 6872, resulted in mean flexural strength values of 638 MPa and 564 MPa, respectively (Della Bona *et al.*, 2007). Yet, investigations of clinically failed all-ceramic restorations have shown that the fracture origin is typically located at the tensile (internal) surface of the crowns, therefore, the ceramic core surface should be placed as the tensile side for flexural testing of multi-layer structures to simulate the clinical situation.

Considering the information presented in this chapter, what is the clinical relevance of mean strength values produced by typical mechanical tests? To answer this question one should take into account that very few clinical fractures result from a single-load application, and most of the *in vitro* tests do not consider the service environment such as the deleterious effects of water and cyclic stress. So, the mean strength values resultant from most tests offer limited clinical information and should be analyzed with caution, but they are part of the materials' characterization process and, coupled with other relevant properties, should suggest the clinical application(s) of the material. Nevertheless, most commercially available ceramics are still marketed based only on "high strength" values!

The failure probability of a brittle material is statistically distributed as a function of the size and spatial distribution of flaws in the material. Failure of ceramic restorations usually originates from the largest flaw oriented within the highest tensile stress field, often located at the surface (Fig. 3.19) and typically induced by machining or grinding. The distribution of number and size of flaws justify the necessity of a statistical approach to failure analysis. Thus, the reliability of ceramics under stress can be based on **Weibull analysis**, where higher values of Weibull modulus (m) correspond to a higher level of structural integrity of the material. Most ceramics have m values in the range of 5 to 15, whereas metals, which can yield plastically during ductile failure, have m values in the range of 30 to 100. This analytical method based on statistical concepts is easily applied when a reasonable number of samples are examined (> 30), and it enables fracture probability to be calculated as a function of applied stress. Yet, Weibull analysis has some limitations that challenge its ability to predict failure of components having complex geometries, especially when they are subjected to a multi-axial stress state, which is the case of dental restorations. Nevertheless, the failure probability of monolithic and laminated ceramic structures can be calculated using Weibull statistics (Della Bona *et al.*, 2003).

In cases where the **Weibull moduli** (m) are similar among experimental structures, a crack size difference does not always explain the strength differences; strength is also a function of the fracture toughness. Thus, the differences in strength may be explained by the differences in toughness

Weibull analysis: The Weibull distribution (named after the Swedish engineer and mathematician Ernst H. Waloddi Weibull) is a continuous probability distribution most often used in survival analysis, reliability engineering and failure analysis. The **characteristic strength** or scale parameter (σ_o) represents the 63.21% of the strength distribution. The **Weibull modulus** (m) is the shape parameter and describes the asymmetrical strength distribution. The scale (σ_o) and the shape (m) parameters are related to the mean value and to the standard deviation for a material with a Gaussian strength distribution, respectively.

that, in turn, are related to the way the materials are processed to produce the final structure. For instance, if the flexural strength and Weibull modulus of a core monolithic ceramic are similar to those of the same core ceramic veneered by a glass and the fracture analysis also shows similar results for these two structures, it can be said that the structural reliability of the veneered core ceramic structure is controlled primarily by that of the core ceramic. Yet, the investigator has to determine the critical core/veneer thickness ratio (t_c/t_v) below which strength and structural reliability become significantly reduced, since this ratio appears to be the dominant factor that controls the failure initiation site in bilayer ceramic structures. In addition, the crack initiation site shifts from veneer to core as the t_c/t_v ratio increases, but the increase in the elastic modulus of the supporting substrate does not affect the crack initiation site. Therefore, the load to fracture initiation is primarily influenced by the thickness of the restoration and, to a lesser extent, the E of the supporting substrate. Using this rationale, the height to width ratio of all-ceramic fixed partial denture (FPD) connectors can be very well related to the fracture strength (Fig. 3.17).

Figure 3.17 - Schematic representation of the height to width ratio (h/b) of FPD connectors plotted against the fracture load. The greater this ratio, the greater the strength of the FPD connector.

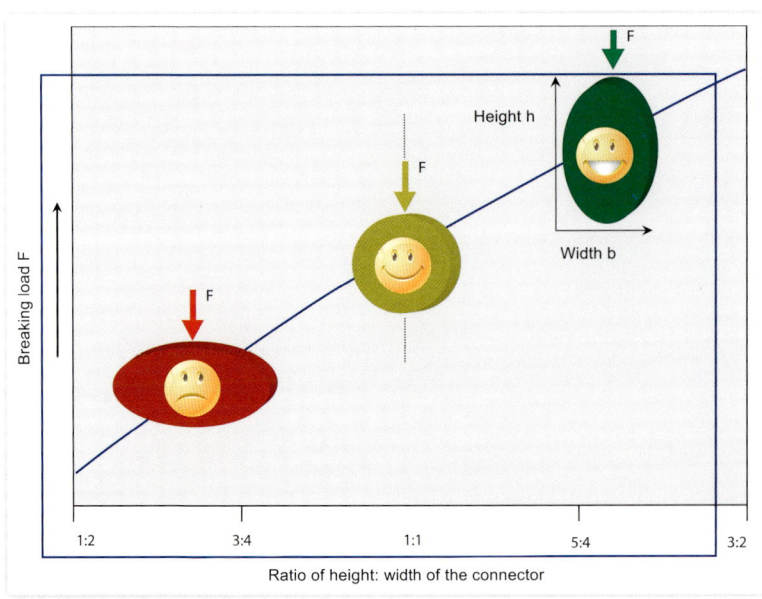

As mentioned, the catastrophic or bulk fracture is the usual failure mode of all-ceramic FPD, and it often initiates in the connector either at core-veneer interface or in the veneer ceramic at the gingival embrasure (Fig. 3.18) (Kelly *et al.*, 1995). So, not all clinical cases are for all-ceramic FPD, it is necessary to have enough tooth preparation height for a clinical acceptable height to width ratio (h/b) (Fig. 3.17).

The geometry of the FPD connectors is also important, that is, the radius of curvature of the occlusal and gingival embrasures should not be small. The smaller the radius of curvature of the embrasure, the higher the **stress concentration**. This information should improve our ability to design all-ceramic prostheses with a sufficiently high margin of safety.

Nevertheless, evaluation of the damage modes in bilayer ceramic structures (disk- and bar-shaped specimens) using an Hertzian contact test has shown that the substrate has a profound influence on the evolution damage from initiation to ultimate failure. Yet, the crack initiation tends to occur from the contact surface (Hertzian cone cracking) in systems having a strong bonded interface and a small elastic-plastic mismatch (*e.g.*, glass/glass-ceramic); whereas in systems with a large mismatch, crack initiation tends to occur at the materials' interface (subsurface radial cracking). So, all these rationale and scientific evidences coupled with (1) the complex geometry of dental ceramic restorations, (2) the composite stresses produced during service (Fig. 3.18), and (3) the challenging intra-oral environment, create a complicated clinical equation of difficult solution when considering just few of the variables. Therefore, researchers and clinicians should improve their interaction in an effort to understand this complex scenario, maximizing the clinical results.

Stress concentration: State of elevated stress in a solid caused by surface or internal defects or by marked changes in contour.

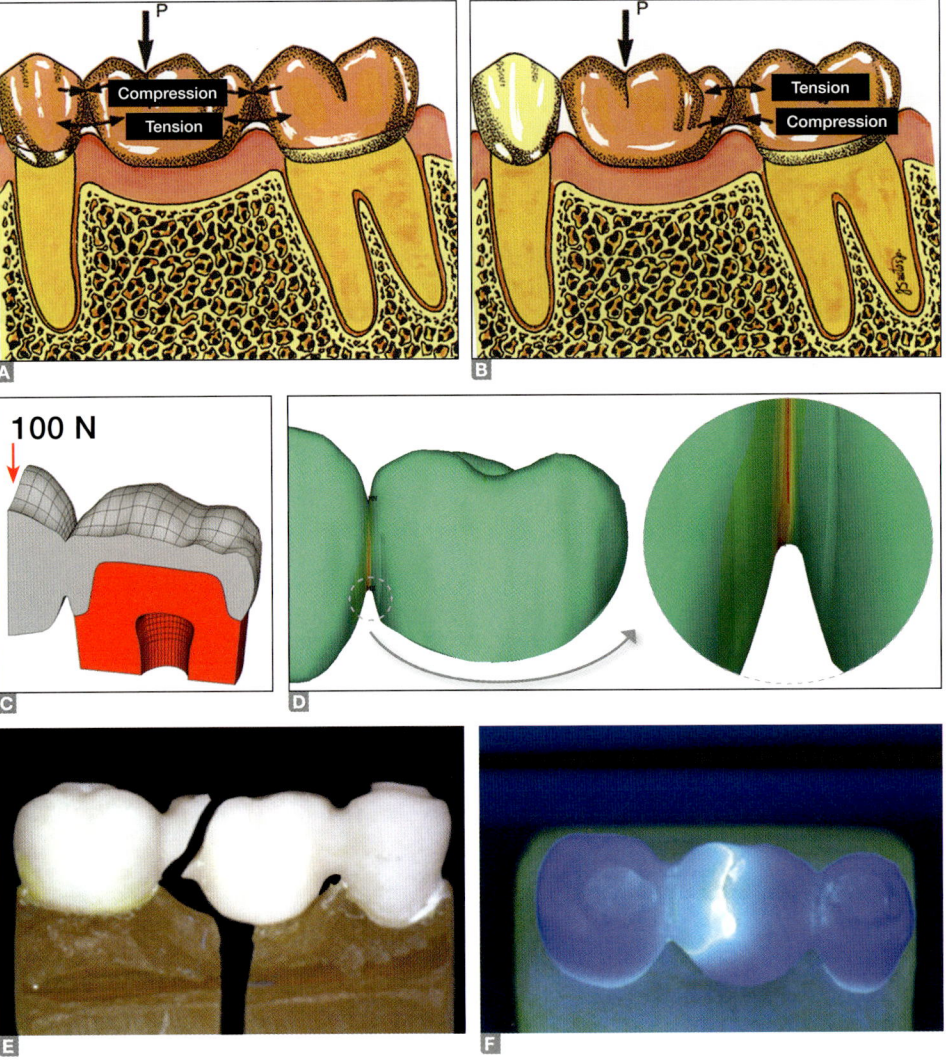

Figure 3.18 - It is known that ceramics are stronger under compression than under tension. This principle was used to improve metal-ceramic (PFM) systems in which the CTE of the ceramic should be slightly lower than the CTE of the metal, placing the metal in tension and the veneer ceramic in compression. This rationale is still sound for all-ceramic systems. Yet, the more similar the CTE values between the core and veneer ceramics, the lower the stresses developed within the system. **A** and **B**- Show schematic illustrations of stresses induced in PFM prostheses by a flexural force (P) at the central fossa of the pontic. Tensile stresses develop on the gingival side of the three-unit bridge (**A**), and on the occlusal side of the two-unit cantilever bridge (**B**). **C** and **D**- Finite element analysis (FEA) simulating a three-unit all-ceramic bridge similar to the one illustrated on **A**. **C**- A cross-sectional perspective view of one-half of longitudinally sectioned 3-D FEA model; simulated loading of 100 N at the central fossa of the pontic. **D**- The FEA image shows the stress distribution at a failure load of 740 N; maximum tensile stress = 156 MPa. **E** and **F**- Images of a fractured three-unit bridge on the working cast (**E**) and examined using a fluorescent liquid under the light (**F**). Note the oblique orientation of fracture path extending from the gingival embrasure to the occlusal contact area. The occlusal embrasure is not included in the fracture path. As mentioned, the geometry of the FPD embrasures is critically important. Courtesy of Dr. Ken J Anusavice.

As ceramic restorations mostly fail by fracture, **fractography** (fracture surface analysis) should be employed to fully understand the failure process. Fractography is well-established as a means of failure analysis in the field of glasses and ceramics and it has been recognized as a powerful analytical tool in dentistry.

The application of fractography is based on the principle that the entire history of the fracture process is encoded on the fracture surface of brittle materials. It has been used to quantitatively relate the stress at failure, the nature of the stress state, and the amount of residual stress relative to the sizes of the initial crack and surrounding topography. Additionally, quantitative fractographic analysis of brittle fracture surfaces shows that there are characteristic markings on the surfaces that are self-similar and scale invariant, implying that **fractal analysis** is also a reasonable approach to analyzing these surfaces (Della Bona *et al.*, 2001; Hill *et al.*, 2001).

Thus, the propagation of preexisting cracks is often the origin of dental ceramic fracture. These cracks can be induced by mechanical means (*e.g.*, grinding or polishing), by processing, or by intrinsic defects (*e.g.*, imperfections in the structure) and can greatly weaken an otherwise strong ceramic. Most evidence shows that crack propagation is determined by varying levels of stress intensity or energy and, because of these relationships, much information is contained within the fracture surface. Therefore, fractographic principles have been used for qualitative analysis of fracture dental restorations confirming the presence of characteristic

Fractography is the study of fracture surfaces of materials. Fractographic methods are routinely used to determine the cause of failure in engineering structures, especially in product failure and the practice of forensic engineering or failure analysis. Fractographic examination can determine the cause of failure by studying the characteristics of a fracture surface. Different types of crack growth produce characteristic features on the surface, which can be used to help identify the failure mode. For brittle materials, such as ceramics, the overall pattern of cracking can be more important than a single crack. An important aim of fractography is to establish and examine the origin of cracking, as examination at the origin may reveal the cause of crack initiation.

Fractal: Term coined by Benoit Mandelbrot (1975), derived from the Latin word "fractus", meaning "broken" or "fractured". It is a rough or fragmented geometric shape that can be split into parts, each of which is (at least approximately) a reduced-size copy of the whole, a property called self-similarity.

Fractal analysis is the modelling of data by fractals. It consists of methods to assign a fractal dimension (D) and other fractal characteristics to a signal, dataset or object which may be sound, images, molecules, networks or other data.

77

Hackle: A line on the crack surface running in the local direction of cracking, separating parallel but noncoplanar portions of the crack surface.

Twist hackle: Hackle separating portions of the crack surface, each of which has rotated from the original crack plane in response to a lateral rotation or twist in the axis of principal tension.

Wake hackle: Hackle mark extending from a singularity at the crack front in the direction of cracking (crack propagation).

markings of the fracture process (Fig. 3.19). Note that the markings are more evident on the fracture surface of amorphous glasses (Fig. 3.19 D) than on crystalline ceramics (Fig. 3.19 A, B, and C). It is evident that the more complex the microstructure the more difficult to identify the characteristic fracture markings and expert knowledge is mandatory.

Most fracture surface observations yield substantial information about the fracture process and enable the calculation of the fracture toughness of the material. In addition, the roughness of the fracture surface gives qualitative information on the extent of crack deflection or other toughening mechanisms.

It is difficult to directly measure the flaw-initiating site, especially in high-strength, fine-grained glass-ceramics, and in cases where failure is caused by poor machining practices. Whenever the flaw itself cannot be measured, the region from which the failure occurred can be determined by observing the patterns on the fracture surface, such as **wake hackle**, coarse hackle, and **twist hackle**. This is the case of the majority of multi-layer structures, such as dental ceramic restorations.

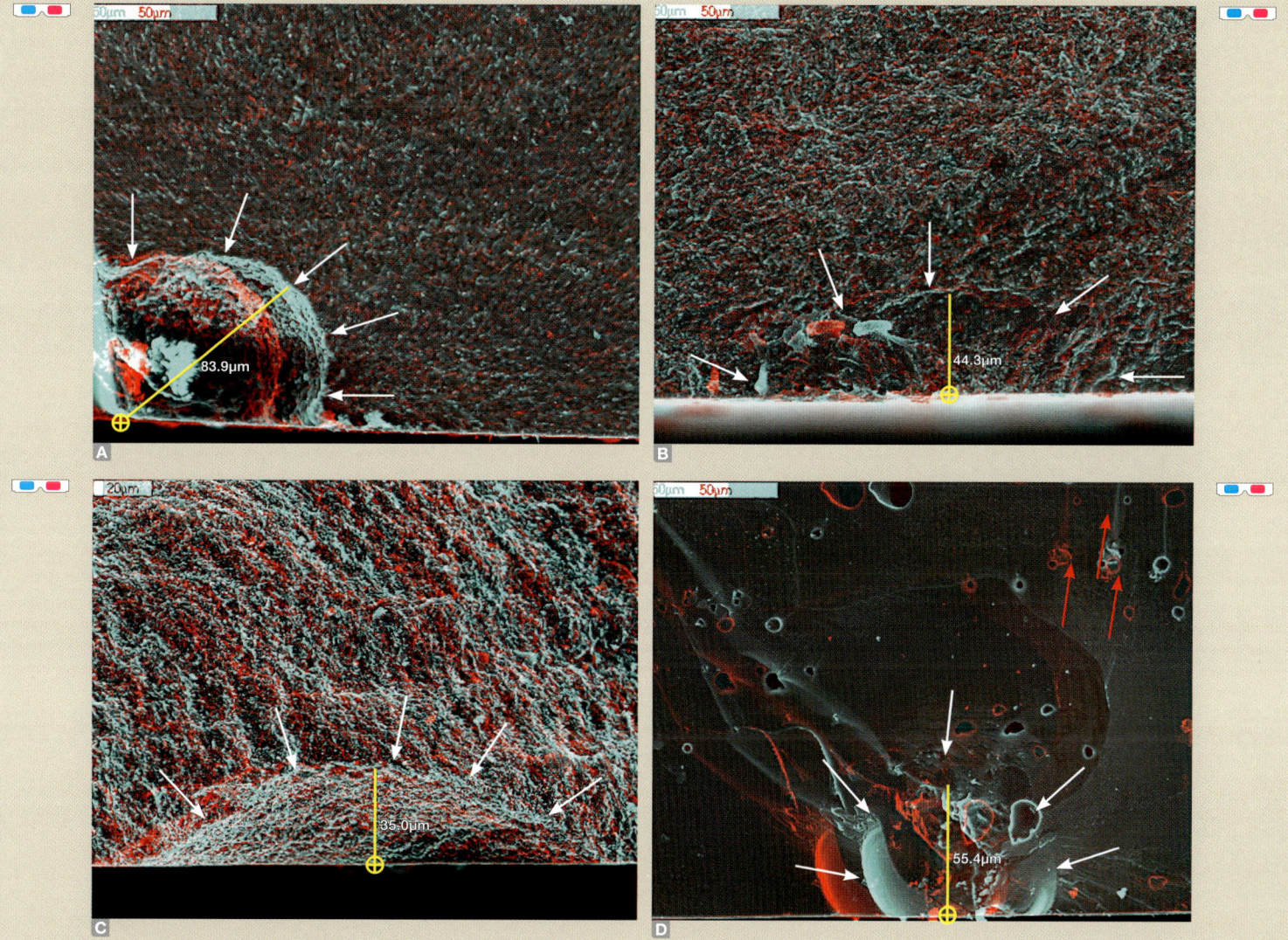

Figure 3.19 - SEI photomicrographs of ceramic fracture surfaces. **A**- Critical flaw (crack) located at the corner (outlined by white arrows) of a leucite-based ceramic (IPS Empress, Ivoclar); line from flaw corner, c = 84 μm (x500). **B**- Semi-circular critical crack outlined by white arrows of a lithium disilicate-based glass-ceramic (IPS Empress2, Ivoclar); measured line represents the semi-minor axis, a = 44 μm (x500). **C**- Semi-circular critical crack outlined by white arrows of a lithium disilicate-based glass-ceramic (IPS e.max, Ivoclar); a = 35 μm (x600). **D**- Amorphous veneering ceramic (IPS Empress2, Ivoclar) showing a critical flaw (crack) outlined by white arrows. Note the wake hackle from little voids (top right) show the direction of crack propagation (red arrows); a = 55 μm (x500).

Dr. Alan Arnold Griffith (1893-1963), worked at the Royal Aircraft Establishment (Farnborough, England). He performed a series of experiments measuring the influence of thickness on tensile strength of glass rods. He showed that as the fiber diameter reduces, the strength increases and at very thin fibers the increase in strength becomes very fast. This phenomenon is directly associated with the number and size of surface cracks, which are reduced as the fiber diameter reduces. As cracks are stress concentrators, the thinner the glass fiber, the fewer and the smaller the cracks, and the stronger the glass fiber. This rationale also helped to explain the difference between the theoretical and typical strength of glasses.

Fracture origin: It is the flaw (crack, defect, discontinuity) from which cracking begins. As it runs, the crack develops a new surface that is perpendicular to the axis of principal tension at its tip. The higher the stress at the crack tip, the faster the crack runs.

The **mirror** region is the smooth portion of the crack surface bounded by **mist hackle**, which are markings on the surface of an accelerating crack close to its effective terminal velocity, observable first as a misty appearance and with increasing velocity revealing a fibrous texture, elongated in the direction of cracking, and coarsening up to the stage at which the crack bifurcates (Fig. 3.21).

Another important material property is the fracture toughness or stress intensity factor. This property has ben extensively used to characterize the fracture resistance of brittle materials. The fracture toughness of ceramics is usually controlled by the fracture in Mode I (opening mode, tensile load) (Fig. 3.20). Irwin (1957) defined failure at the point when the Mode I stress intensity (K_I) reaches a critical value ($K_I \geq K_{IC}$). The critical stress intensity factor (K_{IC}) is in many cases a material constant and it is one measure of the toughness of the material, *i.e.* the resistance to crack propagation. Therefore, the fracture toughness or critical stress intensity factor (K_{IC}) can often be determined using the fractography approach and the **Griffith**-Irwin equation (Fig. 3.21), where "Y" is a geometrical factor that accounts for the location and geometry of the crack and loading (Randall, 1966), "σ_f" is the stress at fracture (also called applied stress "σ_a"), and "c" is the radius of an equivalent semi-circular crack for a semi-elliptical crack of semi-minor axis "a" and semi-major axis "b" (Fig. 3.21) (Mecholsky, 1995a). Fracture toughness is given in units of stress times the square root of crack length (MPa•m$^{1/2}$).

Therefore, the fractography approach to determine fracture toughness involves the identification and measurement of the **fracture origin**, *i.e.* the initial (starting) defect or critical crack (c), using fractographic principles (Fig. 3.21). In case of corner cracks (Fig. 3.19 A), the critical crack (c) size is calculated using the same equation as for the equivalent semi-circular surface crack [c = (ab)$^{1/2}$] (Fig. 3.21). However, "a" is the length of one side of the corner crack and "b" is the length of the other side of the corner crack. So, in this case, (c) corresponds to the distance from the crack corner to the critical flaw-mirror region limit, which corresponds to 84 μm in Figure 3.19 A. For internal flaws, "c" is also calculated by [c = (ab)$^{1/2}$], where "a" is half of the crack minor axis and "b" is half of the crack major axis (Fig. 4.17 C).

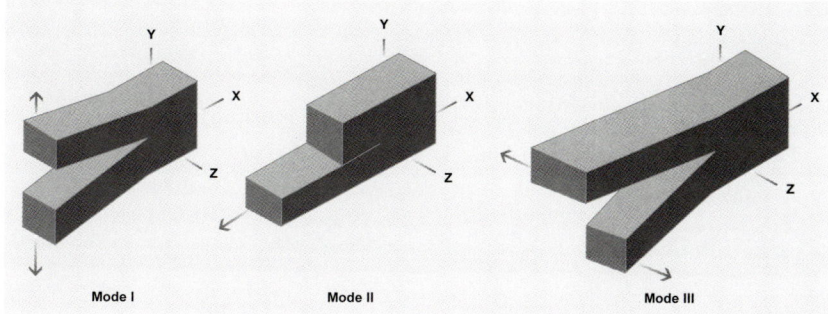

Figure 3.20 - The three modes of crack surface displacement. Mode I is the opening or tensile mode, which is the usual controlling mode in brittle fracture. Mode II is the sliding mode, and mode III is the tearing mode.

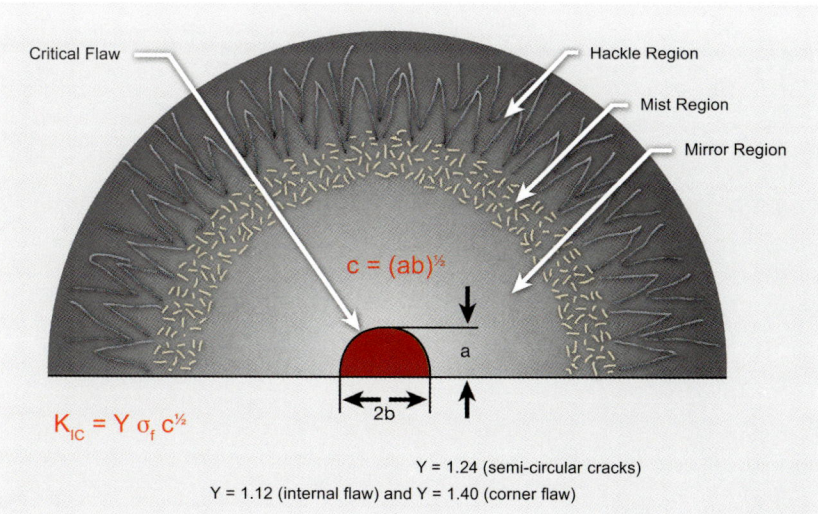

Figure 3.21 - Diagram of the typical brittle fracture surface regions (flaw, mirror, mist, and hackle). The regions are not drawn to scale. Griffith-Irwin equation [$K_{IC} = Y \sigma_f c^{1/2}$] and the approximated "Y" values according to the location of "c" are shown. K_{IC} can be calculated using this fractography approach. Adapted from Mecholsky (1995b).

Fracture mechanics is the field of mechanics concerned with the study of the formation of cracks in materials. It uses methods of analytical solid mechanics to calculate the driving force on a crack and those of experimental solid mechanics to characterize the material's resistance to fracture.

R-curve behavior: An increase in the resistance to crack growth (*i.e.* toughness) during crack extension. The R-curve behavior was originally noted for large-grained ceramics having thermal expansion anisotropy. The increasing resistance to crack extension with crack length was mainly attributed to mechanisms active in the crack wake that shielded the crack tip from the applied stress intensity. In transforming ceramics additional toughening mechanisms contribute to R-curve behavior, with the total available being subdivided into three basic groups: (1) crack deflection and crack branching; (2) contact shielding by wedging and bridging involving broken-out grains or rough crack-wake surfaces and (3) stress-induced zone shielding involving transformation, microcracking and residual stress fields.

To sum up, the complex process of brittle fracture creates at least two new surfaces with distinct topography and texture that can be characterized using principles of fractography. Quantitative fractographic analysis applies the principles of **fracture mechanics** to obtain quantitative information from the fracture surface, such as: the identification of the size and location of the fracture initiating crack or defect; the stress state at failure; the existence, or not, of stress corrosion; a knowledge of local processing anomalies that affect the fracture process; and the calculation of the fracture toughness.

Nevertheless, the transformation toughened ceramics exhibit increased resistance for growth of both short ($\leq 100 \ \mu m$) and long (≥ 0.3 mm) cracks and, for many ceramics, toughness continuing to increase with crack length (**R-curve behavior**) until generally reaching a toughness plateau. These transforming ceramics step away from the simple Griffith dependence on flaw size and many have strengths that depend on the stress needed to trigger transformation rather than being flaw-size sensitive. Quite non-linear behavior is exhibited by the toughest materials bordering on quasi-plasticity with measurable prefailure deformation. Therefore, high strength and high toughness are rarely present in the same material. Remember that the kinetics of transformation are governed by nucleation, with the probability of nucleation enhanced by applied stress and local residual stresses, which scales with grain size. In addition, transformation involves the development of a transformation zone first associated with the crack tip and later becoming a crack wake feature. The size of this zone and features of the

zone microstructure (grain size and microcracking, in particular) control toughening (Kelly and Denry, 2008; Denry and Kelly, 2008).

Thus, under certain service and/or environmental conditions, stable crack extension or slow crack growth can occur at stress intensities that are less than the critical value, K_{IC}. Under such conditions, K_I becomes dependent on the crack growth rate (crack velocity, v) and, hence, the characteristics of the system. The calculation of K_{IC} using the fractography approach in environmental conditions that promote slow crack growth can lead to erroneous values of K_{IC} because of an incorrect assumption of (initial versus final) crack size. Nevertheless, the actual value of K_{IC} should not change due to loading rate or test geometry. If the environment degrades the entire material, then the degraded material is, essentially, a different material. If the environment degrades the local crack, then the crack usually grows and the component is weaker, *i.e.*, lower strength, but also with a larger final crack size, so the toughness of the unaffected region is still the same.

Nevertheless, numerous methods can be used to calculate fracture toughness (K_{IC}). They vary in their degree of difficulty to execute, but the most popular methods are as follows: Single Edge V-Notch Beam (SEVNB; ISO 6872:2008); Single Edge Precracked Beam (SEPB; ISO FDIS 15732); Surface Crack in Flexure (SCF; ISO FDIS 18756); and, Chevron Notched Beam (CNB; ISO CD 24370). Fracture toughness may also be estimated by methods relying on indentation cracks (Indentation fracture, IF, and indentation strength, IS).

Clinically, all-ceramic restorations are susceptible to chemical corrosion and fatigue mechanisms that can considerably reduce their strength over time

Fatigue is the progressive and localized structural damage that occurs when a material is subjected to cyclic loading. The maximum stress values are less than the ultimate tensile stress limit, and may be below the yield stress limit of the material. **Fatigue life** (N_f) is the number of stress cycles of a specified character that a specimen sustains before failure of a specified nature occurs.

Stress corrosion: Degradation caused by the combined effects of mechanical stress and a corrosive environment, usually exhibited as cracking.

and, therefore, reducing their lifetime. Meaning, all-ceramic restorations have to withstand the unfavorable conditions of the oral cavity, with chewing forces from 100 to 700 N applied in a moist ambient at 37°C in more than 10^7 cycles by means of cusps with diameter of 4 to 8 mm, resulting in a mean total contact area of 50 mm^2, and generating stresses from 3,5 to 890 MPa (Peterson *et al*., 1998; Kelly, 1999). One way to improve the mechanical behavior of this type of prosthesis is to use a substructure material with mechanical properties, mainly strength and fracture toughness, similar to the metal alloys used for metal-ceramic restorations (Rekow *et al*., 2006). Following this rationale, zirconia should be the most promising structural material to replace the metal substructure in dental ceramic restorations (Tables 1.1, 2.2, and 3.3).

As explained, the reduction of mechanical strength (σ) due to **fatigue** is caused by the propagation of defects initially present within the ceramic structure. The fatigue behaviour can be determined by subjecting a ceramic material to cyclic loading of a maximum known value and determining the number of cycles required to produce failure. Considering that the rougher the ceramic surface, the greater the number of cracks, and the fewer cycles of stress are needed to fail, the ceramic surface finish is of crucial importance to the restoration lifetime.

In addition, the chemical interaction between the ceramic and the environment at the crack tip can have a major effect on the rate of crack growth. The reaction of water molecules with the oxide bonds (*e.g*., Si-O-Si) at the crack tip further reduce the number of cycles to cause dynamic fatigue failure. So, when these environmental conditions are combined, meaning,

high levels of stress and presence of water, the rate of crack growth is much accelerated and the failure may be resultant from **stress corrosion**.

Thus, crack propagation under subcritical conditions ($\sigma < \sigma_c$; $K_I < K_{IC}$) results from the stress-assisted reaction of water molecules with the ceramic oxide bonds at the crack tip. In the case of toughened ceramics (*i.e.*, zirconia-based ceramics), crack propagation can be further promoted when cyclic stresses are applied. As ceramic restorations are exposed to an aqueous environment and to cyclic loading, the evaluation of the chemical solubility and the fatigue behavior, including subcritical crack growth parameters, is important to estimate the lifetime, and consequently, the clinical success of all-ceramic restorations. The ISO 6872:2008 set the maximum chemical solubility (mass loss) for all types of ceramics (Table 3.2).

Table 3.2 - Classification of ceramics for fixed prostheses by intended clinical use, with required minimum (of mean) flexural strength (σ) and maximum chemical solubility (ML= mass loss), and recommended minimum fracture toughness (K_{IC}) values (according to ISO 6872:2008).

Class	Recommended Clinical Indications	σ (MPa)	ML ($\mu g \bullet cm^{-2}$)	K_{IC} (MPa$\bullet\sqrt{m}$)
1	a. Aesthetic ceramic for coverage of a metal or a ceramic substructure. b. Aesthetic ceramic for single-unit anterior prostheses, veneers, inlays, or onlays.	50	100	0.7
2	a. Aesthetic ceramic for adhesively cemented, single-unit, anterior or posterior prostheses. b. Adhesively cemented, substructure ceramic for single-unit anterior or posterior prostheses.	100	a. 100 b. 2000	1.0
3	Aesthetic ceramic for non-adhesively cemented, single-unit, anterior or posterior prostheses.	300	100	2.0
4	a. Substructure ceramic for non-adhesively cemented, single-unit, anterior or posterior prostheses. b. Substructure ceramic for three-unit prostheses not involving molar restoration.	300	2000	3.0
5	Substructure ceramic for three-unit prostheses involving molar restoration.	500	2000	3.5
6	Substructure ceramic for prostheses involving 4 or more units.	800	100	5.0

Examples of commercially available ceramics: Class 1- VM ceramics (Vita), IPS Empress (Ivoclar); Class 2- IPS Empress (Ivoclar), Cerec Mark II (Vita), OPC (Jeneric-Pentron), Finesse All-ceramic (Dentsply); Class 4- In-Ceram (Vita), IPS Empress2 (Ivoclar), Procera (Nobel Biocare); Class 5- YZ (Vita), Cercon (Dentsply), Lava (3M ESPE).

Table 3.3 - Mean strength (σ) and fracture toughness (K_{IC}) values of most popular ceramics resulted from different testing methods and reported in peer-reviewed published papers.

Core Ceramics	σ (MPa)	K_{IC} (MPa•m$^{0.5}$)
Hot-pressed, leucite-based (IPS Empress, Ivoclar)	85[*w]; 106[§]; 177[§]; 134[β]	1.2[£]; 1.3[#]; 1.7[†]
Hot-pressed, lithia disilicate-based (IPS Empress2, Ivoclar)	215[*w]; 306[§]	2.9[£]; 3.4[#]
Glass-infiltrated alumina-based (In-Ceram Alumina, Vita)	352[β]; 594[§]; 323[§]	4.4[£]; 4.5[†]
Alumina-based (Procera AllCeram, Nobelpharma)	464[§]; 687[β]	4.5[†]
Glass-infiltrated alumina-based zirconia reinforced (In-Ceram Zirconia, Vita)	564[*]; 638[§]; 645[β]	4.8[£]
Y-TZP (YZ, Vita)	900[§]	5.9[γ]
Y-TZP (DC-ZirKon, DCS Dental)	840[§]	7.4[£]
Y-TZP (Lava, 3M ESPE)	786[§]; 1267[β]	-
Y-TZP (Prozir, Norton-St. Gobain)	1450[β]	4.9[♦]; 5.4[†]

§ Three-point bending; * Four-point bending, [w](if tested in 37°C distilled water); ß Biaxial flexural strength; £ Indentation strength; # Fractography approach; † Indentation fracture; ♦ SEPB; γ SEVNB. Y-TZP: yttria tetragonal zirconia polycrystal.

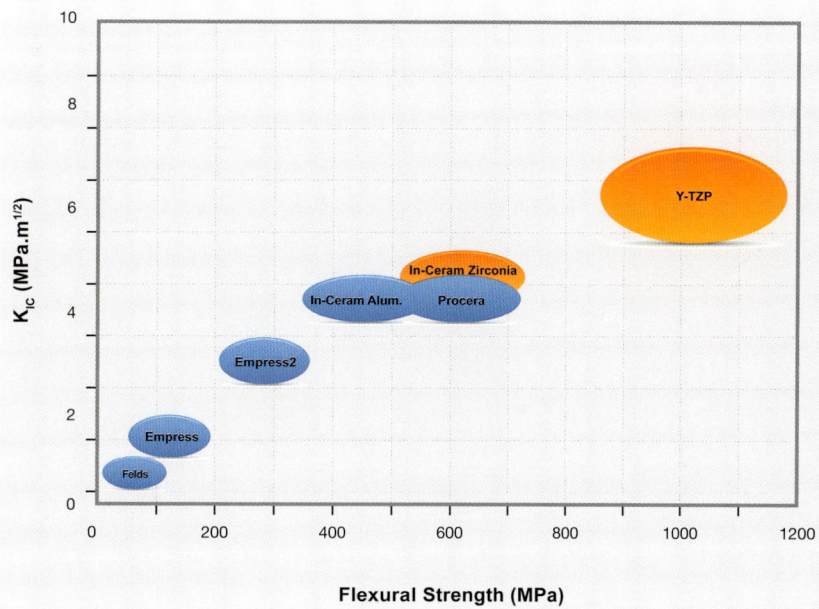

Figure 3.22 - A graph of flexural strength (σ) versus fracture toughness (K_{IC}) based on the results presented in Table 3.3.

This chapter demonstrated that quantitative microstructural analysis can provide an association among the constitution, physical properties, and structural characteristics of materials. It became evident that structural reliability of dental ceramics is a major factor in the clinical success of ceramic restorations. It has been also shown that a complex stress distribution is present in most practical conditions and strength data alone cannot be directly extrapolated to predict structural performance. Additionally, the environmental factors are critically important for the clinical success of ceramic restorations and extrapolation of *in vitro* information to *in vivo* situation should be approached with caution.

Therefore, for the strength test to reflect the variability and time-dependency of a ceramic component in service, the test environment must be similar to the service environment, and the strength-controlling flaw population must be the same as that responsible for failure in service. These factors should be the basis for the selection of a research protocol. As the distribution of strength is a measure of the distribution of the effective flaw sizes leading to failure, fractography principles should be applied for the quantitative and qualitative analyses of fracture surfaces, improving the understanding of the fracture phenomenon, which is, at the end, the most common failure cause of ceramic restorations. Yet, an important question still remains: How strong and tough the dental ceramics need to be (Table 3.3 and Fig. 3.22)?

Selected readings

- Anusavice KJ. *Phillips' science of dental materials*. 11th ed. Philadelphia: W.B. Saunders; 2003.

- Ban S, Anusavice KJ. Influence of test method on failure stress of brittle dental materials. *J Dent Res*, 69:1791-1799, 1990.

- Betamar N, Cardew G, Van Noort R. Influence of specimen designs on the microtensile bond strength to dentin. *J Adhes Dent*, 9:159-168, 2007.

- Betamar N, Cardew G, Van Noort R. The effect of variations in hourglass specimen design on microtensile bond strength to dentin. *J Adhes Dent*, 9:427-436, 2007.

- Callister WD. *Materials Science and Engineering: an Introduction*. 5th ed. New York: John Wiley & Sons, Inc.; 2000.

- DeHoff PH, Anusavice KJ, Hathcock PW. An evaluation of the four-point flexural test for metal-ceramic bond strength. *J Dent Res*, 61:1066-1069, 1982.

- Della Bona A, Hill TJ, Mecholsky JJ. The effect of contour angle on fractal dimension measurements for brittle materials. *J Mater Science*, 36: 2645-2650, 2001.

- Della Bona A, Anusavice, KJ. Microstructure, composition, and etching topography of dental ceramics. *Int J Prosthod*, 15:159–167, 2002.

- Della Bona A, Anusavice KJ, Dehoff PH. Weibull analysis and flexural strength of hot-pressed core and veneered ceramic structures. *Dent Mater*, 19:663-669, 2003.

- Della Bona A, Mecholsky JJ, Anusavice, KJ. Fracture behavior of lithia disilicate- and leucite-based ceramics. *Dent Mater*, 20:956-962, 2004.

- Della Bona A, Donassollo TA, Demarco FF, Barrett AA, Mecholsky JJ. Characterization and surface treatment effects on topography of a glass-infiltrated alumina/zirconia-reinforced ceramic. *Dent Mater*, 23:769-775, 2007.

- Della Bona A, Mecholsky JJ, Barrett AA, Griggs JA. Characterization of glass-infiltrated alumina-based ceramics. *Dent Mater*, 24:1568-1574, 2008.

- Denry I, Kelly JR. State of the art of zirconia for dental applications. Dent Mater, 24:299-307, 2008.

- Fréchette VD. *Failure analysis of brittle materials*. Westerville, OH: American Ceramic Society; 1990.

- Griffith AA. The phenomena of rupture and flow in solids. *Philos Trans R Soc* (London), 221:163-198, 1920.

- Hill TJ, Della Bona A, Mecholsky JJ. Establishing a protocol for measurements of fractal dimensions in brittle materials. *J Mater Science*, 36: 2651-2657, 2001.

- Howard CV, Reed MG. *Unbiased stereology*: three-dimensional measurement in microscopy. Oxford, UK: BIOS Scientific Publishers; 1998.

- Irwin GR. Analysis of stresses and strains near the end of crack transversing a plate. *J Appl Mech*, 24:361-364, 1957.

- Kelly JR. Perspectives on strength. *Dent Mater*, 11:103-110, 1995.

- Kelly JR, Tesk JA, Sorensen JA. Failure of all-ceramic fixed partial dentures in vitro and in vivo: analysis and modeling. *J Dent Res*, 74:1253-1258, 1995.

- Kelly JR. Clinically relevant approach to failure testing of all-ceramic restorations. *J Prosthet Dent*, 81:652-661, 1999.
- Kelly JR, Denry I. Stabilized zirconia as a structural ceramic: an overview. Dent Mater, 24:289-98, 2008.
- Lawn B. *Fracture of brittle solids*. 2nd ed. Cambridge, UK: Cambridge University Press; 1998.
- Kingery WD, Bowen HK, Uhlmann DR. *Introduction to ceramics*. 2d ed. New York: Wiley; 1976.
- Mecholsky JJ. Fractography: determining the sites of fracture initiation. *Dent Mater* 11:113-116, 1995a.
- Mecholsky JJ. Fracture mechanics principles. *Dent Mater*, 11:111-112, 1995b.
- Peterson IM, Pajares A, Lawn BR, Thompson VP, Rekow ED. Mechanical characterization of dental ceramics by hertzian contacts. *J Dent Res*, 77:589-602, 1998.
- Quinn GD. *Fractography of ceramics and glasses*. Washington: National Institute of Standards and Technology (NIST); 2007
- Rahaman MN. *Ceramic Processing and Sintering*. New York: Marcel Dekker, Inc.; 1995.
- Randall PN. Plain strain crack toughness testing of high strength metallic materials. In: Brown Jr. WF, Strawley JE, eds. ASTM STP 410. Philadelphia: *Am Soc Test Mater*, p. 88-126, 1966.
- Rekow ED, Harsono M, Janal M, Thompson VP, Zhang G. Factorial analysis of variables influencing stress in all-ceramic crowns. *Dent Mater*, 22:125-132, 2006.
- Rhee Y-W, Kim H-W, Yan D, Lawn BR. Brittle fracture versus quasi plasticity in ceramics: a simple predictive index. *J Am Ceram Soc*, 84:561-565, 2001.
- Ritter JE. Critique of test methods for lifetime predictions. *Dent Mater*, 11:147-151, 1995.
- Ritter JE. Predicting lifetimes of materials and material structures. *Dent Mater*, 11: 142-146, 1995.
- Studart AR, Filser F, Kocher P, Gauckler LJ. Fatigue of zirconia under cycling loading in water and its implications for the design of dental bridges. *Dent Mater*, 23: 106-114, 2007.

Chapter *4*

Principles of adhesion applied to dental ceramics

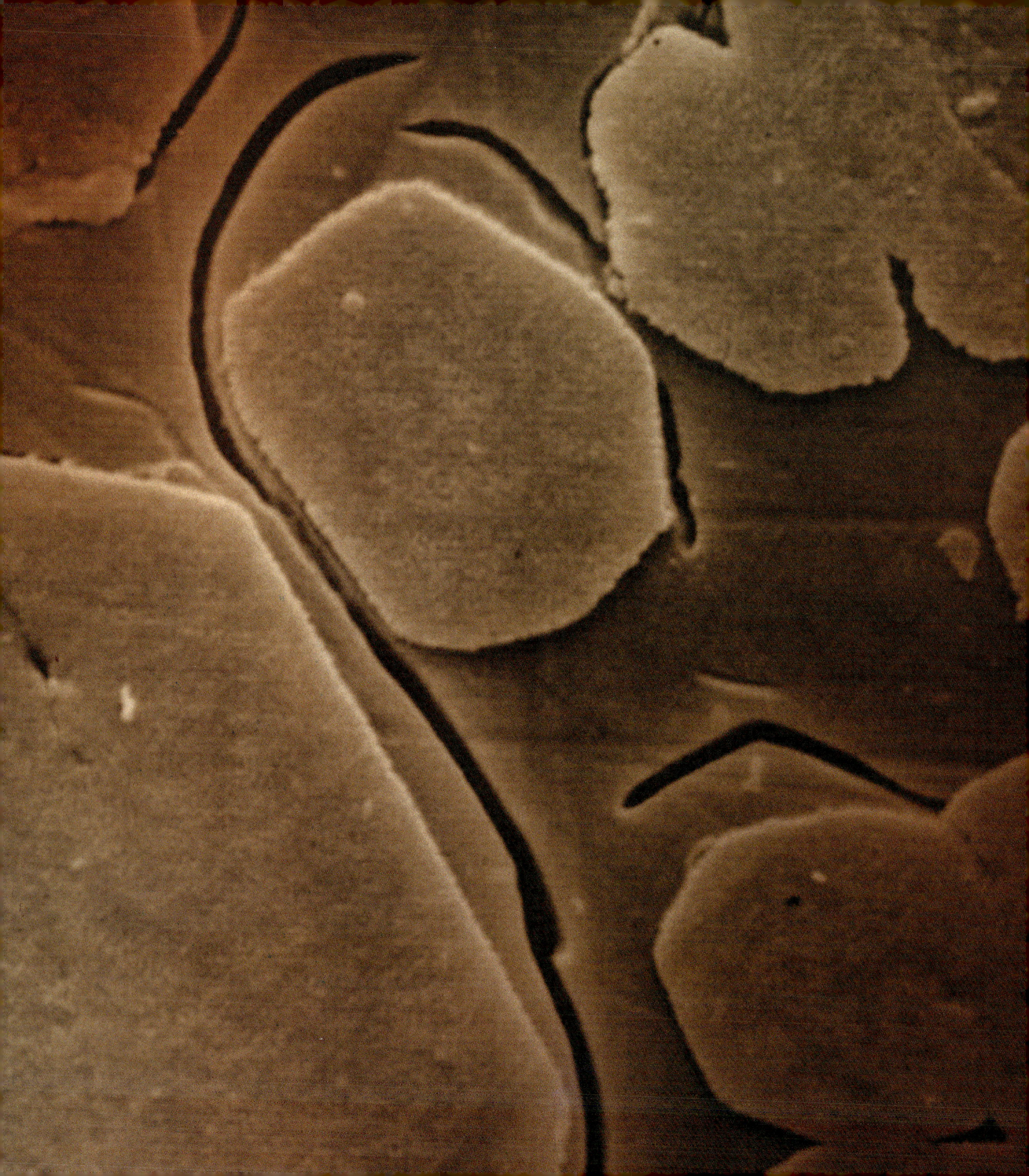

Introduction

Advancing on the rationale presented so far, this chapter introduces the adhesion mechanisms used for ceramic bonding, providing scientific evidences for the clinical success of bonding ceramic restorations, which always require surface treatment(s) to produce an adequate bond to resins. Therefore, the principles associated with the resin-to-ceramic bond phenomenon and the methods to investigate it are also presented.

At first, one could think that the "fragile" ceramic restorations would not withstand the intra-oral service. It could be true if the restoration would not be bonded to the tooth structure or remaining restorative materials (*e.g.*, composites and metals), working as an integrated system where diverse stresses from chewing and para-functional habits (*e.g.* bruxism) are distributed throughout the system due to appropriate bonding (Fig. 4.1). This rationale is so true that the ISO 6872 classified the ceramics according to the intended clinical use and made the distinction between adhesively and non-adhesively cemented restorations (Table 3.2).

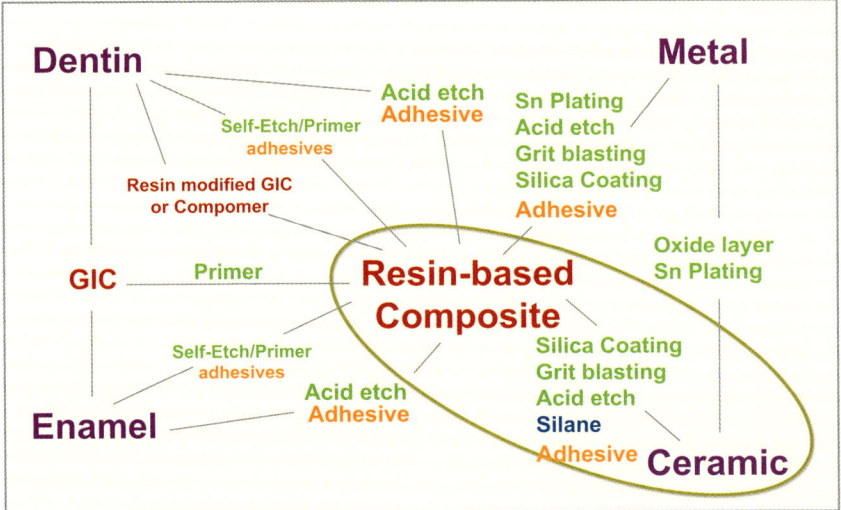

Figure 4.1 - Bonding strategies to tooth structure and dental restorative materials (purple), emphasizing (encircled) the feasible adhesion promoters (surface conditioners) for the bonding interface between ceramics and resin-based composites. The materials are color coded: primers (green); adhesives (orange); coupling agent (blue); luting and restorative bonding composites (red). GIC: glass ionomer cement. Sn: tin.

So, what is adhesion? It can be defined as a molecular (or atomic) attraction between two contacting surfaces (substrates) promoted by the interfacial force of attraction of different molecules (or atoms). This is distinct from cohesion, which is the attraction between same type of molecules within one substance. The adhesion and cohesion concepts are also important for further distinction between adhesive and cohesive failures, discussed later on this chapter. The adhesion phenomenon can occur via **physical**, **mechanical** (structural interlocking) or chemical mechanisms, or a combination of them (Fig. 4.2). Whenever an adhesive agent is used to bond two materials and it solidifies during bonding, the process is called adhesive bonding. Therefore, **adhesives** are substances that promote adhesion between two substrates (**adherends**). In addition, an intermediary substance can be used to enable bonding between adhesive and adherend and such a material is known as a **coupling agent**, *e.g.* silanes (Fig. 4.2 B). Alternatively, the materials used to modify the characteristics of the substrate surface facilitating the adhesion are known as **primers**, *e.g.* phosphoric acid for dental enamel and dentine (Fig. 4.3), and hydrofluoric acid (HF) for ceramics (Fig. 4.2 A). Unfortunately, the distinction between primers and coupling agents is rarely made in the dental literature and the two terms are used interchangeably. A relatively strong bond can result from the synergistic action of a number of bonding mechanisms, such as a large area of intimate contact providing numerous sites for the creation of weak secondary bonds, and the presence of surface undercuts at the microfl.

Adhesive: Substance that promotes adhesion of one substance or material to another.

Adherend: A material substrate that is bonded to another material by means of an adhesive.

Adhesion promoters: Substances that promote bond between two substrates (materials) with no particular affinity for each other and consequently will not wet each other. A **coupling agent** is an intermediary substance used to promote the bond to both of the materials in question (Fig. 4.2 B). Alternatively, **primers** can be used to modify the characteristics of the surface of one of the two materials so that a bond can be created (Fig. 4.2 A).

Acid-etching technique: Process of roughening a solid surface by exposing it to an acid and thoroughly rinsing the residue to promote micromechanical bonding of an adhesive to the surface.

Micromechanical bonding (mechanical interlocking): Mechanical adhesion associated with bonding of an adhesive to a roughened adherend surface (Fig. 4.2 A). A primary condition for this form of adhesion is that the adhesive can penetrate readily into the microscopic undercuts before it begins to set (Fig. 4.10). This condition is determined by the wettability of the adhesive on the substrate, which in turn is governed by the relative surface energies and the resultant contact angle; the ideal situation being that of perfect wetting (Fig. 4.11).

Physical adhesion: When two surfaces are in close proximity, secondary forces of attraction arise through dipole interactions between polar molecules.

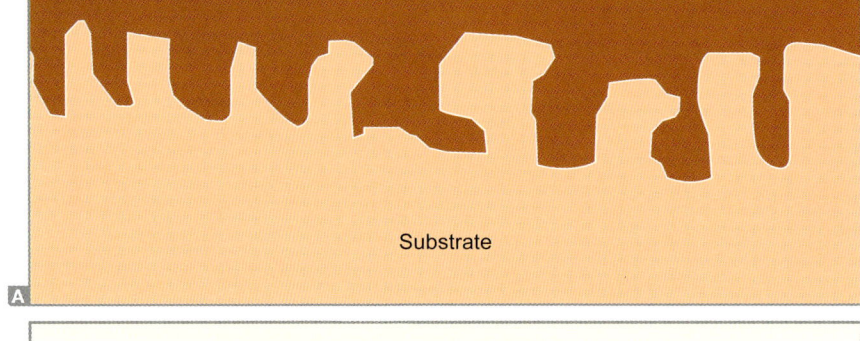

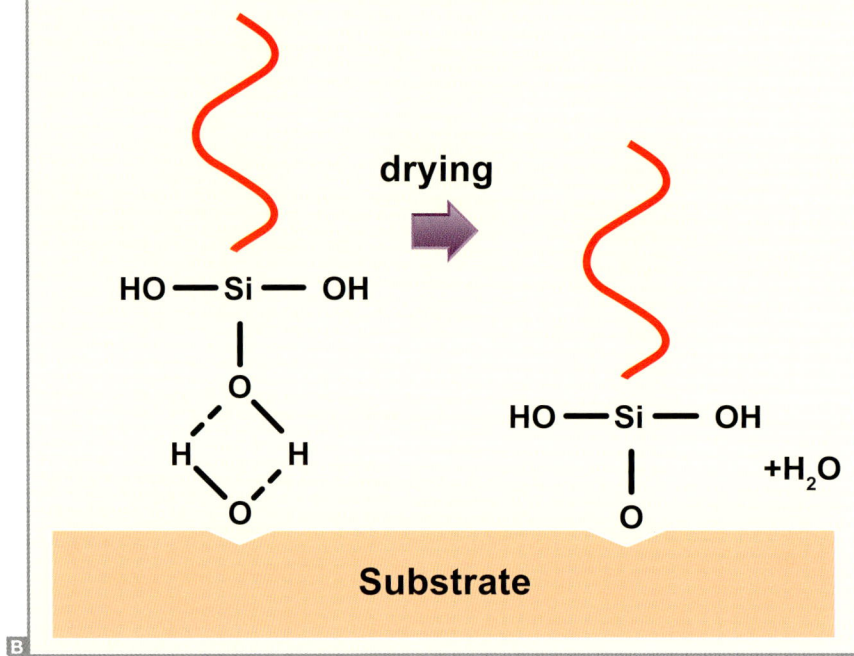

Figure 4.2 - Schematic representations of adhesion mechanisms. **A**- Mechanical interlocking between an adhesive and the treated (primed) substrate (adherend). The most popular methods to produce micromechanical retentive ceramic surfaces are: acid etching, bur abrasion, and airborne particle abrasion. **B**- Hydrogen bond formation between a silane coupling agent and a surface hydroxyl group that, after drying, forms into a covalent bond with the release of water. This chemical mechanism is used to bond resins to glass containing ceramics.

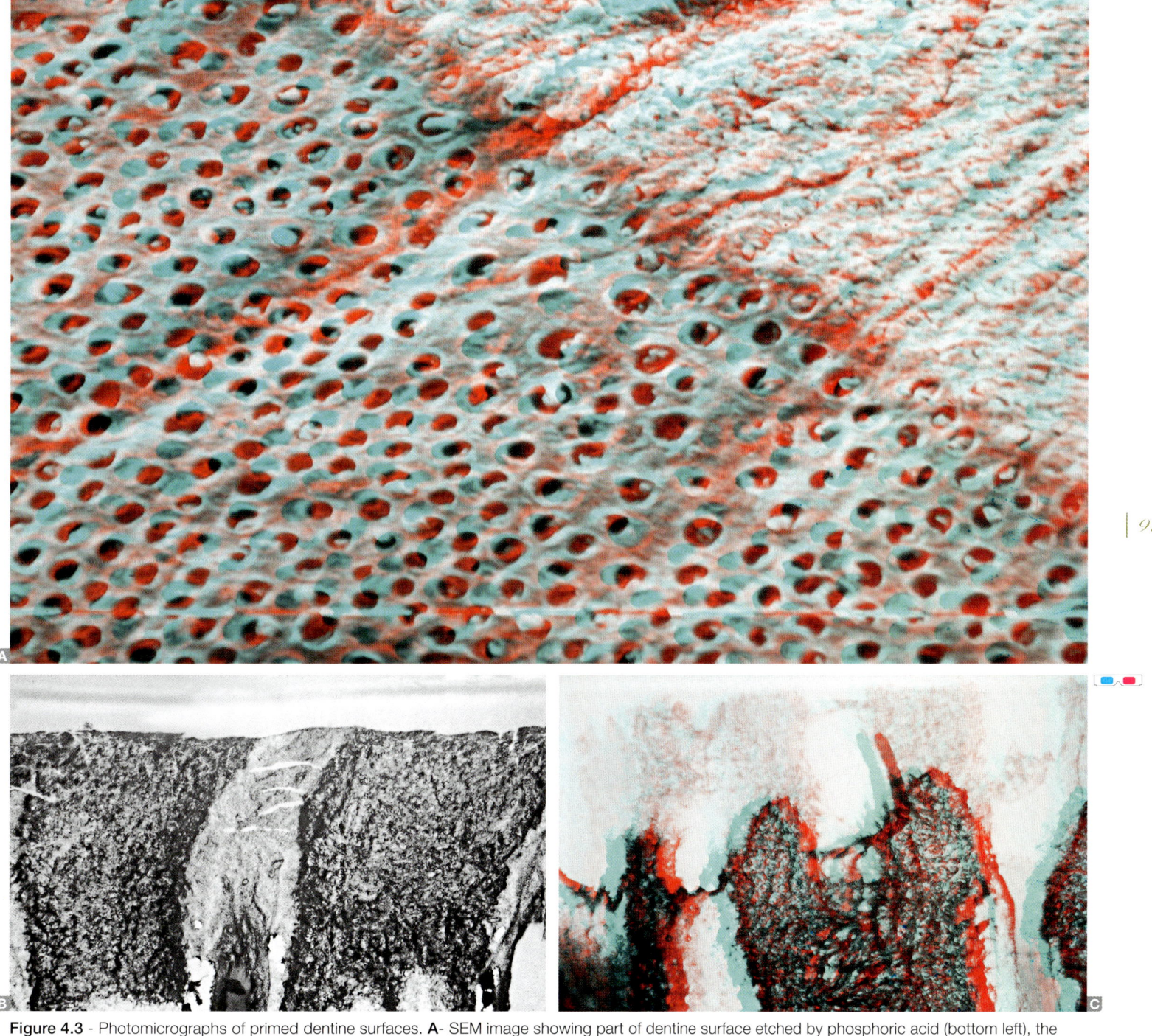

Figure 4.3 - Photomicrographs of primed dentine surfaces. **A**- SEM image showing part of dentine surface etched by phosphoric acid (bottom left), the smear layer was removed and the dentinal tubules are exposed; the smear layer is still present where the acid was not applied (top right). **B**- Transmission Electron Microscopy (TEM) image of the smear layer. **C**- TEM image of primed dentine, leaving the collagen fibers and tubules ready for bonding via molecular entanglement and micromechanical retention.

The adhesive mechanisms to tooth structure (enamel and dentine) are well explored and explained in the dental literature and, therefore, they are not the primary goal of this book. However, the ceramic restorations are bonded to tooth structure and/or other remaining restorative materials (Fig. 4.1) and the clinical procedures will be discussed in chapter 5. Nevertheless, enamel and dentine bonding mechanisms experienced major improvements since Buonocore´s concepts (1955). Different primers and adhesives coupled with specific bonding procedures drastically reduced the microleakage and its consequences (Fig. 4.4). Today, glass ionomer (GIC) and resin-based cements are the primary choices for bonding ceramic restorations to the remaining tooth structure. The GIC and the resin modified GIC (RMGIC) are often selected to cement acid-resistant ceramics because they are very easy to use. Yet, the most popular and effective cements for all types of ceramic restorations are the resin-based composites, specially the systems containing the 10-methacryloyloxydecyl-dihydrogen-phosphate (MDP) monomers, which are often used to cement acid-resistant ceramics.

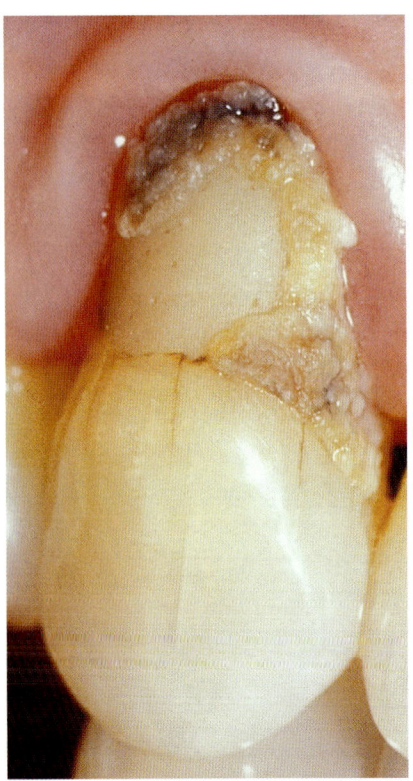

Figure 4.4 - Leakage and plaque retention around a resin composite restoration (1983). The tooth was restored using phosphoric acid to etch enamel and dentine (early total-etch concept) and a bis-GMA-based resin adhesive. The adhesive mechanisms and techniques have improved a lot since that time and the scenario pictured in this figure is seldom experienced in the recent years.

The discovery that most dental ceramics could be acid etched to create a micromechanical bond to resin has led to the development of acid-etched and bonded ceramic restorations. This concept was soon extended to include the repair of fractured (chipped) dental ceramic restorations in the mouth.

Considering the chemical reactivity to acids, the ceramics can be either acid-sensitive or acid-resistant, according to the degree of surface degradation produced by acids. Acid-sensitive ceramics (*e.g.*, feldspar-, leucite-, and lithium disilicate-based ceramics) are readily etched creating micromechanically retentive surfaces (Figs. 3.4 C; 3.9 B; 4.5 B, C and D; 4.6 B, C and D). Acid-resistant ceramics (*e.g.*, glass-infiltrated alumina and zirconia ceramic systems, densely-sintered alumina ceramics, and Y-TZP ceramics) do not show much surface degradation by etching (Fig. 4.9 B), preventing a reliable micromechanical bond to resin.

It has been reported that the clinical success of resin bonding procedures for ceramic restorations and ceramic repairs depends on the quality and durability of the bond between the ceramic and the resin. The quality of this bond depends upon the bonding mechanisms that are controlled in part by the surface treatment that promotes micromechanical and-or chemical bond to the substrate.

Structural and surface analyses of etched ceramics have shown that different etching patterns are created according to the ceramic microstructure and composition (chapter 3), and according to the concentration, application time and type of etchant. Surface defects, often located in the ceramic glass matrix, and phase boundaries of heterogeneous ceramic materials are preferably etched by the acids. Alteration of the surface topography by

Wettability: Relative affinity of a liquid for the surface of a solid.
Wetting: Relative interfacial tension between a liquid and a solid substrate that results in a contact angle of less than 90^0.
Wetting agent: A surface-active substance that reduces the surface tension of a liquid to promote wetting or adhesion.

99

Roughness is a measure of the texture of a surface, It is quantified by the vertical deviations of a real surface from its ideal form. Roughness plays an important role in determining how a real object will interact with its environment. Rough surfaces usually wear more quickly and have higher friction coefficients than smooth surfaces (see tribology). Roughness is often a good predictor of the performance of a mechanical component, since irregularities in the surface may form nucleation sites for cracks or corrosion. There are many different roughness **parameters** in use, but R_a (the arithmetic average of the roughness profile) is by far the most common. Since these parameters reduce all of the information in a profile to a single number, great care must be taken in applying and interpreting them. Small changes in how the raw profile data is filtered, how the mean line is calculated, and the physics of the measurement can greatly affect the calculated parameter. More information can be found in the ISO standards 4287 and 1302.

100

etching results in changes in the surface area and on the **wetting behavior** of the ceramic. This also changes the ceramic surface energy and its adhesive potential to resin. Thus, the ceramic microstructure, composition, and morphology after surface treatment (priming) should yield potentially useful information on the clinical success of the bonding procedures for ceramic restorations and ceramic repairs, justifying the interest of dentists and researchers on potential ceramic surface treatments.

Surface topography changes can be analyzed by profilers that can quantify the **profile parameters**, such as: Ra- average **roughness**; Rq- root-mean-squared roughness; and Rt- maximum height of the profile (peak-to-valley difference).

As discussed in chapter 3, acid-sensitive ceramics are etched by fluoride-containing etchants such as hydrofluoric acid (HF), ammonium bifluoride (ABF) and acidulated phosphate fluoride (APF), producing different surface patterns. HF etching produces a very aggressive effect on the surface of most acid-sensitive ceramics, where porosities are scattered uniformly throughout the ceramic surface. This pattern is more evident for feldspathic, lithia disiliate-based and leucite-based ceramics (Figs. 3.4 C; 3.9 B; 4.5 B; 4.6 B) than for either single-phase (Fig. 4.7 B) or high crystalline content ceramics (Fig. 4.9 B). It is important to remove the surface debris produced after acid etching ceramics. Cleaning under running water or with a blast of air-water seems to be not enough to remove all the debris from the etched ceramic surface (Fig. 4.5 B and C). This cleaning process should be done in a sonic water bath for about 5 min (Fig. 4.6 B and C). Additionally, the precipitation particles resulting from acid etching can be neutralized using a supersaturated solution of sodium bicarbonate and then sonically clean in water.

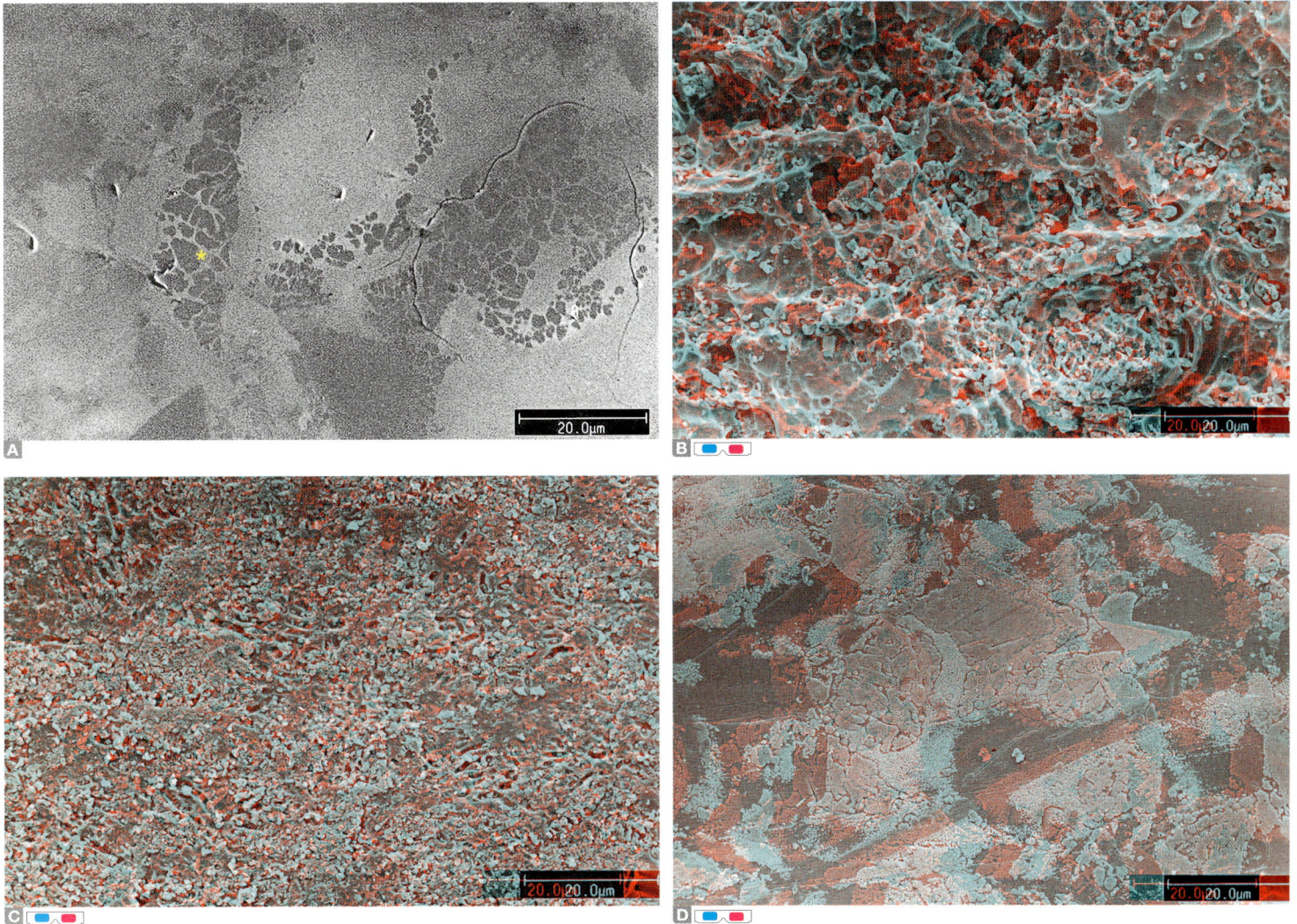

101

Figure 4.5 - Photomicrographs of Vita Omega dentine ceramic.

A- BSI of the microstructure showing clusters of leucite (*) in the glass matrix; cracks can be observed around the leucite clusters. This polished surface presented the following profile parameters: R_a: 95 nm; R_q: 223 nm; and R_t: 16 μm.

B- Ceramic surface etched with 9.6% buffered HF for 2 min; R_a: 1.4 μm; R_q: 2.1 μm; and R_t: 40 μm.

C- Ceramic surface etched with 10% ABF for 1 min; Ra: 197 nm; R_q: 398 nm; and R_t: 31 μm.

D- Ceramic surface etched with 4% APF for 2 min; R_a: 120 nm; R_q: 204 nm; and R_t: 10 μm. Acid etched surfaces were not sonically cleaned in a water bath. (x1000).

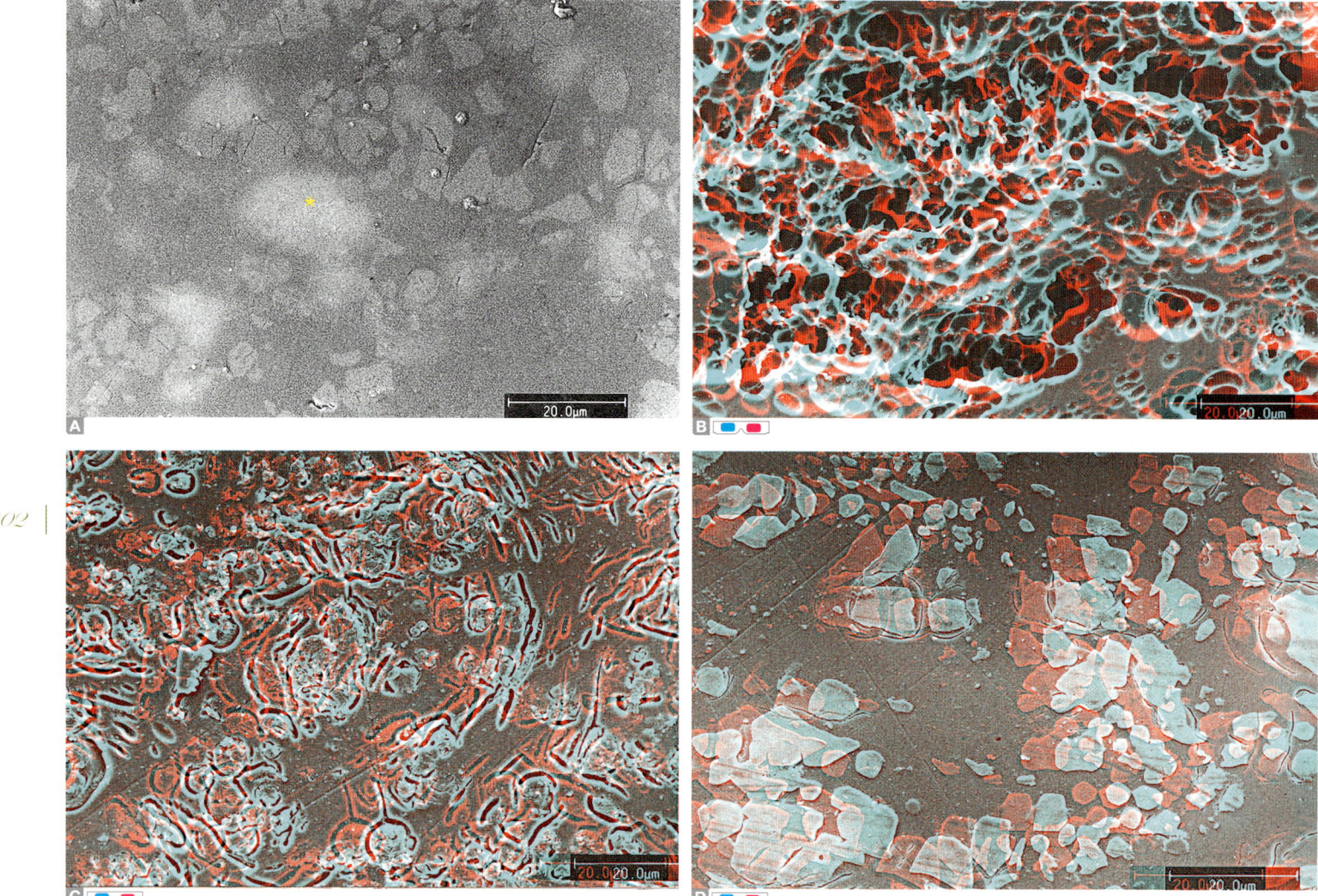

Figure 4.6 - Photomicrographs of Ceramco II ceramic.

    A- BSI of the microstructure showing leucite (*) in the glass matrix. This polished surface presented the following profile parameters: R_a: 85 nm; R_q: 130 nm; and R_t: 6 μm.

    B- Ceramic surface etched with 9.6% buffered HF for 2 min; R_a: 1 μm; R_q: 1.4 μm; and R_t: 39 μm.

    C- Ceramic surface etched with 10% ABF for 1 min; grooves are created around the leucite particles; R_a: 317 nm; R_q: 588 nm; and R_t: 37 μm.

    D- Ceramic surface etched with 4% APF for 2 min; surface deposits were created on the leucite crystals; R_a: 176 nm; R_q: 420 nm; and R_t: 16 μm. (x1000).

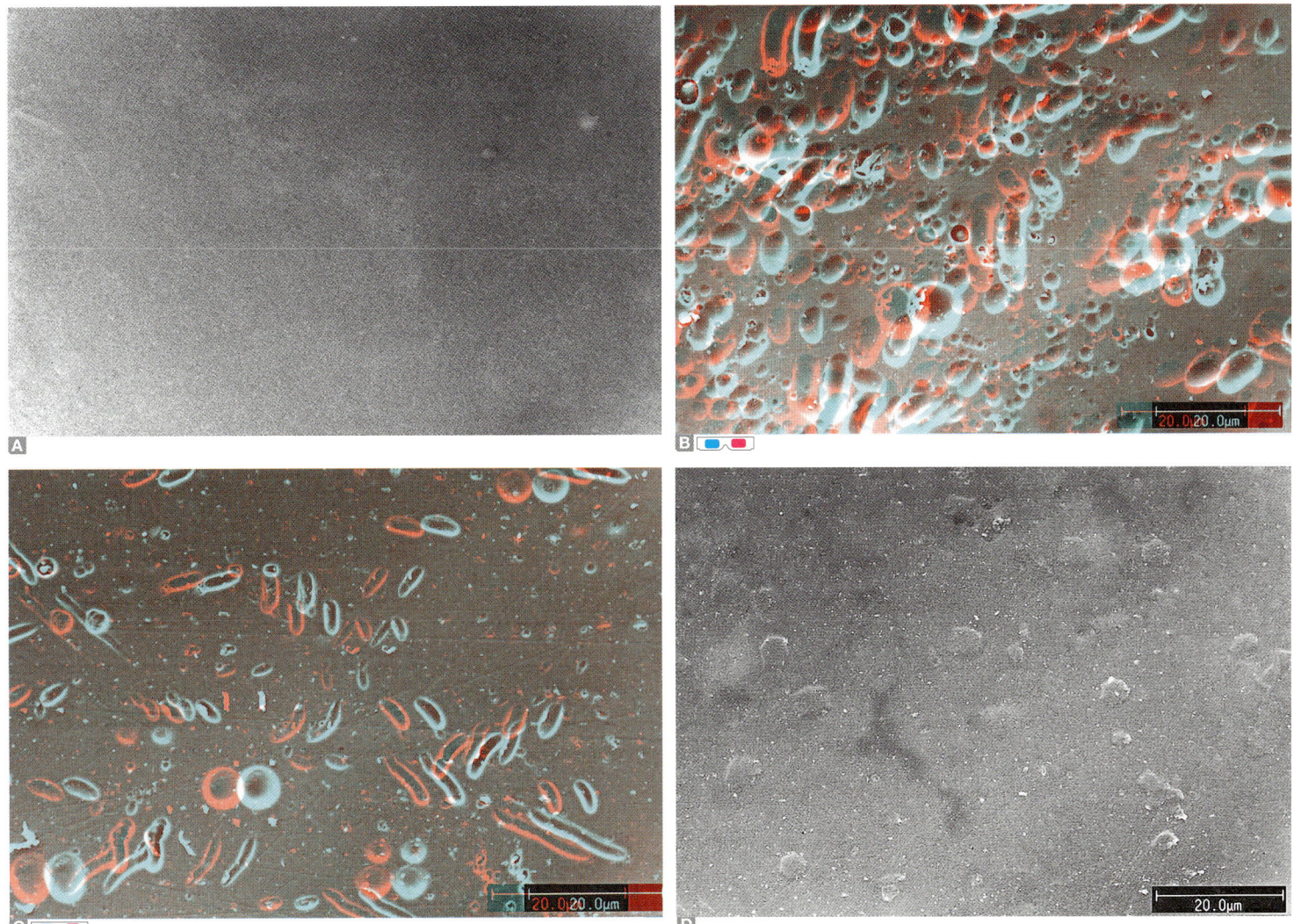

Figure 4.7 - Photomicrographs of Duceram LFC ceramic (Ducera).

    A- BSI of the polished surface of this single-phase glass; R_a: 90 nm; R_q: 190 nm; and R_t: 8 μm.

    B- Glass surface etched using 9.6% buffered HF for 2 min; R_a: 0.9 μm; R_q: 1.3 μm; and R_t: 36 μm.

    C- Glass surface etched using 10% ABF for 1 min; R_a: 297 nm; R_q: 568 nm; and R_t: 34 μm.

    D- Glass surface etched by 4% APF for 2 min; R_a: 100 nm; R_q: 184 nm; and R_t: 9 μm. (x1000).

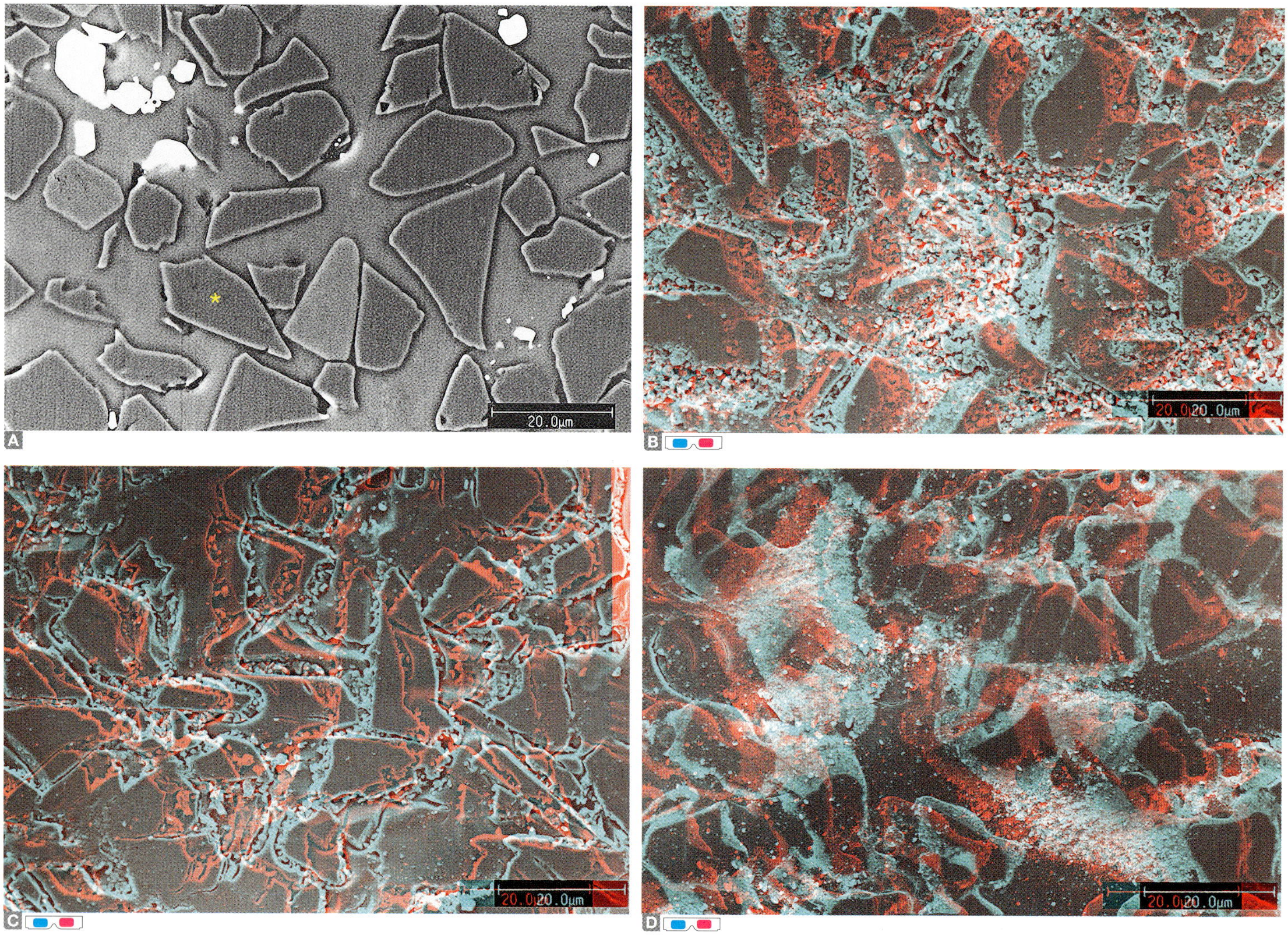

Figure 4.8 - Photomicrographs of Vitadur-N core ceramic (Vita).

    A- BSI of the microstructure showing particles of alumina (*) in the glass matrix; the bright particles are zirconia.

    B- Ceramic surface etched by 9.6% buffered HF for 2 min.

    C- Ceramic surface etched by 10% ABF for 1 min.

    D- Ceramic surface etched by 4% APF for 2 min. (x1000).

ABF etching produces mostly linear defects (grooves) that are primarily formed because of the acid attack on existing surface cracks, leucite-induced cracks, and phase boundaries (Figs. 4.5 C; 4.6 C; 4.7 C; 4.8 C). This etching pattern is also observed after using HF for reduced times and/or at lower concentrations, as for SEM preparation for microstructural observations (Fig. 3.4 B), suggesting that ABF acts as a low power HF etchant.

The APF etchant seems to build up surface deposits preferentially on the leucite crystal phase (Figs. 4.5 D; 4.6 D). Several studies demonstrated that treating the ceramic surface with APF alone produces an insufficient and inconsistent micromechanically-retentive surface and, as a consequence, the lowest bond strength values for resin-based composites. Nevertheless, APF is most often the active product used for preventive dentistry (fluoride application) and it can produce surface changes on composite and ceramic restorations.

Treating the ceramic surface with HF produced a substantial and consistent roughness on acid-sensitive ceramics, mainly because of its action on defects and phase boundaries (Figs. 3.4 C; 3.9 B; 4.5 B; 4.6 B; 4.8 B). In addition, surface preparations prior to HF etching appear to be needless because this etching process produces a new surface pattern. In contrast, the APF etching builds up on the roughened pre-treated surface. Therefore, it may be important that the ceramic surface is first roughened either with a diamond bur or by grit blasting to enhance the resin bond to APF-treated ceramic.

106

Airborne-particle abrasion (air abrasion; grit blasting; sand blasting): the process of altering the surface of a material through the use of abrasive particles propelled by compressed air or other gases.

The chemical reactivity of single-phase materials depends on crystallographic orientation (Fig. 4.7). In polycrystalline materials, etching characteristics vary among crystal types. Atoms along the grain (crystal) boundaries are more chemically active and dissolve at a greater rate than those within the exposed grain resulting in the formation of small grooves after etching. This explains the presence of grooves between phases (leucite and glass) or along the grain boundaries (Figs. 3.4 B; 4.6 C).

Therefore, differences in ceramic microstructure and ceramic composition are controlling factors in the development of micromechanical retention produced by etchants on acid-sensitive ceramics, and the etching mechanism is different for all acids, with HF producing the most aggressive etching pattern on most acid-sensitive ceramics.

Some clinicians also use coarse diamond rotary instruments or oral gritblaster (**airborne particle abrasion** systems) as the first step in the repair of fractured ceramic restorations. It has been shown that other than the scalloped surface created by the rotary instrument, both procedures produce a similar topography. In addition, these methods tend to create more stress and sharp cracks in the ceramic surface, and these are readily attacked by acids and may weaken the ceramic. Yet, for bonding to acid-resistant ceramics, such as Vita In-Ceram Zirconia, the airborne particle abrasion methods using alumina particles or silica modified alumina particles (silica coating) produced greater Ra values and the silica coated surfaces showed a significant increase (76%) in the concentration of silicon, which should also enhance bonding to resin via silane coupling agents (Fig. 4.9 and Table 4.1).

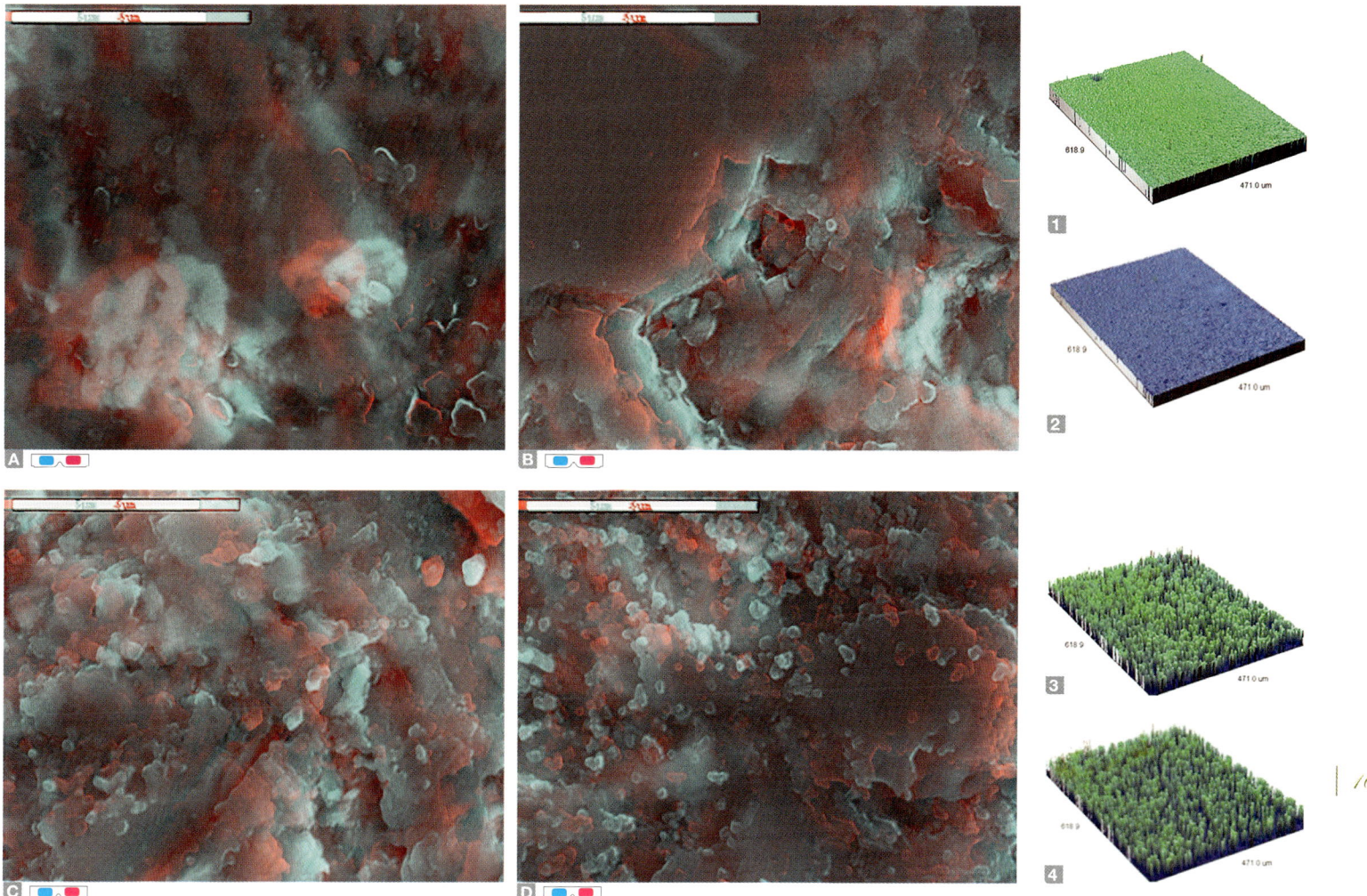

Figure 4.9 - SEM photomicrographs (left; x5000) and surface roughness profiles (right; optical profilometry, x10) of Vita In-Ceram Zirconia (IZ) ceramic.

    A and 1- IZ ceramic surface polished through 1 μm alumina abrasive.

    B and 2- 9.5% HF-treated IZ ceramic surface (etching time: 90 s).

    C and 3- IZ surface grit blasted with 25 μm alumina particles for 15 s.

    D and 4- Silica coated IZ ceramic surface using 30 μm silica modified alumina particles blasted for 15 s. The roughness parameters created by these treatments are presented in Table 4.1.
    From Della Bona *et al.*, 2007a.

Table 4.1 - Mean values of roughness parameters, statistical grouping for R_a, and the amount of silicon on the IZ ceramic surface after different treatments (Della Bona *et al.*, 2007a).

Surface treatments	R_a *	R_q	R_t	Si (K) element %
1. As-polished	207 ± 17 nm [b]	321 ± 14 nm	12.5 ± 3.4 μm	1.25
2. Hydrofluoric acid (HF)	231 ± 14 nm [b]	330 ± 10 nm	24.2 ± 3.1 μm	0.87
3. Grit blasting using alumina particles	1.0 ± 0.2 μm [a]	1.6 ± 0.5 μm	63 ± 4 μm	0.98
4. Silica coating	836 ± 49 nm [a]	1.6 ± 0.1 μm	55 ± 2 μm	2.21

* Different superscription letters indicate statistical significant differences (p < 0.05).

A **condensation reaction** is a chemical reaction in which two molecules or functional groups combine to form one single molecule, together with the loss of a small molecule. When this small molecule is water, it is known as a dehydration reaction. When two separate molecules react, the condensation is termed intermolecular. If the union is between atoms or groups of the same molecule, the reaction is termed intramolecular condensation, and in many cases leads to ring formation.

The increase of crystalline content (alumina and zirconia particles) in dental ceramics significantly improved the mechanical properties of these materials, allowing for a more predictably use of all-ceramic restorations. Nevertheless, the increase in crystalline content resulted in acid-resistant ceramics, which have greater structural performance than the acid-sensitive ceramics, but they can not be etched to promote an adequate bond to resin (Figs. 4.8 B; 4.9 B). To overcome this problem, silica coating (silicatization) systems (*e.g.*, Rocatec and Cojet, 3M ESPE) have been used to create a silica layer on metal and ceramic surfaces through high-speed surface impact of the silica-modified alumina particles that can penetrate up to 15 μm into ceramic and metal substrates (Fig. 4.9 D). This tribochemical effect may be explained by two bonding mechanisms: (1) the creation of a topographic pattern via airborne particle abrasion allowing for micromechanical bonding to resin; and (2) the promotion of a chemical bond between the silica coated ceramic surface and the resin-based material, via a silane coupling agent (Fig. 4.9 D; Table 4.1).

Silane has been used to enhance the bonding between organic adhesives and ceramics or metals in various industries since the 1940s. The technology of organosilane coating of inorganic filler particles has improved their bonding to matrix resins causing a major influence on the manufacture of resin composite materials. This technology also improves the chemical adhesion of ceramic bonded restorations and resin-bonded ceramic repairs.

Silane coupling agents bond to Si-OH on ceramic surfaces by **condensation reactions** (Fig. 4.2 B) and the methyl methacrylate double bonds provide bonding to the adhesive. As long as there are adequate Si-OH sites on the ceramic surface, satisfactory bonding should be achievable. Therefore, if the goal is to obtain a thin silane coating on any ceramic surface, the protocol should consider the various ceramic microstructures and silane types, and mechanisms to reduce the silane coating thickness, such as heat treatment.

In addition, the type of resinous adhesive also plays and important role on the bond to high crystalline content ceramics. It has been reported that the chemical bond to these ceramics is improved by using adhesive resin systems containing the phosphate (MDP) monomers.

Therefore, the adhesion between dental ceramics and resin-based composites is the result of a physico-chemical interaction across the interface between the resin (adhesive) and the ceramic (substrate). The physical contribution to the adhesion process is dependent on the surface treatment and topography of the substrate and can be characterized by its surface energy. Alteration of the surface topography by etching and airborne particle abrasion results in changes on the surface area and on the wettability of the substrate, which are related to the surface energy and the adhesive potential. In addition, the surface energy of a solid is greater than that of its interior where the interatomic distances are equal, and the energy is minimal (chapter 3). Similarly, at the surface of the lattice, the energy is greater because the outermost atoms are not equally attracted in all directions. This increase in energy per unit area of surface (J/m^2 or N/m) is referred to as the surface energy (γ), or **surface tension** for liquids.

Surface tension (γ): Interfacial tension, usually between a liquid and a solid surface, which occurs because of unbalanced intermolecular forces. The amount of work necessary to create a unit area of air/liquid interface ($mN/m = mJ/m^2 = dynes/cm$).

109

> ❧❧
>
> **Viscosity** (η)- Resistance of a fluid to flow. The viscosity is controlled by frictional forces within the liquid. Thus, viscosity is a measure (in MPa/s or cP) of the consistency of a fluid and its inability to flow. A highly viscous fluid flows slowly. The study of the deformation and flow characteristics of materials is the basis for the science of **rheology**.
>
> ❧❧

Therefore, the surface atoms of a solid tend to form bonds to other atoms in close proximity to the surface, reducing the surface energy of the solid. Again, achieving an energy balance or the lowest energy state is the driving force for the chemical bond between the adhesive and the adherend. Yet, the surface energy and the adhesive qualities of a given solid can be reduced by any surface impurity or contaminate, such as human secretions and air voids. The functional chemical groups available or the type of crystal plane of a space lattice present at the surface also affect the surface energy.

A fundamental requirement of adhesion is the intimate molecular contact. It seems simple, but regardless of how smooth the contacting surfaces may appear, they are likely to be very rough at microscopic level. Therefore, when the surfaces are brought into contact, only the peaks of the asperities are in contact and an adhesion between the surfaces is virtually impossible (Fig. 4.10 A). In addition, the attraction is negligible when the surface molecules of the attracting substances are separated by distances greater than 0.0007 μm (0.7 nm). So, an adhesive that flows into the surface irregularities of the adherend is often used to overcome this problem (Figs. 4.2 A; 4.10).

A clean (no contaminants) and dry surface ensures that the adhesive has the best possible chance of creating a proper bond with the adherent (Fig. 4.10 C). In addition, the wettability of the adherend by the adhesive, the **viscosity** of the adhesive, and the morphology of adherend surface influence the ability of the adhesive to make intimate contact with the adherend.

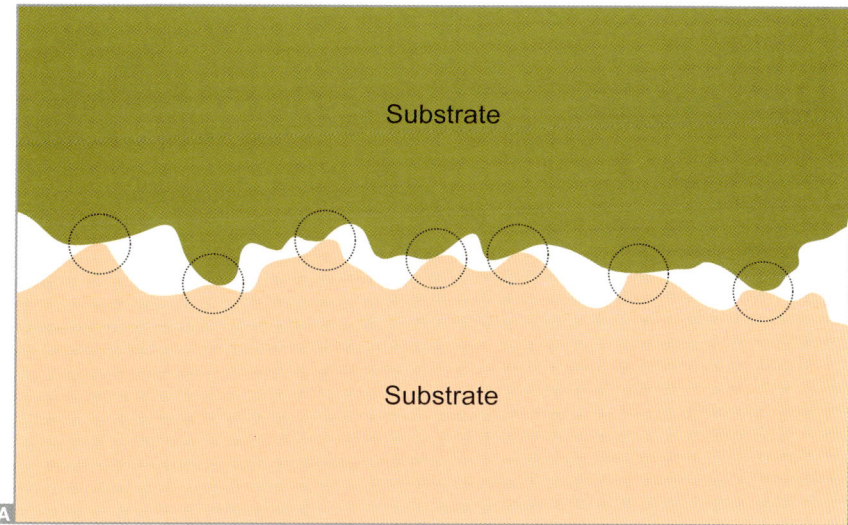

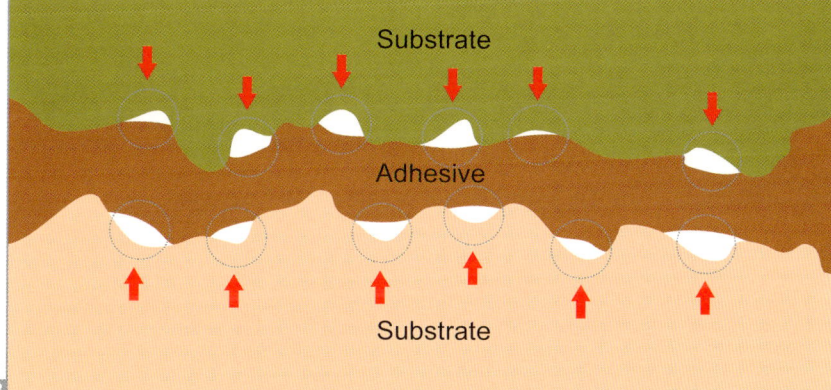

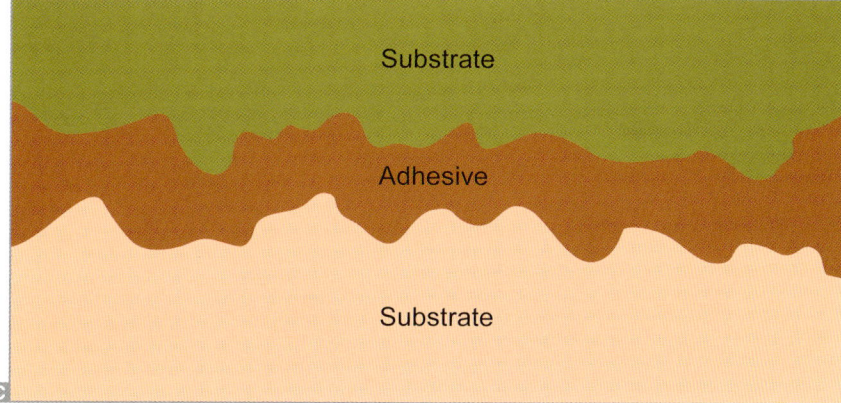

Figure 4.10 - Schematic representations of two contacting solid surfaces at microscopic level.
A- There are only few contact points between the two surfaces; actually, only the peaks of the asperities contact.
B- Air bubbles (voids) created in surface irregularities (red arrows); they act as stress concentrators, contributing to crack propagation and failure.
C- The adhesive spreads well on the rough surface (perfect wetting).

Contact angle (θ): Angle of intersection between a liquid and a surface of a solid that is measured from the solid surface through the liquid to the liquid/vapor tangent line originating at the terminus of the liquid/solid interface; used as a measure of wettability, whereby no wetting occurs at a contact angle of 180⁰ and complete wetting occurs at an angle of 0⁰.

Considering the adhesion phenomenon, wettability is the ability of an adhesive to contact a substrate. Wetting is the relative interfacial tension between an adhesive and a solid adherend, resulting in a **contact angle** (θ) of less than 90⁰. Perfect wetting is the fluid ability to cover the substrate completely, so that the maximum benefit is obtained from whichever adhesive mechanism is activated (Fig. 4.11). In case of good surface wetting, adhesive failures should not occur. Failure, in such a case, actually occurs cohesively within the adherend or in the adhesive itself, not along the adherend-adhesive interface (information on bonding tests and fracture analyses made at the end of this chapter should be considered).

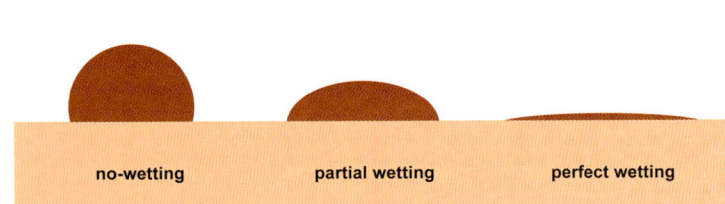

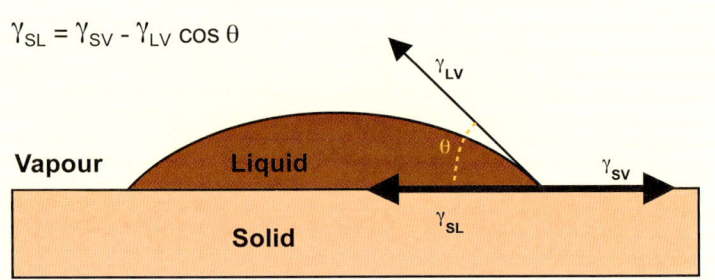

$$\gamma_{SL} = \gamma_{SV} - \gamma_{LV} \cos \theta$$

Figure 4.11 - Wetting characteristics for liquids on an adherend surface. A perfect wetting is reached when a liquid spreads freely over the entire solid surface. If the liquid does not wet the surface of the adherend, adhesion between the liquid and the adherend will be negligible or nonexistent and a large contact angle (θ) is formed.

Figure 4.12 - Schematic illustration of the sessile drop technique, which is a test performed to determine the chemical affinity that a liquid (adhesive) has to a solid (adherend). A drop of liquid is placed (allowed to fall from a certain distance) onto a solid surface. When the liquid has settled (become sessile) the drop will retain its surface tension. The figure shows the energy vectors and contact angle (θ), where γ_{SV} is the surface energy of the solid (at the solid-vapour interface), γ_{LV} is the surface tension of the liquid (at the liquid-vapour interface), and γ_{SL} is the surface energy between the solid and the liquid. Because the tendency for the liquid to spread increases as the θ decreases, the θ is a useful indicator of the surface wettability. As the θ increases from 0 to 90 degrees, the value of cos θ decreases from 1 to 0. The relationship among the γ parameters can be used to determine the γ_{SL} according to the Young equation ($\gamma_{SL} = \gamma_{SV} - \gamma_{LV} \cos\theta$) and the work of adhesion ($W_A = \gamma_{SV} + \gamma_{LV} - \gamma_{SL}$). Combining these two equations yields the Dupré equation [$W_A = \gamma_{LV} (1 + \cos\theta)$].

The adhesive-adherend interaction is governed by (1) a driving force associated with their surface energies that tend to spread the adhesive over the adherend, and (2) resistance to **spreading** that depends upon the viscosity of the adhesive, the surface irregularities and the presence of contaminants. So, a low surface tension liquid will readily spread over a high surface energy substrate, because the substrate surface is replaced by a lower surface energy surface. For instance, teflon (PTFE-polytetrafluoroethylene: $\gamma = 18$ mJ/m^2) is often used to prevent the adhesion of fluids (*e.g.*, water: $\gamma = 73$ mJ/m^2) to a surface (no wetting, Fig. 4.11). Conversely, metals (*e.g.*, steel: $\gamma = 230$ mJ/m^2) that have higher surface energy interact strongly with liquid adhesives (*e.g.*, liquid resin: $\gamma = 40$ mJ/m^2). The greater the surface energy, the greater the capacity for adhesion.

As "flat" surfaces are not actually planar and the surface imperfections present a potential impediment to reach a good bond (Fig. 4.10 A), the fluidity (viscosity- η) of the adhesive influences the extent to which the surface irregularities are filled. This liquid ability of filling the surface irregularities (*e.g.*, cracks, crevices, pores) can be quantified by the penetration coefficient (PC $= \gamma \cos\theta / 2\eta$).

Air pockets (voids) may be created during the spreading of the adhesive, preventing a complete wetting of the adherend surface (Fig. 4.10 B). When the adhesive interfacial region is subjected to thermal changes and mechanical stresses, the voids act as stress concentrators (Fig. 4.10 B). The generated stress may become so great that it initiates a separation in the adhesive bond adjacent to the void. This crack may propagate from one void to the next, and

Spreading is what happens when a liquid already in contact with a solid spreads. The spreading coefficient (S) is a widely used means of characterizing spreading problems with one overall value. It is defined thermodynamically as
[$S = \gamma_S - \gamma_{SL} - \gamma_L$]; where $\gamma_S =$ the surface energy of the solid, $\gamma_{SL} =$ the interfacial tension between the spreading liquid and the solid, and L = the surface tension of the spreading liquid. The general rules of thumb are:
(1) If S is calculated to be less than 0, then no spreading will occur.
(2) If S is calculated to be between 0 and 10, then spreading will occur to an extent related to the value of S. The higher S is, the greater the extent of spreading.
(3) If S is greater than 10, complete spreading will occur.

113

the joint may separate under stress. Thus, the extent to which an adhesive wets the surface of an adherend may be determined by measuring the θ between the adhesive and the adherend. The smaller the θ, the better the wettability, and the better the adhesive potential.

Experimentally, the above concepts can be demonstrated using either the sessile drop method (pendant drop method) (Fig. 4.12), the bubble pressure technique, or the Wilhelmy plate method (dynamic contact angle - DCA) (Fig. 4.13). Usually, the wettability of surfaces is quantified using high purity water as the probing liquid. This practice is valid for analyzing differences between substrates; however, the W_A based on water wettability has no clinical significance for resin bonding to ceramic (Fig. 4.12). Instead, an adhesive-equivalent liquid resin should be used as the probing medium to characterize the changes in the wetting behavior of treated ceramics surfaces. So, the W_A and the wetting behavior of the resin on treated ceramic surfaces can be characterized using DCA analysis, contact angle and surface energy data (Figs. 4.12; 4.13). This research protocol was used to determine the W_A of resin on treated lithia disilicate-based ceramic (IPS Empress2, Ivoclar). The ceramic specimens were examined as-polished (control) and after acid etching using either 9.5% HF for 1 min or 4% APF for 2 min (Fig. 4.14 A and B). These three ceramic surfaces were also examined after the application of a silane coupling agent (8% methacryloxypropyltrimethoxy silane - MPTMS). Advancing and receding contact angles (θ_a and θ_r) were measured using HPLC water (γ=72.6 mJ/m^2) and liquid resin (γ=39.7 mJ/m^2) as probing media. The results are summarized in Table 4.2.

between the adhesive and the composite within which molecular interaction and chemical bonding occur between the two materials; (2) the adhesive; and (3) the interfacial region between the adhesive and the ceramic, including the treated ceramic surface region where micromechanical and/or chemical bonding occurs (Fig. 4.15).

As for the monolithic materials, the evaluation of the structural reliability of the adhesion zone by Weibull analysis is also an important component for an integral analysis of the bonding interface (chapter 3). Again, the bond strength values resultant from any bond test, including the microtensile bond strength test, can only be considered a reliable indicator of the resin-ceramic bond quality if the fractures occur within the adhesion zone (Figs. 4.16 and 4.17).

Although the mode of failure is an important aspect of bond strength tests, it is not commonly reported. A detailed inspection of the fractured surfaces can indicate the failure mode of a bonded assembly. The fracture behavior of adhesive interfaces depends on the stress level, the flaw distribution, material properties, and environmental effects. Therefore, fracture surface characterization combined with analyses of fracture mechanics parameters (chapter 3) are of great importance to understand and predict bonded interface reliability and also to reduce the risk for data misinterpretation such as the inference that the bond strength must exceed the cohesive strength of the ceramic when the fracture initiates within the ceramic material and away from the interface. Therefore, the classification of the modes of failure based on principles of fractography (Figs. 4.16; 4.17; 4.18) should assist researchers to correctly interpret the fracture phenomena.

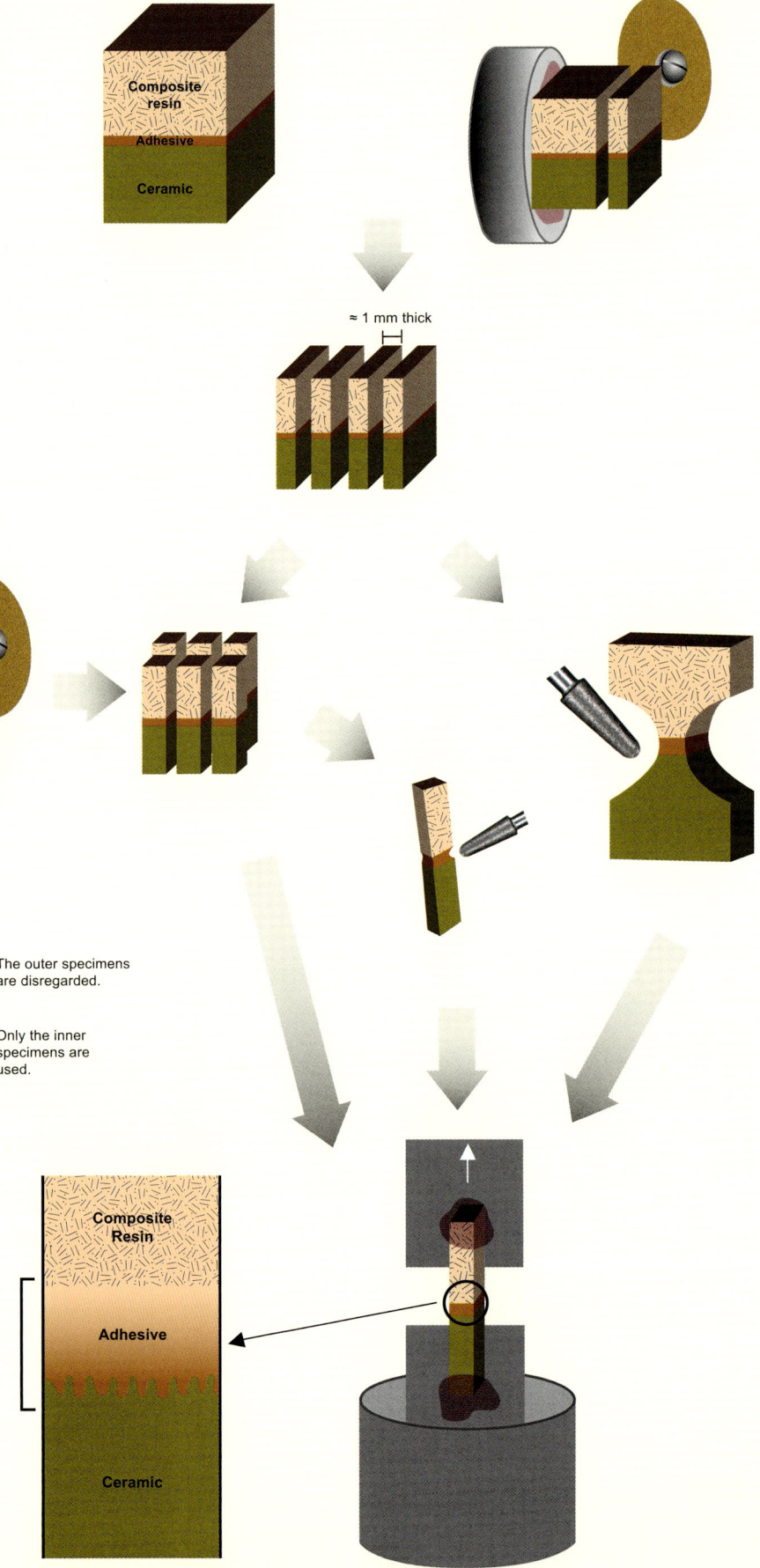

Composite resin

Adhesive

Ceramic

≈ 1 mm thick

The outer specimens are disregarded.

Only the inner specimens are used.

Composite Resin

Adhesive

*Adhesion Zone

Ceramic

Figure 4.15 - Schematic representation of the typical methods of preparing specimens for the microtensile test. Blocks of materials (substrates) can be fabricated from commercial products (*e.g.* ceramics, metals and composites) or from natural tissues (*e.g.* teeth), or even built up in layers on the top of other block (*e.g.* light cured resin-based composites). A surface of the block(s) is treated following the research protocol and the opposing material is bonded; in this case, a resin-based composite block is bonded to a surface treated ceramic block. A slow-speed diamond wheel saw is used to cut the blocks. The first cut produced slabs (slices) approximately 1 mm in thickness that can be either trimmed to obtain dumbbell shaped specimens or rotated 90⁰ and a second set of cuts is made to produce the non-trimming bar shaped specimens. As the bar specimens are not trimmed, the specimens located at the outside surface (outer) have to be discarded. There are also a third specimen design that can be fabricated from the bar specimen, which is trimmed at the adhesion zone (*) to a kind of dumbbell shape. All specimens have to be examined for flaws using light microscopy (x20), excluding from the experiment the specimens with visible flaws. The specimens are attached, *i.e.* glued using cyanoacrylate adhesive (*e.g.* Zapit, Superglue, and Superbonder), to the flat aligned grips of the universal testing machine and loaded to failure in tension (cross-head speed: 0.5-1 mm/min). The load at fracture (P, in N) and the specimen bonding area (A, in mm²) are used to calculate the bond strength value (in MPa). The resultant fracture surfaces have to be examined using fractographic principles.

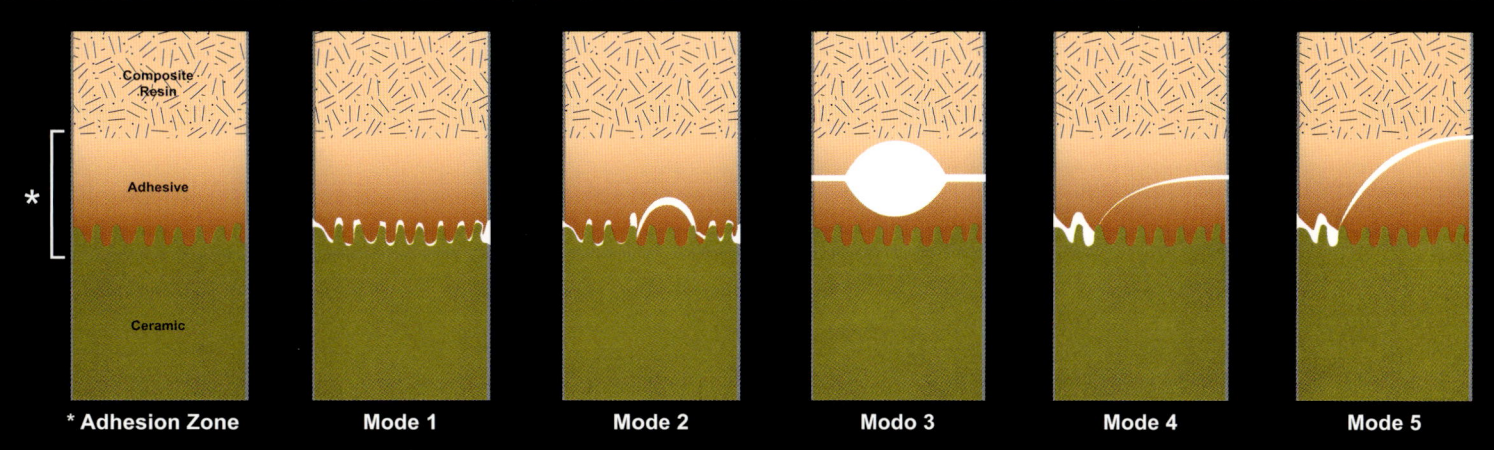

Figure 4.16 - Schematic representation of the modes of failure for the microtensile bond strength test of ceramic bonded to resin composite, based on crack initiation and principles of fractography.
    Mode 1: adhesive separation at the ceramic-adhesive resin interface (adhesive failure).
    Mode 2: failure starts at the ceramic-adhesive interface, goes into the adhesive resin and returns to the interface.
    Mode 3: failure from internal flaw (penny-shape internal crack).
    Mode 4: failure starts at the ceramic-adhesive interface propagates through the adhesive resin.
    Mode 5: failure starts at the ceramic-adhesive interface, goes through the adhesive resin to reach the composite-adhesive interface.
        Modes 2-5 are examples of cohesive failures. The adhesive-ceramic interface seems to be the weakest link of the system.
        From Della Bona *et al.*, 2003.

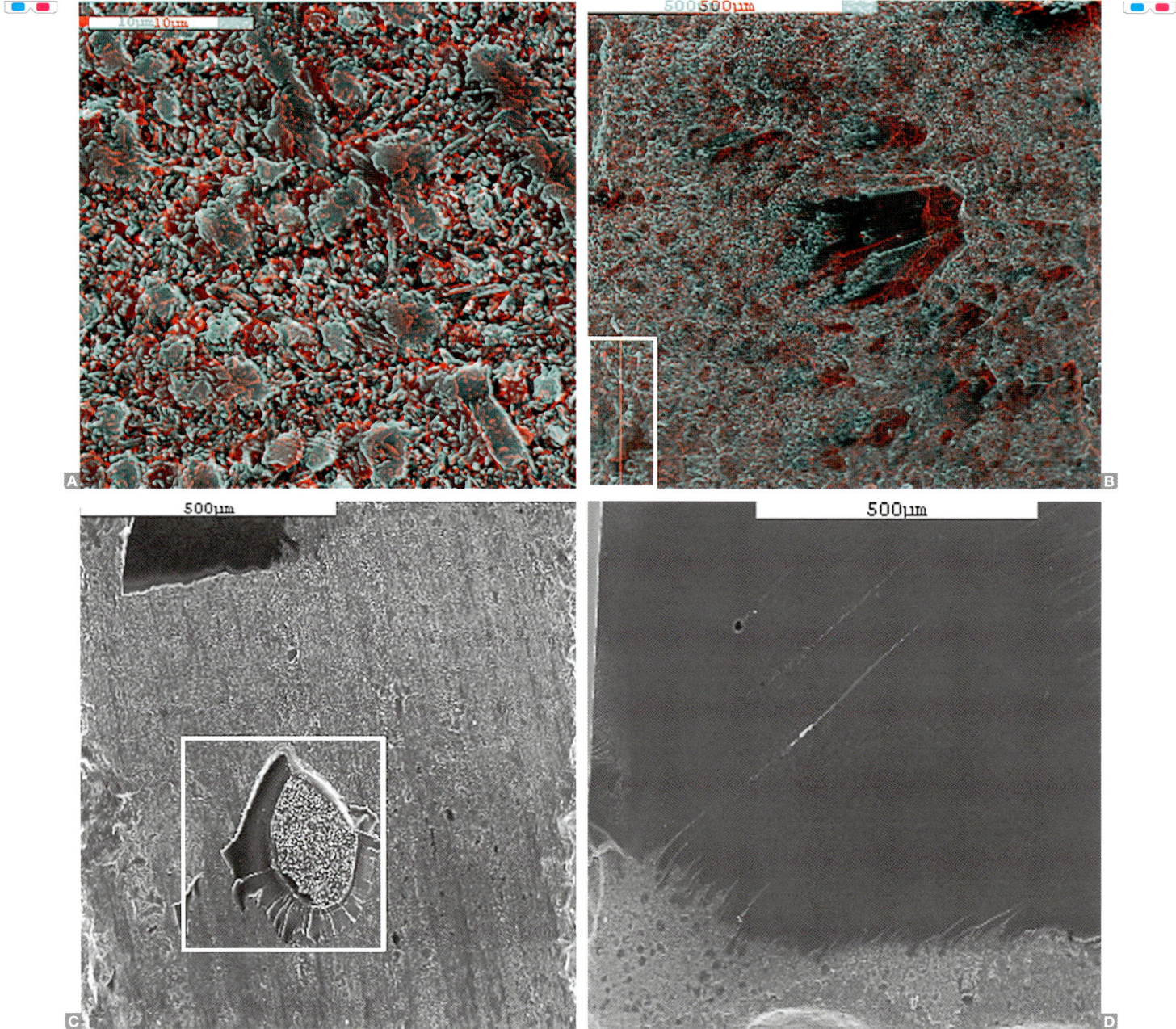

Figure 4.17 - Representative SEM micrographs of the modes of failure, schematically illustrated in Fig. 4.16. **A**- Fracture surface of APF-treated IPS Empress2 bonded to resin; no trace of other substrate was found on the surface (Mode 1- adhesive failure) (x3000). **B**- Semicircular flaw is the crack origin (in the white box); the adhesive resin island in the middle of the fracture surface represents what has been characterized as failure mode 2 (x80). Additionally, the fracture markings are easier observed on the adhesive resin areas. **C**- Internal flaw (in the white box) is the crack origin characterizing failure mode 3 (x80). **D**- Failure starts at the ceramic–adhesive interface as a corner flaw (lower left) and propagates through the adhesive resin (Mode 4) (x80). From Della Bona *et al.*, 2003.

Despite of the variable fracture surface morphology, the ceramic-adhesive interface seems to be the weakest link of this system, and each ceramic surface treatment has a failure trend. Adhesive failure (mode 1) is not a common outcome during microtensile bond strength testing. This mode of failure normally occurs during specimen cutting procedures, i.e. during specimen preparation, suggesting a weak bond (Fig. 4.17 A). HF-treated ceramic specimens usually produces failure that starts at the ceramic-adhesive interface and either propagates through the adhesive (mode 4), or reaches the adhesive-composite interface (mode 5) or returns to the ceramic-adhesive interface (mode 2) (Fig. 4.17 B and D).

Therefore, optical microscopy observation is often not enough to determine the mode of failure of bonding interfaces. A thorough SEM examination of the fracture surfaces following the principles of fractography and confirmation of surface composition through the use of **X-ray elemental map** analyses (Fig. 4.18) produce a more consistent and complete description of the fracture process and the modes of failure. These analyses would avoid simplistic comments such as the "mixed mode of failure" that often follows the "adhesive and-or cohesive" unscientific observations. Thus, when fractography is correctly used to determine the fracture origin, a proper scientific statement on the mode of fracture can be formulated (chapter 3).

Elemental mapping is a microscopic technique where the distribution of elements over the surface of a sample is determined. It requires the use of an **electron microprobe**, using EDS or WDS (Fig. 4.18).

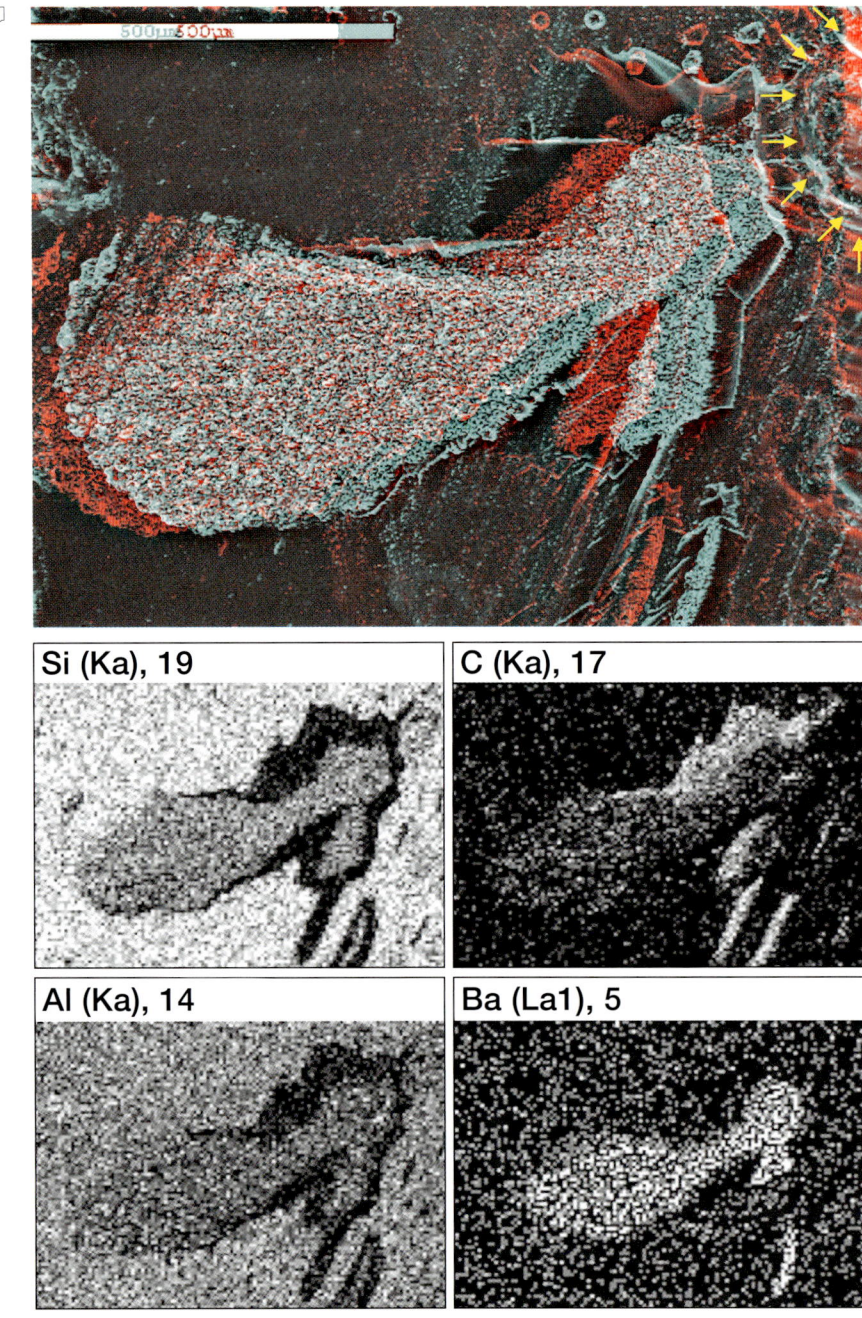

Figure 4.18 - A fracture bonding interface surface examined using SEM to determine the mode of failure, which was confirmed using X-ray dot mapping. Two-dimensional scanning using X-ray dot mapping involves taking the output of the single-channel analyzer and using it to modulate the brightness of the cathode ray tube (CRT) during normal secondary-electron raster scanning. Each X-ray photon detected appears as a dot on the CRT, with regions of high concentration characterized by a high dot density. This figure shows a SEM image (top) and X-ray elemental maps of fracture surface of IPS Empress ceramic (Ivoclar) bonded to a resin-based composite (Z100, 3M). The label at the top of X-ray maps indicates the elements and their intensity. The critical flaw is indicated by the yellow arrows at the top right corner of the SEM micrograph (x100). The fracture starts along the ceramic-adhesive interface, propagates through the adhesive resin to reach the composite-adhesive interface (Failure Mode 5). From Della Bona *et al.*, 2003.

As commented and demonstrated by finite element analyses (FEA) of stresses, the non-uniformity of the interfacial stress distribution generated during conventional tensile and shear bond strength testing may lead to fracture initiation from flaws at the interface or within the substrate at areas of high localized stress. Thus, to test the integrity of bonded interfaces one can subject a bonded assembly to a variety of loading conditions to control the crack path along the interface or within the interfacial region. Additionally, one can promote crack initiation within the adhesion zone and use an interfacial toughness test coupled with fracture mechanics and fractographic principles to estimate the apparent interfacial fracture toughness (K_A), as suggested by Della Bona *et al.*, 2006. Strictly speaking, measurement of the toughness at the bonding interface in terms of K_{IC} (chapter 3) is undefined. However, tensile tests can be performed in which an inserted crack or defect is the source of failure. Therefore, the K_A can be calculated from the size of the defect and the strength with the appropriate geometric factor. Thus, the apparent fracture toughness value (K_A) reflects the ability of a material to resist unstable crack propagation at the interface.

Usually, in order to maintain equal compliances of the specimen halves, *i.e.* for the two halves to have equal strain energy, most interfacial fracture toughness tests require $E_1 t_1^3 = E_2 t_2^3$, where E_1 and t_1 are the elastic modulus and the thickness, respectively, for one specimen half (*e.g.* ceramic); and E_2 and t_2 are the elastic modulus and the thickness, respectively, of the other specimen half (*e.g.* resin-based composite). As the microtensile test is uniaxial, there is no need to balance the compliance for the two materials

129

to measure K_A. Even so, because the fracture toughness in this form is really a pseudocritical stress-intensity factor, *i.e.* apparent toughness (K_A), and considering the fact that it is difficult to define a stress intensity at an interface, one must still determine an effective modulus for the materials. Nevertheless, it has been reported a positive correlation between the W_A, the tensile bond strength (σ), and the K_A, that is, the higher the mean W_A value, the higher the mean σ and K_A values.

Another appropriate way to assess the interfacial bond is to analyze the energy per unit crack surface area, G_I, that is required for a crack to advance in the bond plane. The toughness is related to the critical strain energy release rate (G_{IC}) and is a measure of the resistance of the bond to fracture, since G_{IC} represents the relative energy required to create the new surfaces.

In summary, this chapter explained how the clinical success of either a repaired ceramic restoration or a resin cemented ceramic restoration depends on the quality and durability of the adhesive-ceramic bond interface, which is the main focus of this book. The quality of this bond depends upon the bonding mechanisms that are controlled in part by the specific surface treatment used to promote micromechanical and/or chemical retention to the substrate(s). However, the quality of this bond should not be assessed based on bond strength data alone. Structural and surface analyses of treated ceramics showed that different surface patterns are created according to the type of ceramic and type of primer (*e.g.* acids, airborne particle abrasion, silica coating). The concentration, application time and type of acid are also critical factors for priming acid-sensitive ceramics. Additionally, silica coating acid-resistant ceramics is important to improve bonding to resin and this concept may be essential for further developments on adhesion to acid-resistant ceramics. Thus, it is important to know the ceramics microstructure and composition (previous chapters), the morphology and wettability after surface treatment/activation that provide fundamental understanding of the surface ability for micromechanical retention and chemical adhesion. This information coupled with the knowledge on the mode of failure, can yield relevant information on the clinical performance of all-ceramic restorations, which is the ultimate test for any adhesive system.

This chapter completed a series of concepts, experimental procedures and rationale on adhesion to ceramics, developing the fundamental basis to understand the clinical performance of bonded all-ceramic restorations, the possible failure causes, and the principles to improve the adhesion mechanisms of resin-based composite bonded to dental ceramics.

Selected readings

- Anusavice KJ. *Phillips' science of dental materials*. 11th ed. Philadelphia: W.B. Saunders, 2003.
- Ban S, Anusavice KJ. Influence of test method on failure stress of brittle dental materials. *J Dent Res*, 69:1791-1799, 1990.
- Della Bona A, van Noort R. Shear versus tensile bond strength of resin composite bonded to ceramic. *J Dent Res*, 74:1591-1596, 1995.
- Della Bona A, Anusavice KJ, Shen C. Microtensile strength of composite bonded to hot-pressed ceramics. *J Adhes Dent*, 2:305-313, 2000.
- Della Bona A, Anusavice KJ. Microstructure, composition, and etching topography of dental ceramics. *Int J Prosthodont*, 15:159-167, 2002.
- Della Bona A, Anusavice KJ, Hood JAA. Effect of ceramic surface treatment on tensile bond strength to a resin cement. *Int J Prosthodont*, 15:248-253, 2002.
- Della Bona A, Anusavice KJ, Mecholsky Jr JJ. Failure analysis of resin composite bonded to ceramic. *Dent Mater*, 19: 693-699, 2003.
- Della Bona A, Shen C, Anusavice KJ. Work of adhesion of resin on treated lithia disilicate-based ceramic. *Dent Mater*, 20:338 - 344, 2004a.
- Della Bona A, Mecholsky Jr JJ, Anusavice KJ. Fracture behavior of lithia disilicate- and leucite-based ceramics. *Dent Mater*, 20:956 – 962, 2004b.
- Della Bona A, Anusavice KJ, Mecholsky Jr JJ. Apparent interfacial fracture toughness of resin/ceramic systems. *J Dent Res*, 85:1037 - 1041, 2006.
- Della Bona A, Donassollo TA, Demarco FF, Barrett AA, Mecholsky Jr JJ. Characterization and surface treatment effects on topography of a glass-infiltrated alumina/zirconia-reinforced ceramic. *Dent Mater*, 23:769 - 775, 2007a.
- Della Bona A, Borba M, Benetti P, Cecchetti D. Effect of surface treatments on the bond strength of a zirconia-reinforced ceramic to composite resin. *Braz Oral Res*, 21:10 - 15, 2007b.
- Kitasako Y, Burrow MF, Nikaido T, Harada N, Inokoshi S, Yamada T, Takatsu T. Shear and tensile bond testing for resin cement evaluation. *Dent Mater*, 11:298-304, 1995.
- Pashley DH, Carvalho RM, Sano H, Nakajima M, Yoshiyama M, Shono Y, et al.. The microtensile bond test: a review. *J Adhes Dent*, 1:299-309, 1999.
- Phoenix RD, Shen C. Characterization of treated porcelain surfaces via dynamic contact angle analysis. *Int J Prosthodont*, 8:187-194, 1995.
- Quinn GD. *Fractography of ceramics and glasses*. Washington: National Institute of Standards and Technology (NIST); 2007
- Sano H, Shono T, Sonoda H, Takatsu T, Ciucchi B, Carvalho R, Pashley D. Relationship between surface area for adhesion and tensile bond strength- Evaluation of a micro-tensile bond test. *Dent Mater*, 10: 236-240, 1994.
- van Noort R, Noroozi S, Howard IC, Cardew G. A critique of bond strength measurements. *J Dent*, 17: 61-67, 1989.
- van Noort R, Cardew GE, Howard IC, Noroozi S. The effect of local interfacial geometry on the measurement of the tensile bond strength to dentin. *J Dent Res*, 70:889-893, 1991.
- van Noort R. *Introduction to dental materials*. 3rd ed. London: Mosby, 2007.
- Versluis A, Tantbirojn D, Douglas WH. Why do shear bond tests pull out dentin? *J Dent Res*, 76:1298-1307, 1997.

Chapter 5

Clinical applications of adhesion to cement and repair dental ceramic restorations

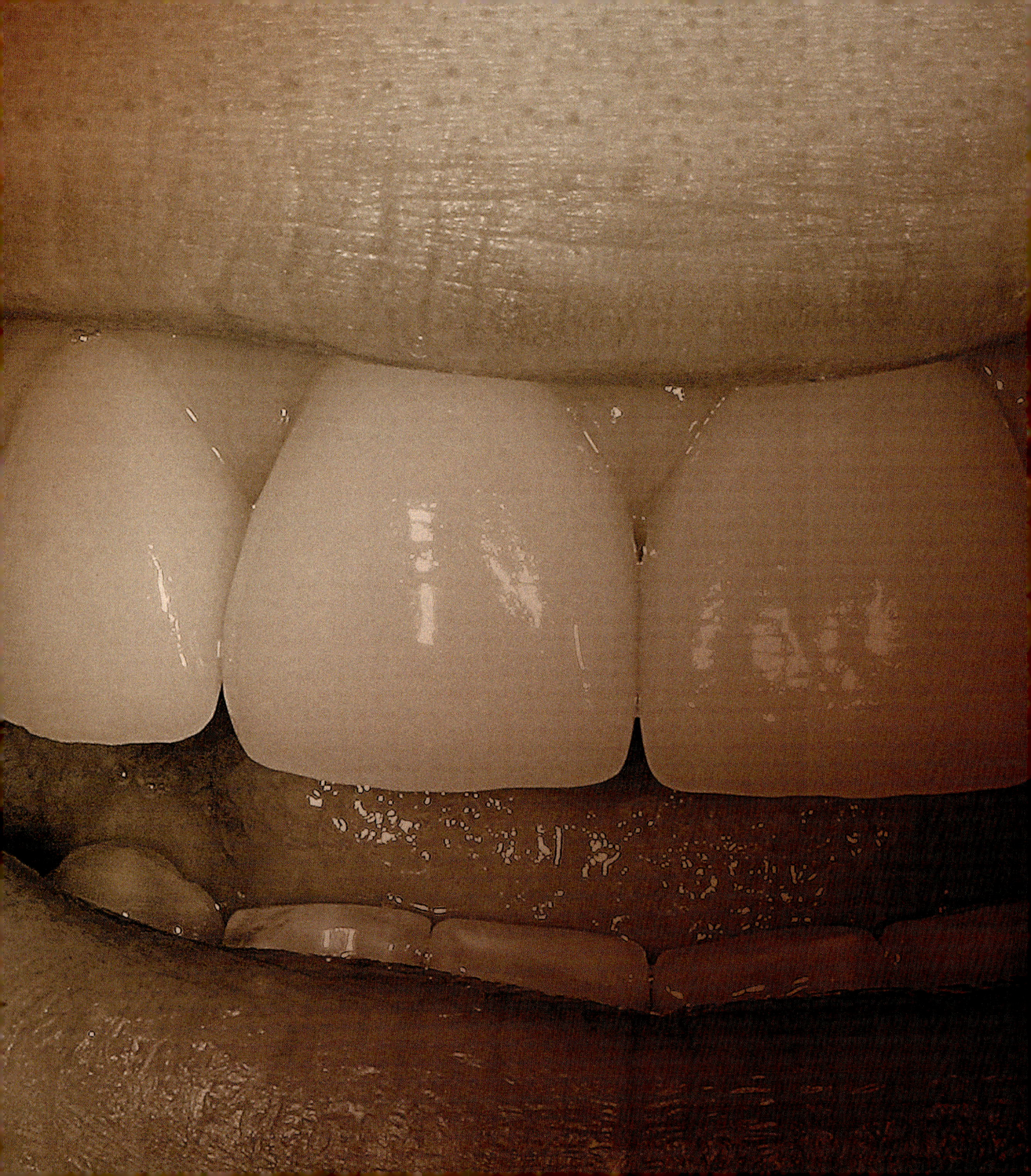

Introduction

Why are we so interested in dental ceramic restorations? There is a very simple answer: long-lasting esthetics. The ceramic restorations look good for years, and no other dental material can surpass that! So, long-lived esthetics and biocompatibility are the promise of all-ceramic restorations.

The new polycrystalline dental ceramics are stronger and tougher, but have to be veneered for pleasant esthetics. Additionally, these restorations have to be bonded to teeth to have greater survival rate.

This chapter presents the clinical applications of resin adhesion for cementing and repairing dental ceramic restorations, illustrating the concepts and phenomena explained in previous chapters.

Evidence-based dentistry: The process of systematically finding, appraising, and using contemporaneous research findings as the basis for clinical decisions. Evidence-based dentistry asks questions, finds and appraises the relevant data, and harnesses that information for everyday clinical practice. It should follow four steps: formulate a clear clinical question from a patient's problem; search the literature for relevant clinical articles; evaluate (critically appraise) the evidence for its validity and usefulness; implement useful findings in clinical practice.

Secondary or recurrent caries: Caries that appears at a location with a previous history of caries. This is frequently found on the margins of fillings and other dental restorations. On the other hand, **incipient caries** describes decay at a location that has not experienced previous decay. **Arrested caries** describes a lesion on a tooth which was previously demineralized but was remineralized before causing a cavitation.

Microleakage: Flow of oral fluid and bacteria into the microscopic gap between a prepared tooth surface and a restorative material.

An endless dynamic evolution in ceramic materials and technology has sustained a progressive research interest on dental ceramic restorations. This constant improvement is based on the excellent ceramic properties, discussed in previous chapters, and on **evidence-based dentistry** that is presented in this chapter. Notwithstanding, all-ceramic restorations may also fail and the most frequently reported failures are bulk fracture (Fig. 5.1), chipping (Fig. 5.2), debonding, and **secondary caries**. As mentioned, failures due to fracture are mostly related to the brittle nature of ceramic materials and inadequate restorative design. Secondary caries and periodontal support are biological responses not related to the ceramic materials. In fact, there is no evidence to say that marginal gap is clinically related to secondary caries. On the contrary, it is more related to the caries susceptibility of the patient. Additionally, resin-bonding decreases the **marginal leakage** of ceramic restorations, improving the overall strength of the restoration (Albert and El-Mowafy, 2004; Magne, 2005; Magne *et al.*, 2007). So, this chapter suggests procedures to minimize failures in all-ceramic restorations, highlighting the importance of case selection, tooth preparation, material selection, restoration design, cementation technique, occlusion equilibration, and patient proservation.

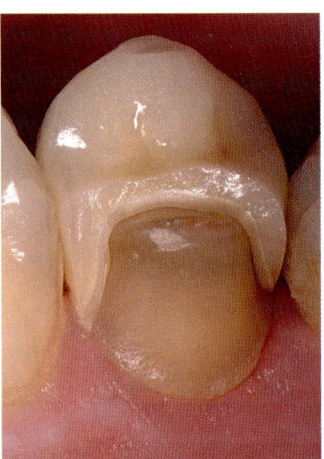

Figure 5.1 - A catastrophic fracture of a resin bonded all-ceramic crown (Procera Alumina, Nobel Biocare) on a premolar. The restoration was replaced.

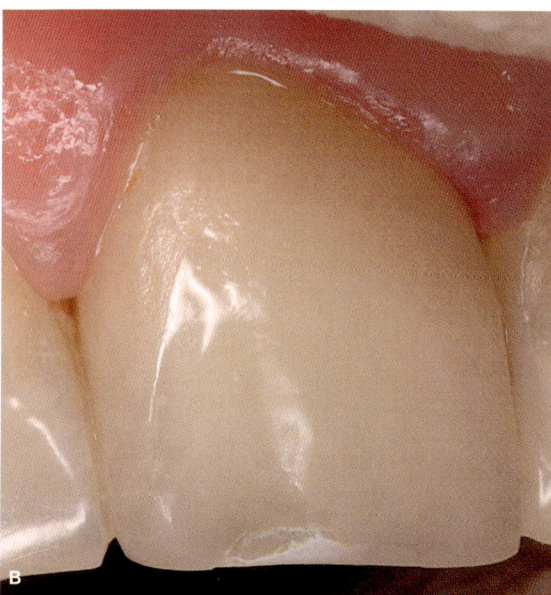

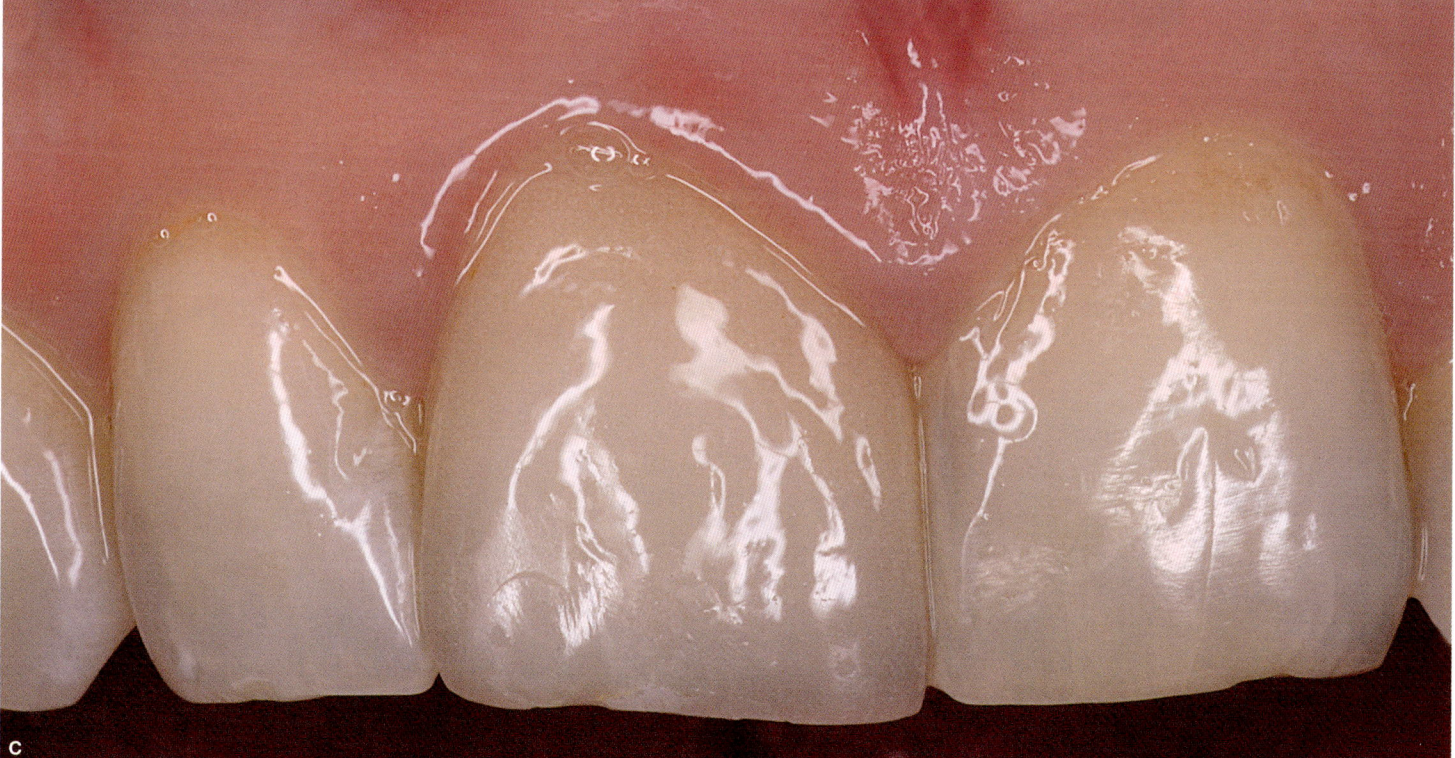

137

Figure 5.2 - Recurrent ceramic chipping and resin-based composite repair of a resin bonded leucite-based ceramic crown (IPS Empress, Ivoclar) on upper central incisor. **A**- The image shows a recurrent fracture (chipping) on the labial aspect slightly distal to the previous resin-based composite repair to the incisal edge, which is now more visible lingually. **B**- Fractured area was etched using 9.5% hydrofluoric acid (HF) for 90 s. Note the HF effect (white area) on the composite filler particles, which were etched away. **C**- A silane coupling agent and a resin-based adhesive system were used for the second resin-based composite repair. The crown fractured catastrophically after 3 years in service and it was replaced. Courtesy of Dr. Simon E Northeast.

Opalescence is a type of dichroism seen in highly dispersed systems with little opacity. The material appears yellowish-red in transmitted light and blue in the scattered light perpendicular to the transmitted light. The phenomenon is named after the appearance of opals.

Opacity is the measure of impenetrability to electromagnetic or other kinds of radiation, especially visible light. In radiative transfer, it describes the absorption and scattering of radiation in a medium, such as a plasma, glass, etc. An opaque object is neither transparent (allowing all light to pass through) nor translucent (allowing some light to pass through).

It is necessary to have some knowledge about the ceramic systems and processes available on the market to plan any all-ceramic restorative treatment.

As explained in chapter 3, dental ceramics can be either polycrystalline, particle-filled glass or mostly glass (Fig. 3.3). We have known that highly esthetic dental ceramics are predominantly glasses with very small amounts of particles (oxides) to control optical effects such as **opalescence**, color and **opacity**. They are the best material to mimic the optical properties of enamel and dentin. They are usually referred as veneering materials or glasses and most of them come paired with their appropriate substructure ceramic. Some veneering materials are single phase silica-based glasses and acid etching does not result in a very effective retentive surface for bonding to resins (Fig. 4.7), which is much improved by the chemical bonding mechanism via silane coupling agents.

Higher amounts of filler particles can be added to the glass (particle-filled glasses) to improve properties such as strength and coefficient of thermal expansion. The fillers usually are crystalline particles (*e.g.* leucite, Figs. 3.4; 3.8; 4.5; 4.6) or phase(s) of a higher melting glass (Fig. 5.3). These heterogeneous materials facilitate etching at grain boundaries. In addition, the leucite reacts and-or dissolves in contact with fluorine-based acids (Figs. 4.5; 4.6) resulting in micromechanical retentive ceramic surfaces, improving bonding to resin-based adhesive systems.

The filler particles can be mechanically added as powder or precipitated within the starting glass by special nucleation and growth heating treatments as for glass-ceramics (chapter 3). Representative examples of such material are the Ivoclar Vivadent ceramics containing high concentrations of lithium disilicate crystals (IPS Empress 2, Fig. 3.9; e.maxPress and e.maxCAD) and the mica-filled material (Dicor, Dentsply Inc.) that is no longer on the market (Fig. 5.25). The In-Ceram system (Vita Zahnfabrik) is another example of high crystalline content ceramic where the filler particles and the glass phases are both continuous in space, with the filler being either alumina (In-Ceram Alumina; Figs. 3.5; 3.12 A, B; 5.26; 5.30), magnesium aluminate spinel (In-Ceram Spinell) or a 70-30% mixture of alumina-zirconia (In-Ceram Zirconia; Figs. 3.7; 5.29) (Fig. 5.4). As for the lithia disilicate crystals (Fig. 3.9 B), the alumina and zirconia particles are not dissolved by acids, and most of the mechanical retention is resultant from the acid reaction with the glass phase (Figs. 4.8; 4.9). Therefore, for these ceramic systems, the greater the amount of the glass phase, the rougher the etched ceramic surface, wich improves the resin adhesive potential.

139

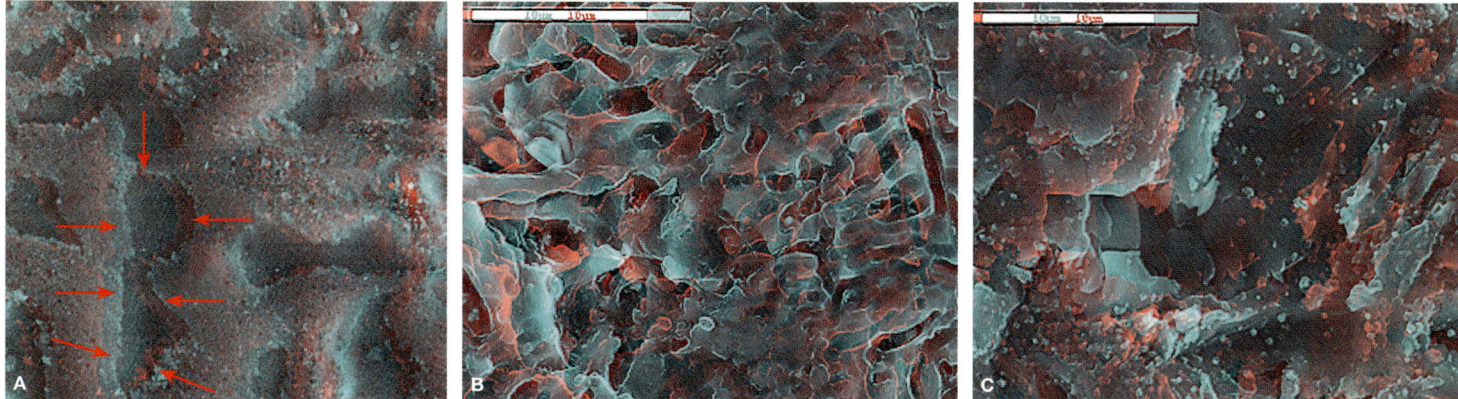

Figure 5.3 - Representative SEM images of a feldspathic glass (VM7, Vita). **A**- The material has no crystalline phase but two glass phases (red arrows are showing a darker glass phase surrounded by a lighter glass phase, both have similar composition). **B**- Retentive grooves are created on the VM7 surface treated with hydrofluoric acid (HF). **C**- Silica coating using airborne-particle abrasion (Cojet system, 3M ESPE) resulted in deposition of silica-modified alumina particles on the VM7 surface. (x5000). However, silica coating is not the pre-treatment of choice for resin bonding to glasses and low-crystalline ceramics, which have enough silica for the chemical bond via silane coupling agents (Boscato *et al.*, 2007).

The increase in crystalline content to fully polycrystalline reduced crack propagation, originating high strength and tougher substructure ceramics (Fig. 5.4). However, they are difficult to cut and well-fitting restorations were not practical prior the introduction of computer-aided manufacturing (CAM). In general, the computer-aided systems use a 3-D data set representing either the prepared tooth or a wax model of the desired substructure. The data set is used to produce either an enlarged die upon which ceramic powder is packed (Procera, Nobel Biocare) or to machine (Fig. 5.5) an oversized structure from partially fired ceramic powder (ZirCAD, Ivoclar Vivadent; Cercon, Dentsply Prosthetics; Lava, 3M ESPE; In-Ceram YZ, Vita Zahnfabrik). Both approaches rely upon well-characterized ceramic powders for which firing shrinkage can be predicted accurately. As these ceramic substructures are relatively opaque, the restorations have to be veneered to enhance esthetics.

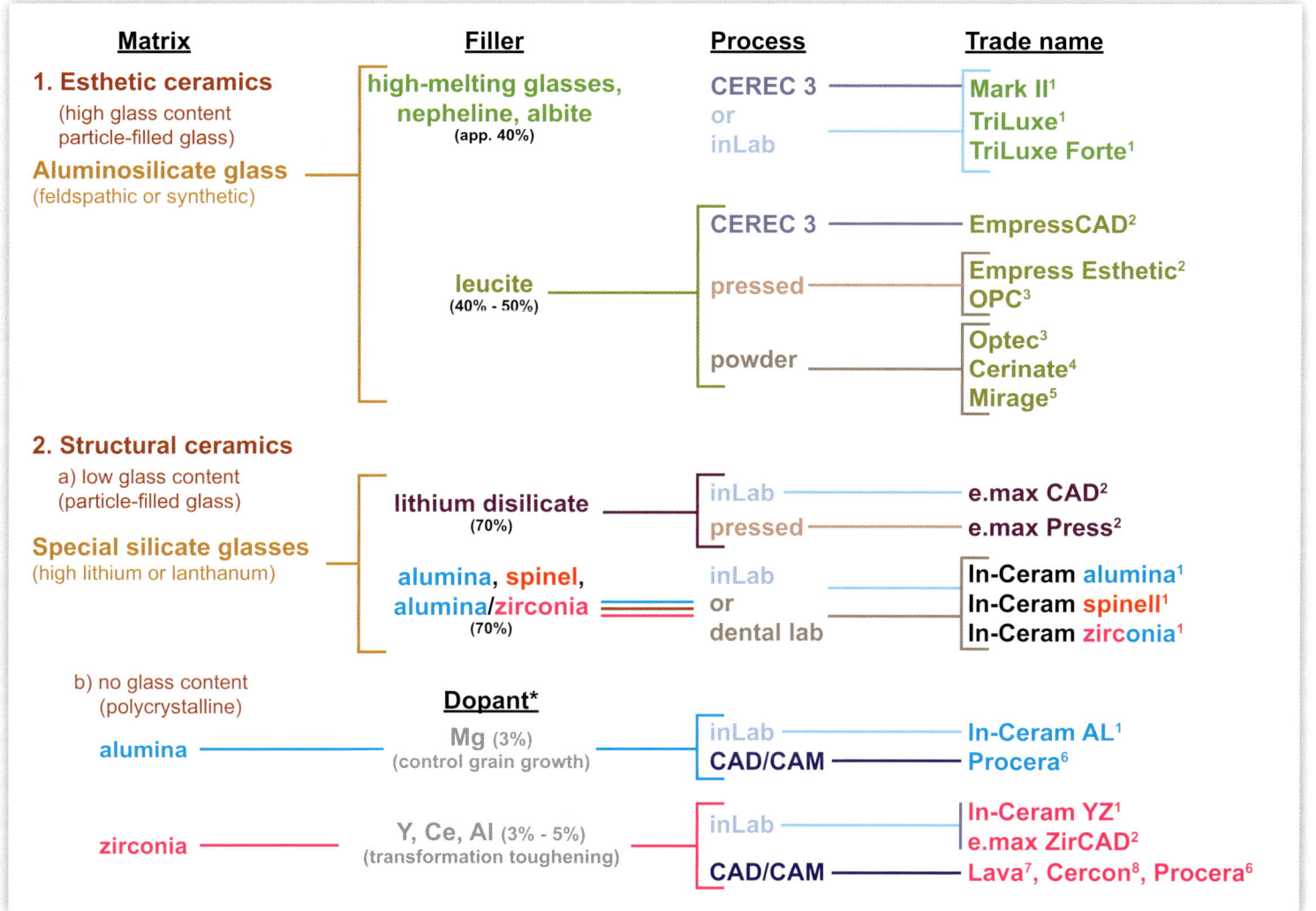

141

Figure 5.4 - Chart of commercially available dental ceramic systems for all-ceramic restorations based on the matrix material, filler concentration and type, fabrication process and trade name. For polycrystalline ceramics containing no glass (2.b), the main phase ("matrix") is either alumina or zirconia and the "fillers" are not particles but modifying atoms called "dopants or stabilizers". Cerec 3, for dentists, and inLab, for dental laboratory technicians, are types of **CAD-CAM** systems. There are some ceramic systems made for specific CAD-CAM machines, such as Cerec 3 and inLab (Sirona). The figure is color coded: **brown** - classes of ceramics; **blue** - alumina-based ceramics; **pink** - zirconia-based ceramics; **purple** - lithium disilicate-based ceramics; **red** - spinel; **lime** - leucite-based ceramics; **dark green** - glasses. The superscripted numbers relate to manufacturers: 1- Vita Zahnfabrik; 2- Ivoclar Vivadent; 3- Pentron; 4- Den-Mat; 5- Chameleon Dental Products; 6- Nobel Biocare; 7- 3M ESPE; 8- Dentsply Prosthetics. Adapted from Kelly (2006), with permission of Quintessence.

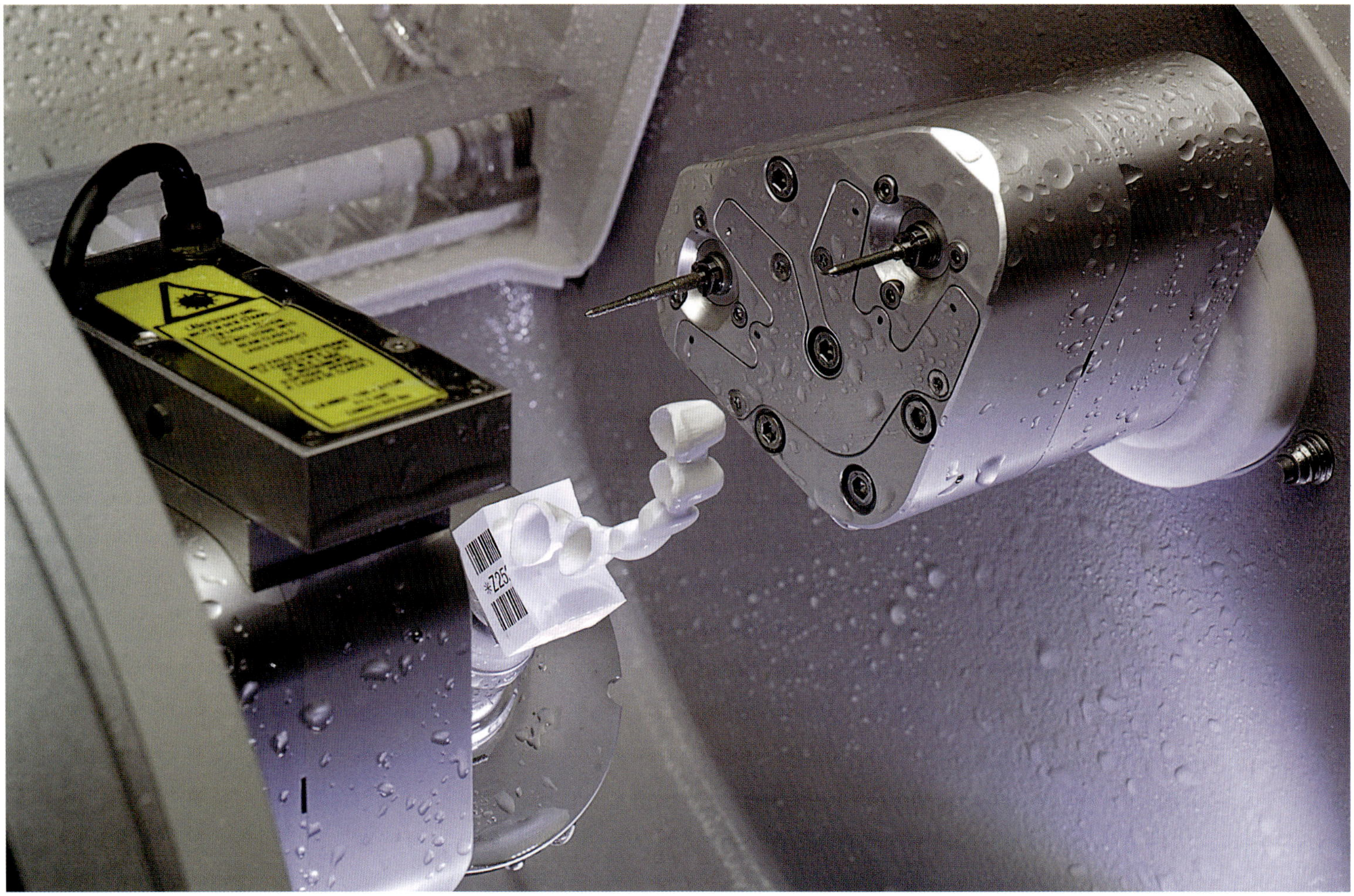

Figure 5.5 - Cerec inLab MC XL milling unit (Sirona Dental Systems) cutting a zirconia-based ceramic block (Vita In-Ceram YZ). The system improved tremendously from the first generation machines introduced in 1985. Courtesy of Sirona AG, Germany.

Ceramic blocks for CAD-CAM processing can be fabricated by extrusion molding (*e.g.* Vitablocks Mark II), dry pressing (*e.g.* all Vita In-Ceram blocks and Vitablocks TriLuxe), or **hot isostatic pressing** (HIP) procedures. For the extrusion molding process, the ceramic powder is mixed with plasticizing agents and water. The plasticized ceramic mixture is pressed into a screw extruder and through a nozzle that gives the material its form. To prevent crack formation, drying of the material takes place over several days under controlled ambient conditions before firing the blocks to over 1000^0C. In the dry pressing procedure the ceramic powder is filled into a mold and compacted by the stamping press. The Vita In-Ceram blocks, for example, are porously sintered spinel ($MgAl_2O_4$), alumina (Al_2O_3) and zirconia reinforced alumina (Al_2O_3-ZrO_2) either for glass-infiltration (respectively, In-Ceram Spinell, In-Ceram Alumina, and In-Ceram Zirconia) or for densely sintering. A shrinkage factor must be considered for the densely sintered blocks (In-Ceram AL and In-Ceram YZ), which have a bar code containing information on the shrinkage factor that is identified by the CAD-CAM scanner and taken into account during the machining process (Table. 5.1). Yet, no shrinkage occurs during glass infiltration, which may result in better marginal fit of the glass-infiltrated In-Ceram ceramic restorations.

Hot isostatic pressing (HIP) is a manufacturing process used to reduce the porosity of metals and influence the density of many ceramic materials. This improves the mechanical properties, workability and ceramic density. The HIP process subjects a component to both elevated temperature and isostatic gas pressure in a high pressure containment vessel. Pressure is applied to the material from all directions (hence the term "isostatic").

143

Table 5.1 - Clinically and laboratory relevant features, properties and indications for the ceramic blocks from Vita.

Ceramic blocks (Vita)†	Special Features	Relevant Properties	Clinical Indications	Sirona System
Vitablocs™ Mark II	Monochromatic, tooth-colored block	• Fine-structure feldspathic ceramic; • Mild to the opposing teeth; very good esthetics; • Customizable and reduced wear of milling tools	Inlays, onlays, veneers and crowns in the anterior and posterior areas	• Cerec 3, Cerec MC XL; • inLab, inLab MC XL
Vitablocs™ TriLuxe	Smooth shade transition to simulate tooth thirds (incisal/occlusal, middle and cervical)			
Vitablocs™ TriLuxe Forte	• Finer nuances of the shade transition; • Chroma was added to the cervical area; • Fluorescence was increased in the middle-to-cervical area			
In-Ceram™ Spinell*		Excellent translucency and esthetics	Anterior crown substructure	inLab, inLab MC XL
In-Ceram™ Alumina*	• No shrinkage process; • Individual coloring in four shades and glass infiltration in one step	Good combination of strength and esthetics	Substructure for anterior crowns and 3-unit FPD	
In-Ceram™ Zirconia*		Very good strength and ability to mask discolored preparations	Substructure for anterior and posterior crowns and 3-unit FPD	
In-Ceram™ AL**		Very good strength	Primary components. Substructure for anterior crowns and 3-unit FPD and posterior crowns	inLab, inLab MC XL
In-Ceram™ YZ**	Individual coloring in five shades can be done prior dense sintering.	Greatest strength and ability to mask discolored preparations	Primary components. Substructure for anterior and posterior crowns and multi-unit FPD	

† Trade names follow same color code as for Figure 5.4. * Infiltration ceramic; ** Sinter ceramic.

As mentioned in chapters 2 and 3, the zirconia (ZrO_2) has to be stabilized by a dopant (stabilizer), which usually is either ceria (CeO_2), as for Vita In-Ceram Zirconia fabricated by slip casting (Fig. 3.7) and dry pressed, or yttria (Y_2O_3) (Fig. 2.6 B), as for In-Ceram YZ (Vita) and Cercon (Dentsply Prosthetics) (Fig. 3.10).

Having introduced the most popular ceramic systems (Fig. 5.4), treatment planning should start by giving the patient all the possible treatment options, including the most conservative and less expensive ones, which, some times, are just perfect for the patient (Figs. 5.6; 5.7; 5.8). It is certainly noteworthy, that one study reported that the primary reason for replacing direct restorations (amalgams and resin-based composites) is due to a patient changing dentists (Bogacki *et al.*, 2002). Dentists should be mindful and judicious not to follow that same thought pattern with regard to indirect restorations.

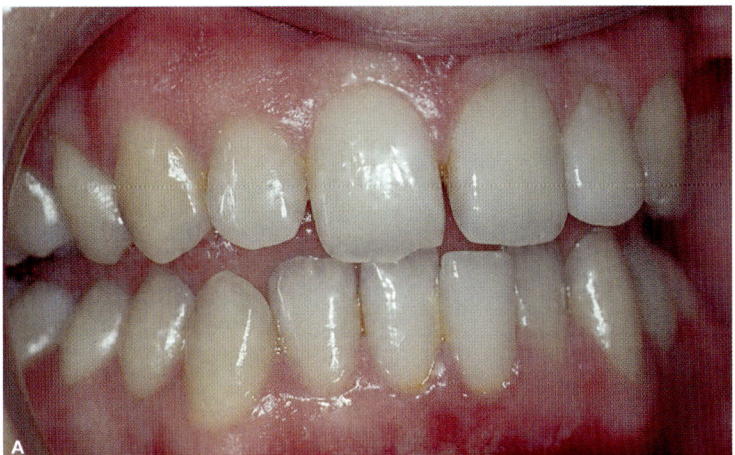 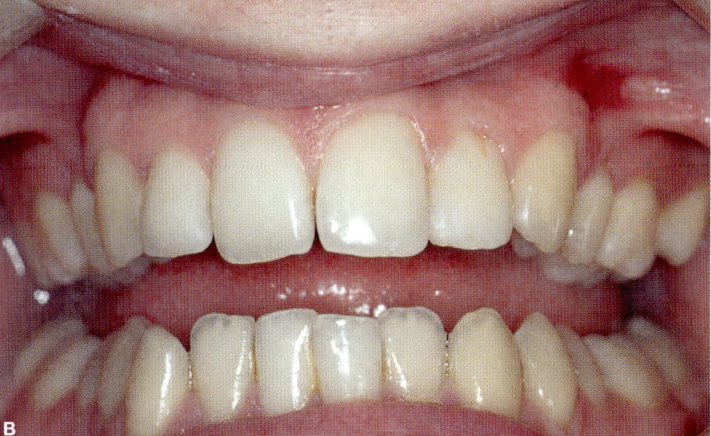

Figure 5.6 - Young male patient wishing to improve anterior esthetics. **A**- treatment plan involved closure of small diastema and change the shape of lateral incisors. **B**- A low cost and conservative direct restorative procedure using resin-based composites was sufficient to meet the expectations of the patient.

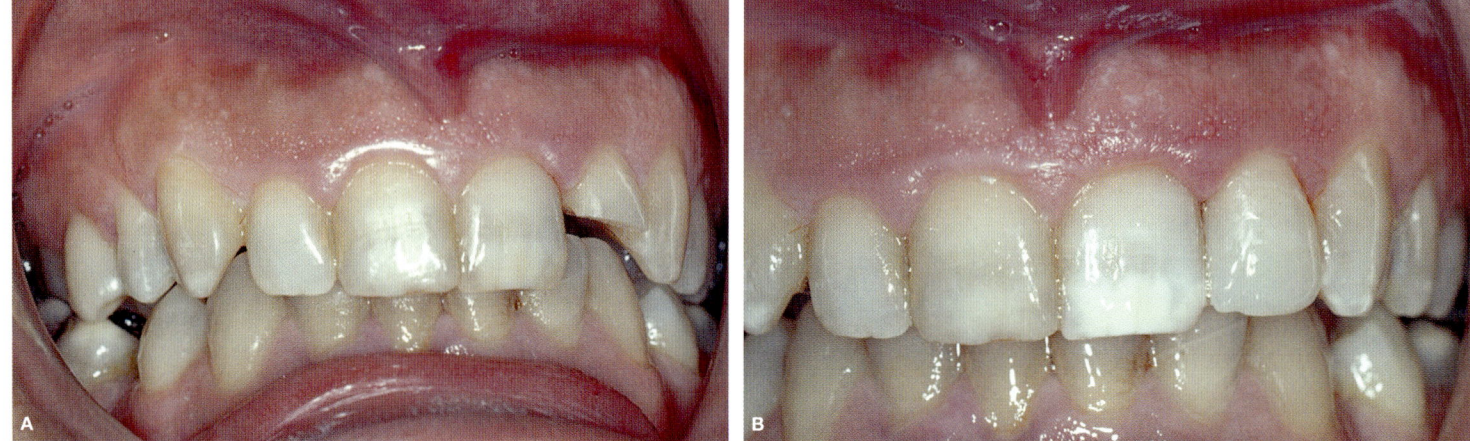

Figure 5.7 - **A**- Adult female patient with a fractured lateral incisor resulting from a frontal impact. **B**- A conservative direct restorative procedure using resin-based composites was the emergency treatment, which is still in place 8 years later.

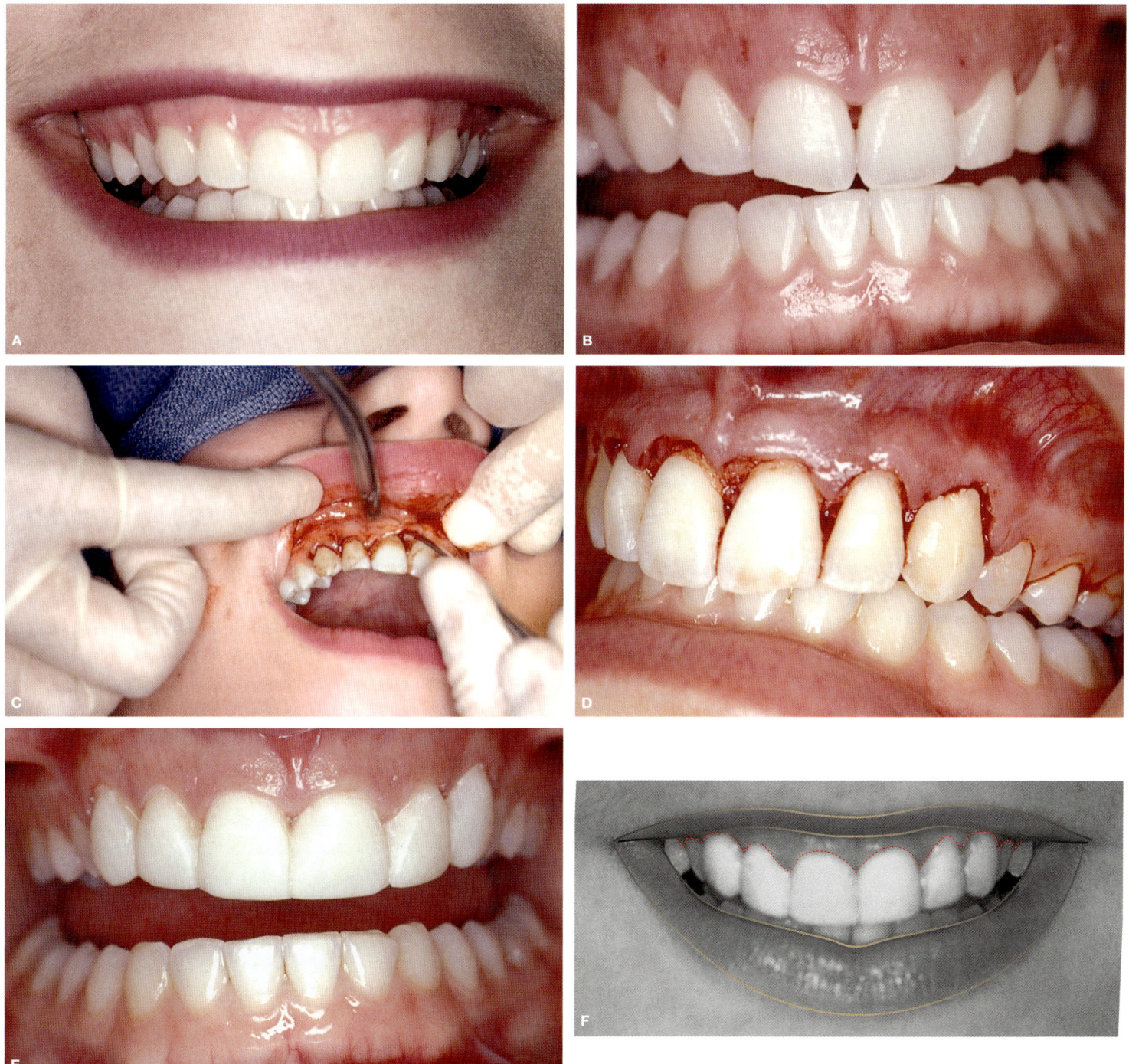

Figure 5.8 - Short clinical crowns resulting from excess gingival coverage. **A**- A close-up image of the initial case. Study casts and diagnostic wax-up simulations were done. After measuring the crowns and gingiva and imaging simulations, the esthetic crown lengthening (gingivoplasty) was performed (**B**, **C**, **D**). **E**- Oral tissues were completely recovered after 15 days. **F**- Comparing with the initial case (**A**) and having Fig. 5.16 as a reference, a satisfactory smile line was achieved with esthetic crown lengthening only (one month after surgery). No restorative dentistry procedure was needed, as initially intended by the patient.

Veneer restoration (laminate veneer): A superficial or attractive display in multiple layers. A thin sheet of material usually used as a finish. A protective or ornamental facing.

Kaplan-Meier statistics: It is a life-table statistical analysis that fairly represents the actual amount of time each restoration has spent in service.
Simple survival statistics can significantly inflate survival percentages.

Amelogenesis imperfecta: An autosomal dominant or X-linked disorder in which there is faulty development of the dental enamel owing to agenesis, hypoplasia, or hypocalcification of the enamel. It is marked by enamel that is very thin and friable and frequently stained in various shades of brown.

Enamel hypoplasia: A form of amelogenesis imperfecta characterized by incomplete formation of the dental enamel and transmitted as an X-linked or autosomal dominant trait. It is also associated with vitamin A, C, or D deficiency, infectious disease, prematurity, birth injury, Rh incompatibility, trauma, or local infection. Small grooves, pits, and fissures are seen in mild cases, deep horizontal rows of pits in severe cases, or absence of enamel in extreme cases.

Diastema: An abnormal opening or fissure between two adjacent teeth.

Bruxism: A disorder characterized by grinding and clenching of the teeth.

148

However, in most cases, more elaborated and complex restorative treatments are necessary to solve functional and esthetical problems, and, at same time, fulfilling the patient expectations. These treatments often involve all-ceramic restorations such as veneers, inlays, onlays, crowns and bridges (FPDs).

In a recent comprehensive review on the clinical success of all-ceramic restorations, Della Bona and Kelly (2008) compiled and compared clinical evidence for the treatment of teeth using all-ceramics. They mentioned that ceramics are particularly suited for **veneer restorations**, which have failure rates, including loss of retention and fracture, of less than 5% after 5 years in service. One of the first clinical studies, examining 83 Empress veneers (now named Empress Esthetic, Ivoclar Vivadent), reported a success rate of 99% at 6 years (Fradeani, 1998). Two other reports on feldspathic porcelain veneers (n=3045 and n=1826) showed very similar long-term survival rates (**Kaplan-Meier**) starting on 96% at 5 years, 93% at 10 years, 91% at 12 years in one study (Layton and Walton, 2007), and 94% at 12 years in another study (Fradeani *et al.*, 2005). Mechanical and biological problems that occured were associated with esthetics (31%), mechanical complications (31%), periodontal support (12.5%), loss of retention (12.5%), caries (6%), and tooth fracture (6%).

The classic clinical indications for esthetic treatment using ceramic veneers (porcelain veneers or laminate veneers) are tetracycline-stained teeth (Figs. 5.9; 5.22), defects resulted from **amelogenesis imperfecta/enamel hypoplasia** (Figs. 5.21), large **diastema** (Figs. 5.10; 5.26), small teeth (Fig. 5.10), peg-shaped (cone-shaped) teeth (Fig. 5.11), twisted teeth (Fig. 5.12), reconstruction of worn canine guidance because of **bruxism** (Fig. 5.13), substituting old resin-based composite veneers (Fig. 5.14) and masking old composite restorations (Fig. 5.15).

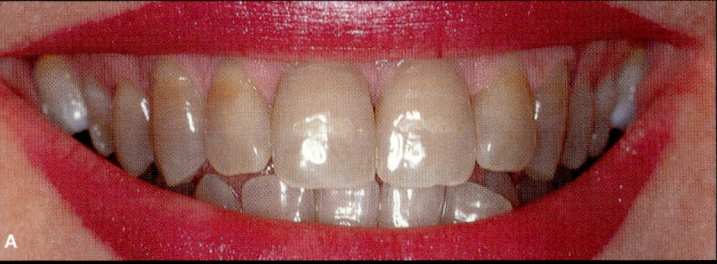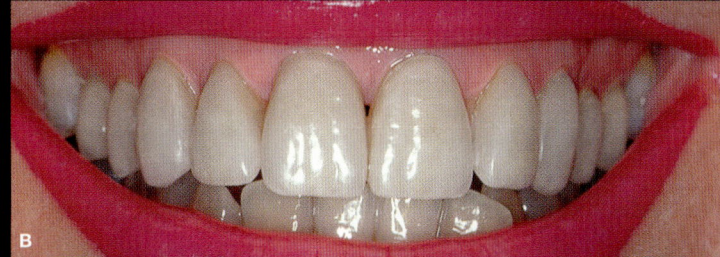

Figure 5.9 - A- Female patient with mild stained teeth and few events of mild enamel hypoplasia that were restored with ceramic veneers (**B**). Complete clinical case described in figure 5.22.

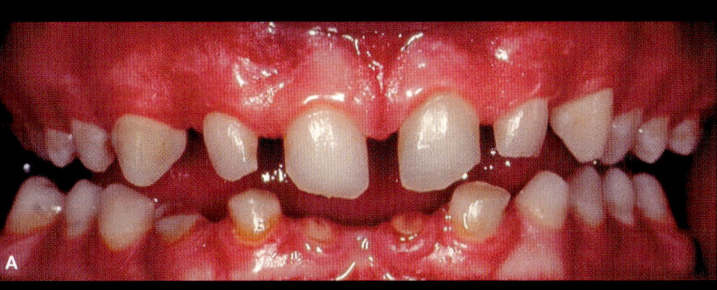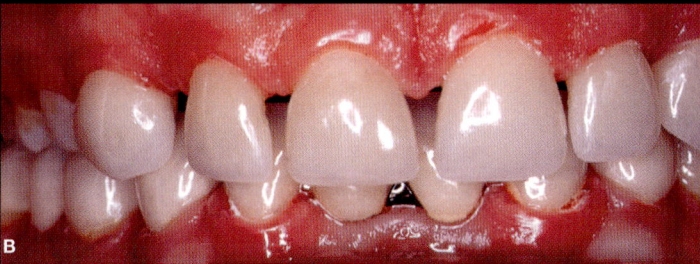

Figure 5.10 - A- Adult male patient with small teeth. **B-** Teeth were enlarged using ceramic veneers and lower anterior crowns.

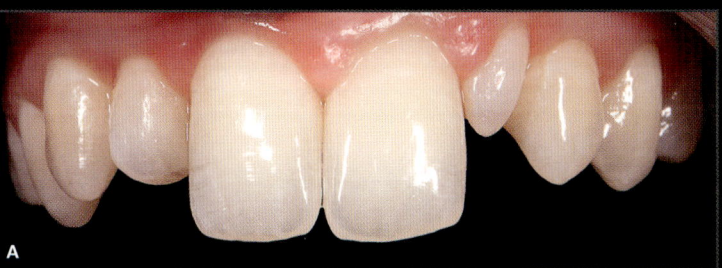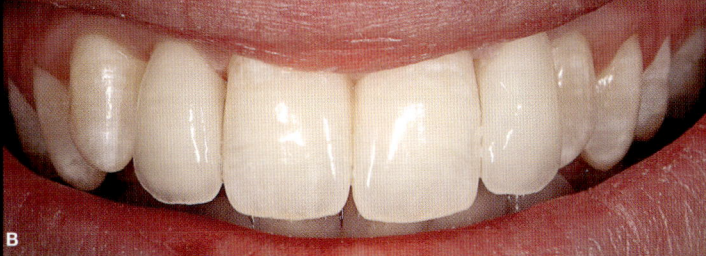

Figure 5.11 - A- Patient with peg-shaped lateral incisors. **B-** Ceramic veneers (e-max, Ivoclar) were made to restore the lateral incisors shape. Courtesy of Dr. Simon E Northeast.

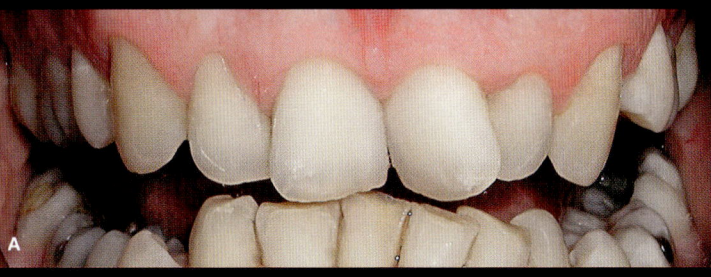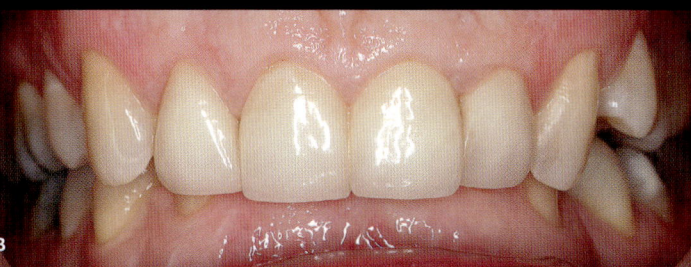

Figure 5.12 - A- Patient with crowding and twisted upper anterior teeth that were restored using ceramic veneers (Mirage, Chameloen Dental Products) (**B**). Courtesy of Dr. Simon E Northeast.

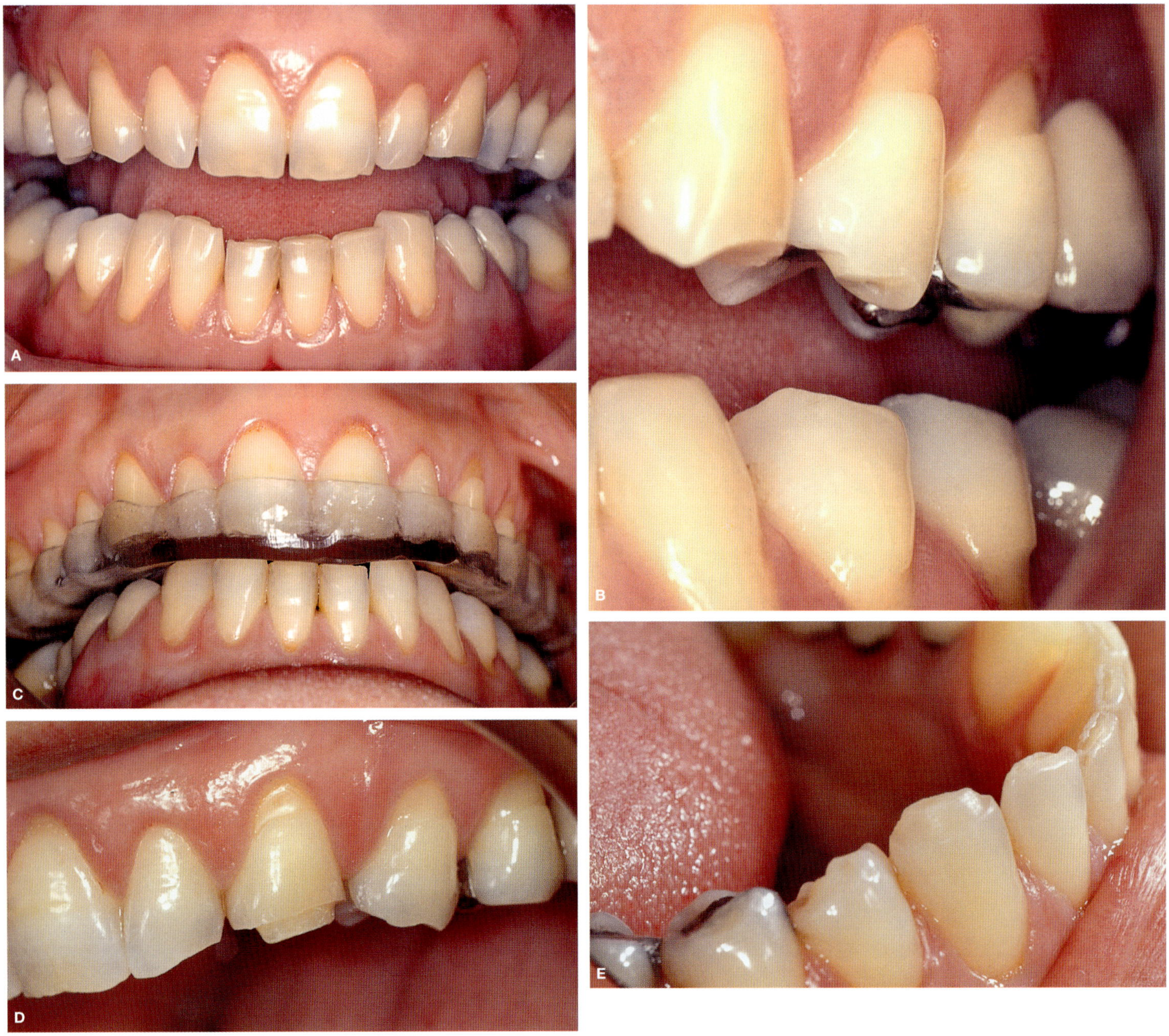

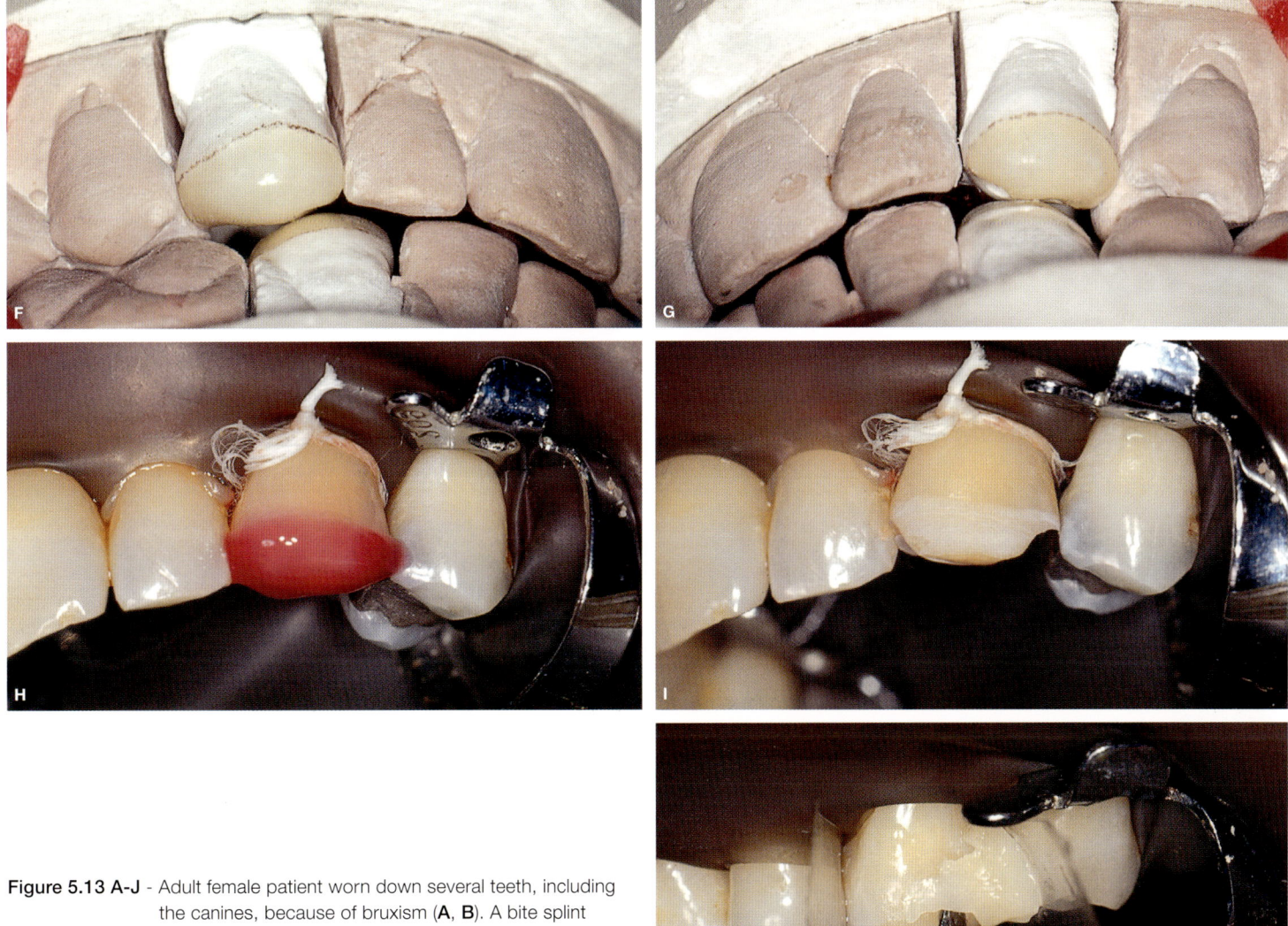

Figure 5.13 A-J - Adult female patient worn down several teeth, including the canines, because of bruxism (**A**, **B**). A bite splint was fabricated (**C**) and canine teeth were prepared (**D**, **E**) for ceramic restoration (**F**, **G**). The preparations included the canine contacts and guidance pathways. Teeth were isolated using rubber dam and preparations were etched with phosphoric acid (**H**, **I**). Ceramic veneers (Vitadur Alpha, Vita) were HF-etched, silane-treated and resin bonded in place. The excess dual-cured resin-based composite cement was removed with a scalpel blade and light cured (**J**).

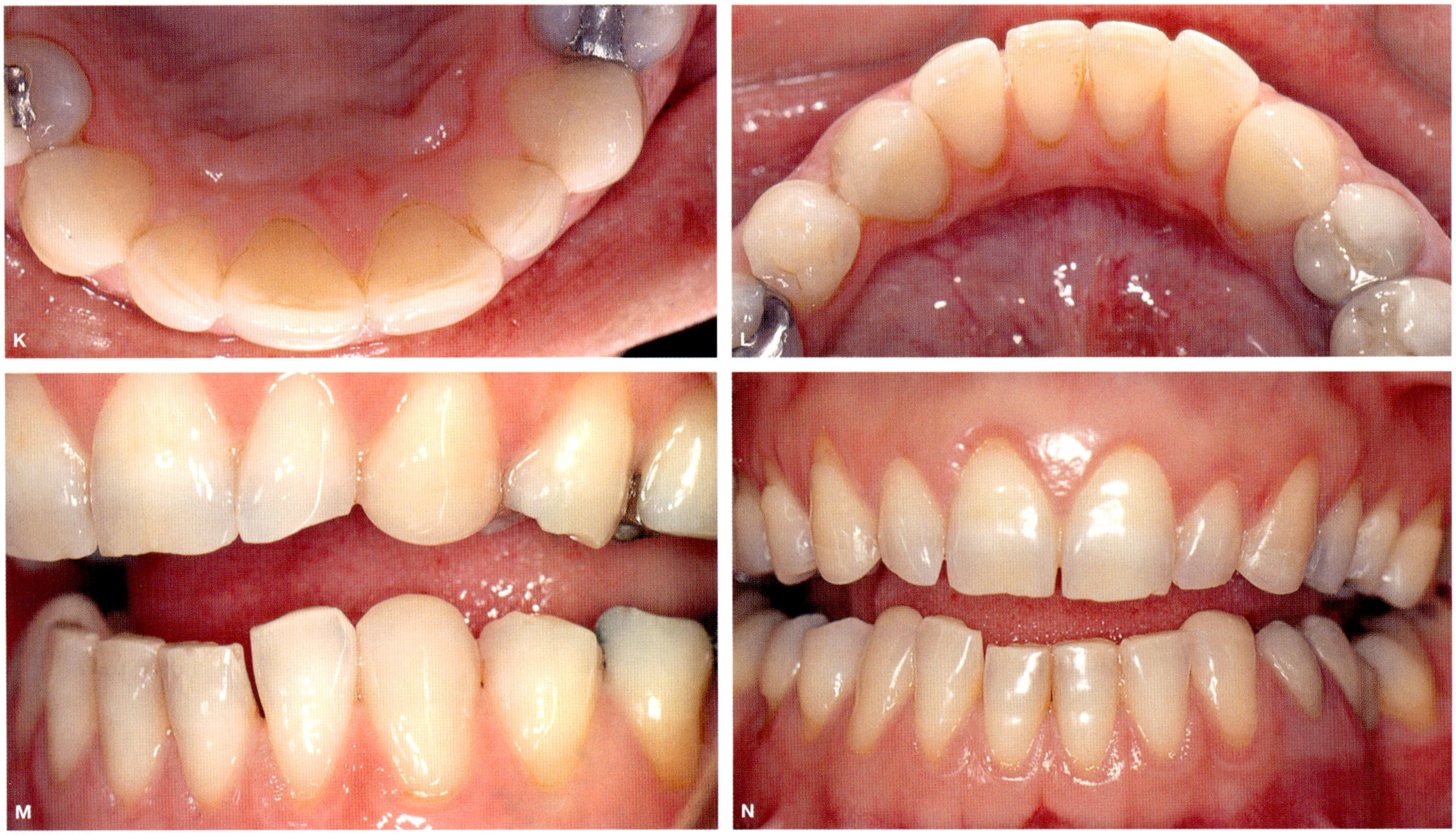

Figure 5.13 K-N - Tooth anatomy was restored and protected with a bite splint (**K, L, M, N**).

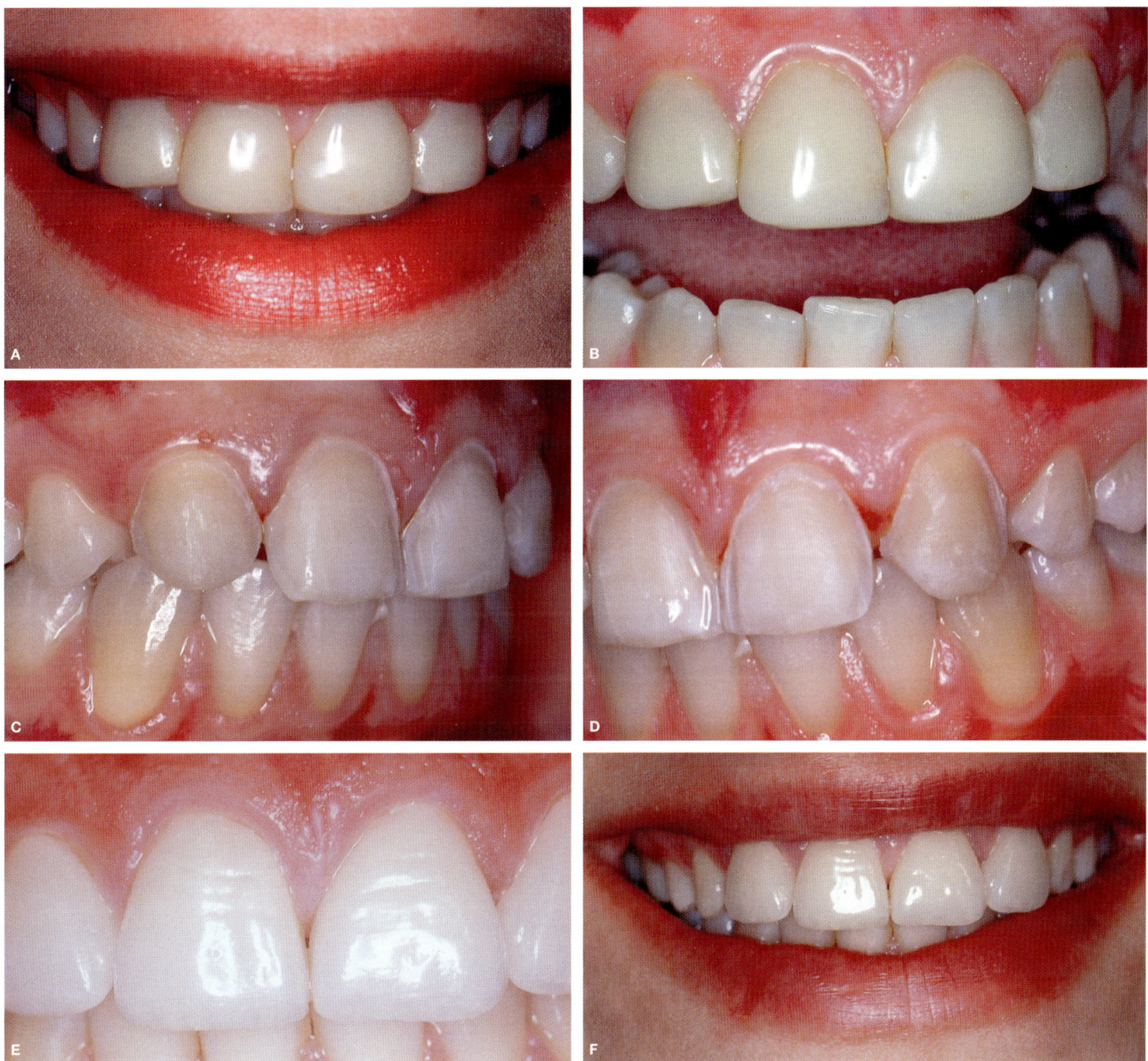

Figure 5.14 A-F - Adult female patient with missing upper lateral incisors and old resin-based composite veneers on the upper anterior teeth (**A**, **B**). The old composite veneers were removed and teeth were prepared for ceramic veneers (**C**, **D**). The restorations (VM7, Vita) were HF-etched, silane-coated and resin bonded in place (**E**, **F**).

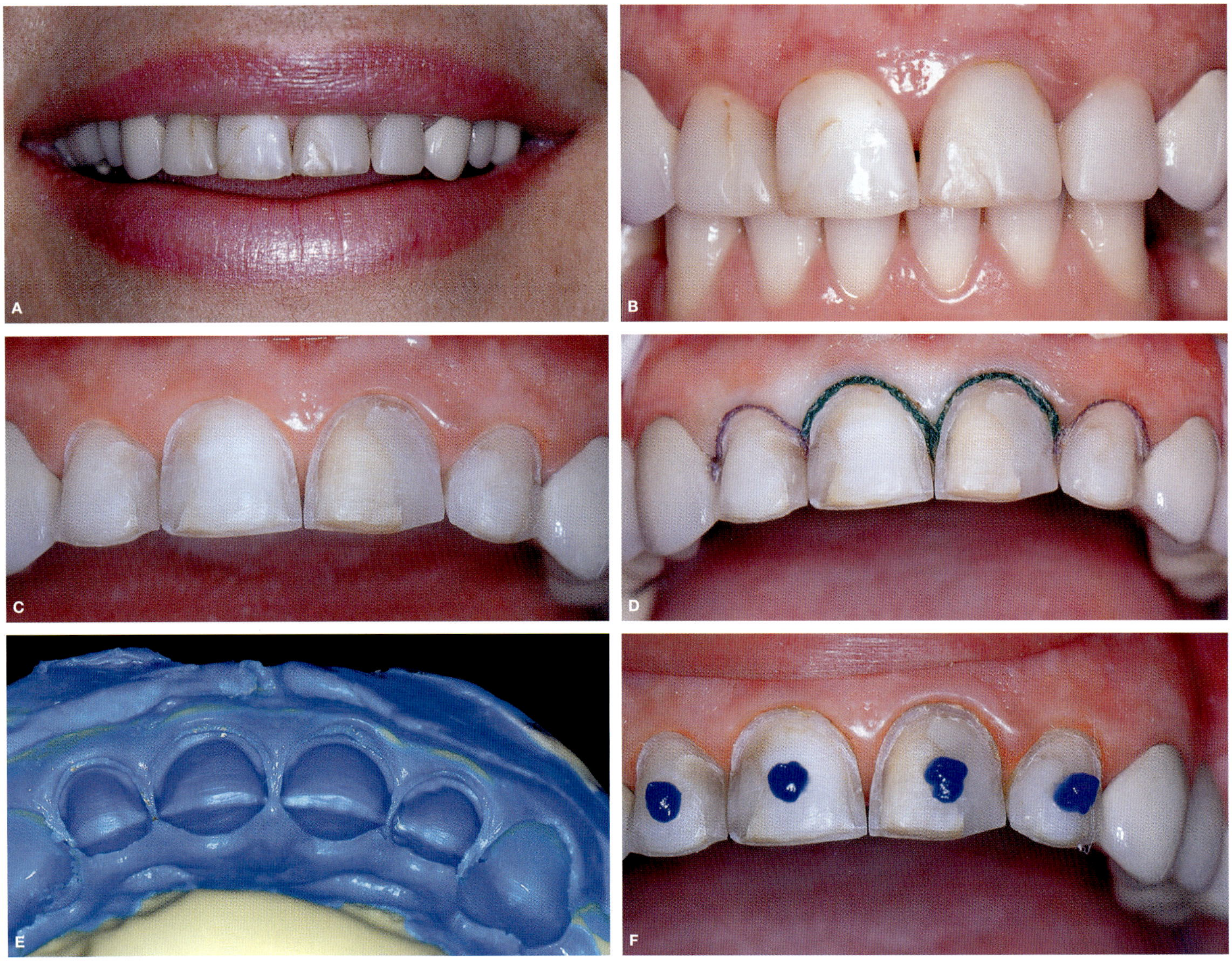

Figure 5.15 A-F - Adult female patient with several labial stained resin-based composite restorations (**A**, **B**). Teeth were prepared (**C**), gingival retraction cords (Tissue Management kit, Ultradent) were placed (**D**) and silicone impressions were made (**E**). A small, centered area of the preparations was acid etched with 30% phosphoric acid (spot etched) (**F**).

incisal edge are more difficult to orient correctly during bonding and it is very difficult to match the optical properties of the remaining incisal edge because of insufficient ceramic thickness.

In order to have adequate optical properties incorporated in the incisal third of the ceramic veneer restoration, the tooth preparation should allow for an incisal ceramic thickness of 1.5-2.0 mm (Fig. 5.19). The most popular veneer preparation flattens the incisal edge, leaving a butt finishing line configuration on the lingual surface (Figs. 5.18 C; 5.19). The overlap preparation (Fig. 5.18 D) places the finishing line on the lingual face, which is a high tensile stress area of the upper teeth and may weaken the restoration. However, these two preparations (Fig. 5.18 C and D) offer great orientation during bonding and allow for the best esthetic results. Yet, the incisal-to-gingival path of insertion resulted from the overlap preparation (Fig. 5.18 D) may produce an undesirable shade effect because of mixing tints within the cement during the bonding procedure. Tints or pigments can be added to the resin-based composite cement to either mask unpleasant tooth shades or characterize different areas of the tooth.

The preparation should preserve the interproximal contact if the dental enamel is sound and the contact area is in the correct place. In this case, the preparation should follow the papilla and extend slightly under the interproximal contact to ensure coverage of the tooth in this area. In cases of diastema, the preparation should pass the interproximal contact position, having always in mind the restoration path of insertion.

It is important to round all angles within the preparation, specially the facio-incisal angle, to prevent stress concentration that can lead to ceramic failures.

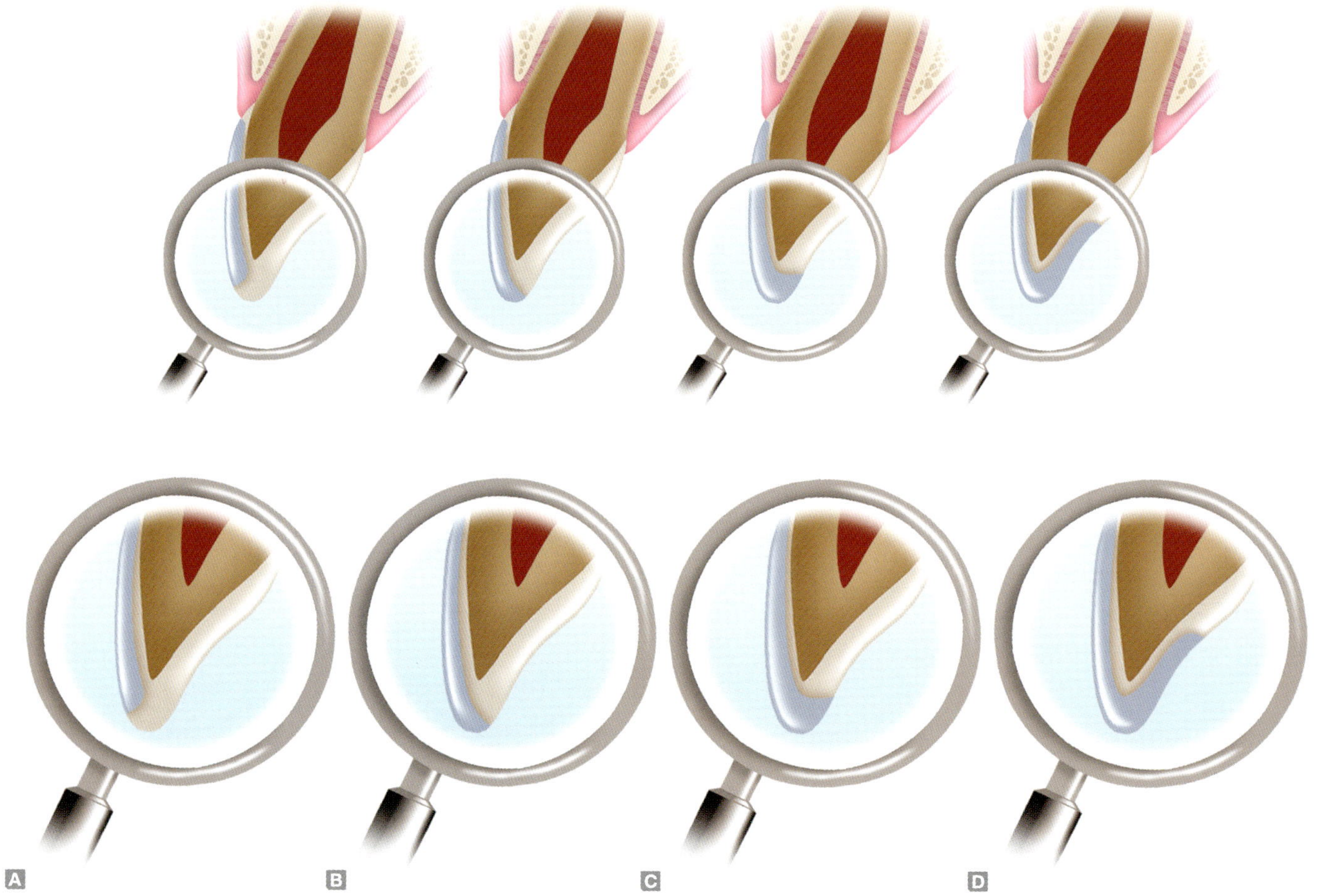

Figure 5.18 - Four types of ceramic veneer preparation. They basically differ on the incisal reduction. (**A**) Window preparation; (**B**) feather preparation; (**C**) flat, butt finishing line preparation; (**D**) overlap preparation.

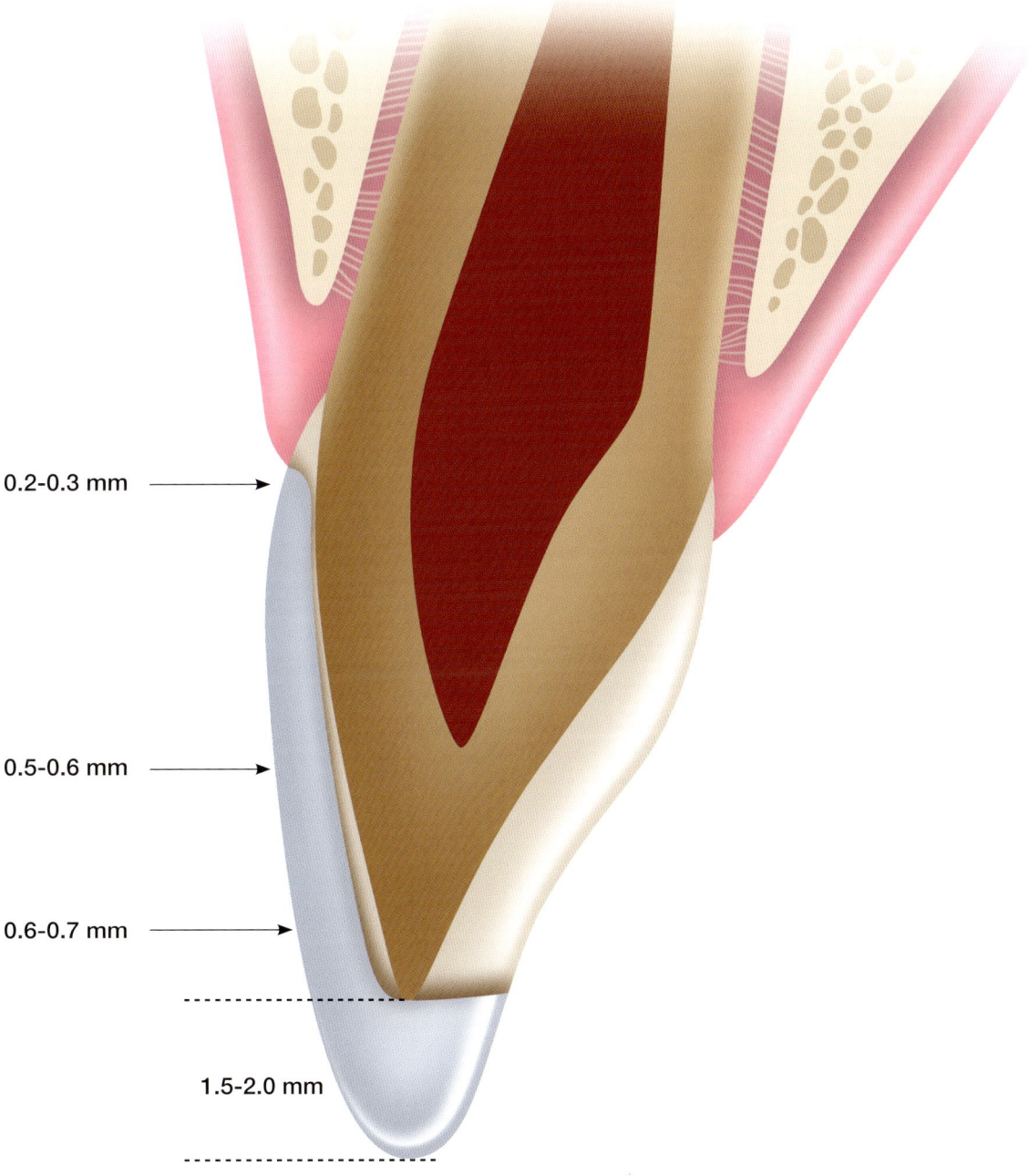

0.2-0.3 mm

0.5-0.6 mm

0.6-0.7 mm

1.5-2.0 mm

Figure 5.19 - Typical veneer preparation. The ideal enamel reduction for the ceramic veneer preparation per tooth third is as follows: gingival- 0.2-0.3 mm; middle- 0.5-0.7 mm; and incisal- 1.5-2.0 mm.

Some studies have suggested an immediate dentin sealing (IDS) after tooth preparation. A literature review suggested the need for a revision in the dentin bonding procedure, recommending an immediate application and polymerization of a dentin bonding agent to the freshly cut dentin, before taking impression (Magne, 2005). This procedure appears to achieve improved bond strength, fewer gap formations, decreased bacterial leakage, and reduced dentin sensitivity. A three-step total-etch or a 2-step self-etching dentin bonding agent with a filled adhesive resin is recommended for this specific purpose. This approach to adhesion also has a positive influence on tooth structure preservation, patient comfort, and long-term survival of indirect bonded restorations (Magne *et al.*, 2007).

After tooth preparation, retraction cord is placed to expose gingival margins and final impressions are made using accurate impression materials (addition silicone or vinyl polysiloxane, and polyether) (Fig. 5.15 D and E). Provisional restorations are usually made with resin-based composites using clear plastic or silicone matrix, or even directly built on the tooth preparation. It is important that the provisional restorations are very well polished to avoid any excess dental plaque build-up and gingival irritation.

Ceramic veneers are usually fabricated using feldspathic or leucite-reinforced ceramics, which are acid-sensitive ceramics and offer the best optical properties. Once the ceramic veneers are fabricated and received by the dentist, the clinical procedures for bonding the restorations are as follow (Table 5.2):

Table 5.2 - Clinical procedures for resin bonding acid-sensitive ceramic restorations.

1- Investigate the ceramic restorations for any defect and check them for fit on the master cast (dies).

2- Carefully remove the provisional restorations and any remaining resinous material from the bonding area.

3- Clean the tooth preparation with oil-free pumice paste.

4- Try in the restorations individually, then all together. Interproximal contact areas may be adjusted with a microfine diamond bur or disk.

5- If the laboratory did not acid etch the bonding surface of the restorations, the dentist has to do it using a buffered hydrofluoric acid (HF) gel according to the manufacturer's instructions. Hold the ceramic restorations with plastic tweezers to avoid any other unwanted HF reaction. After acid etching the ceramic surface, wash it with oil-free water spray for 20 s and dry it completely observing the opaque appearance resultant from acid etching.

6- Select the shade of resin-based composite cement or water-soluble try-in paste, place on the treated ceramic surface and try in the restoration. If try-in paste is used, wash the restoration with water and dry it before the next bonding step. If a resin-based cement is used, remove it from the restoration with acetone in a sonic bath for 5 min. To prevent fracture of ceramic margins during the sonic bath, place the restoration on a gauze pad in a glass beaker with acetone. The bulk of the resin composite is removed with a brush during the sonic bath. The ceramic restoration has to be transfer to another beaker with clean acetone for final cleaning (Della Bona and Barghi, 1993). This try-in/cleaning step is repeated until selection of the correct shade is completed.

7- Apply silane coupling agent to the etched ceramic surface and allow it to dry for 5 min, then completely dry the surface using oil-free air.

8- Clean the tooth preparation with oil-free pumice paste. In case of restoring both central incisors, the bonding procedure has to start with them.

9- Place clear plastic matrix or dead-soft metal matrix on the proximal aspects of the preparation. In case of veneering both central incisors, place the matrix on distal aspects of the preparations.

10- Etch the preparation(s) with 30-40% phosphoric acid for 20 s, wash and blot out the excess water. Remove the matrix(es).

11- Apply an appropriate adhesive system on the treated ceramic surface and on tooth preparation, following the manufacturer's instructions for each substrate.

12- Place a dental floss on the proximal surfaces of the preparation(s) and leave it on the papilla. In case of veneering both central incisors, place the dental floss on midline papilla.

13- Turn off the operatory light, use a handle (Pic-n-stic, Pulpdent) to hold the restoration (mainly for veneers and onlays/inlays) and place the selected shade of the resin-based composite cement on the treated ceramic surface.

14- Gently place the restoration onto preparation and tease into place. Visually inspect the restoration to ensure it is in the correct place. In case of restoring multiple teeth, including both central incisors, start the cementation procedure from them making sure that the mesial surfaces are in contact. Excess cement should come out from all margins.

15- Light-cure the restoration(s) for 5-10 s and remove the excess resin cement with a scalpel blade and using the dental floss previously placed on the papilla. Both ends of the dental floss should be brought together; holding both ends, pull the floss lingually.

16- Complete light-curing of the resin cement for 40 s from each tooth face. In case of cementing ceramic veneers start light-curing from the lingual surface.

17- Be sure to remove all excess resin cement from the proximal aspects of the restorations.

18- Repeat all the steps for each restoration being placed.

19- In case of veneers, remove excess resin cement from lingual surfaces using an egg- or flame-shaped, 12-fluted carbide bur and polishing points or disks.

20- If gingival margins require any finishing and polishing, carefully use finishing diamond or 12-fluted carbide burs.

21- Finish the proximal areas using finishing and polishing strips.

22- Reshape incisal edges and embrasures with finishing diamond burs and appropriate abrasive points.

23- Final polish with silicone points and diamond polishing paste on a wet felt wheel and prophylaxis cup.

24- Check for occlusal contacts, carefully eliminating the occlusal interferences created by the restorative treatment.

25- Patient has to return in one week for any minor reshaping and polishing. A healthy gingiva should be present, otherwise inspect for any overcontoured and/or rough margin.

26- Recall the patient every 6 months.

The bonding mechanisms to all substrates are explained in chapter 4 and summarized on Fig. 4.1. The materials used to bond a ceramic restoration (veneer) to a prepared tooth surface are schematically presented in Fig. 5.20 and illustrated clinically in several Figures throughout this chapter.

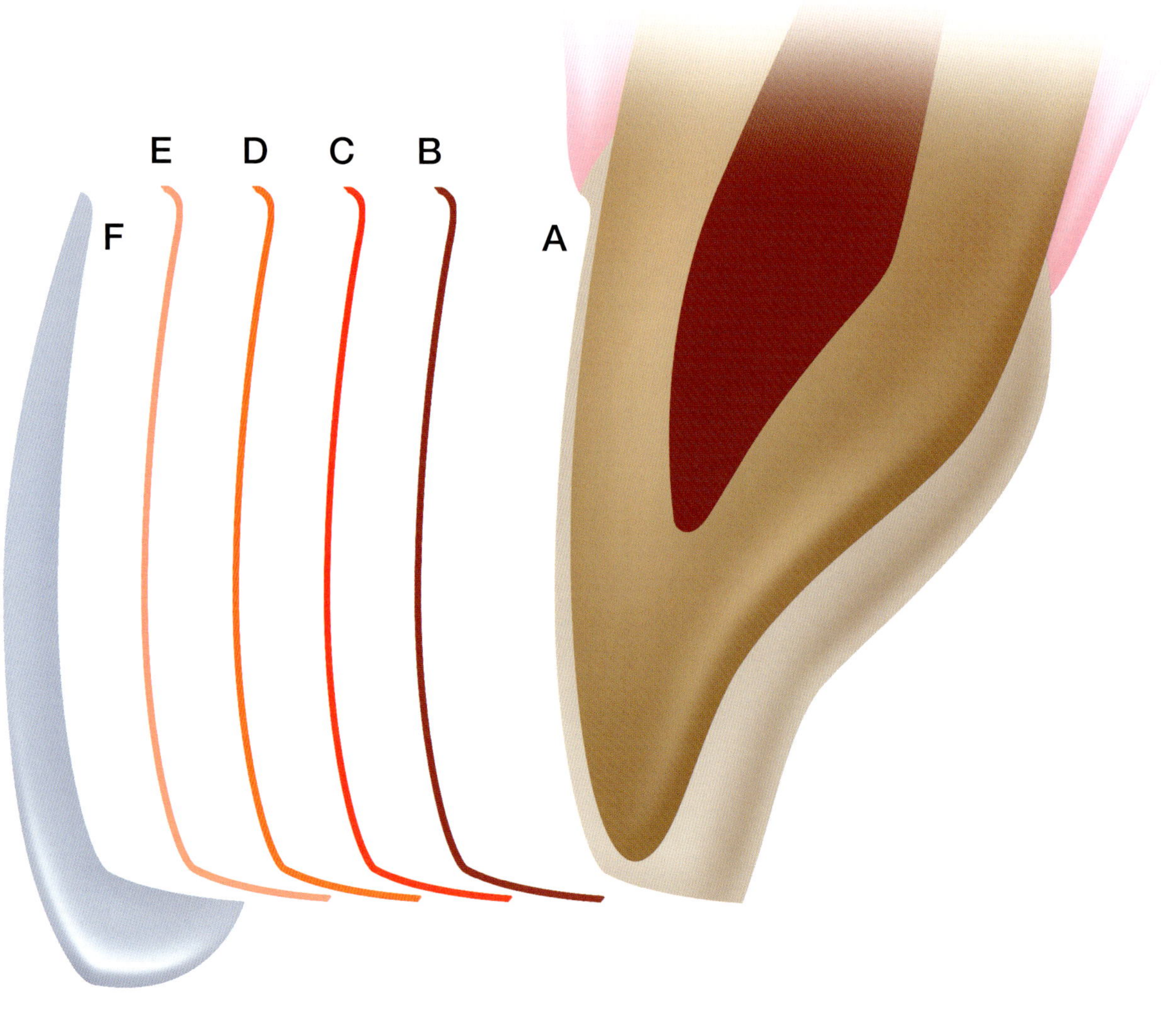

Figure 5.20 - Typical surface treatment for ceramic veneer bonded to tooth enamel: **A**- Etched enamel; **B**- Adhesive resin; **C**- Resin-based composite cement; **D**- Adhesive resin; **E**- Silane coupling agent; **F**- Etched ceramic veneer.

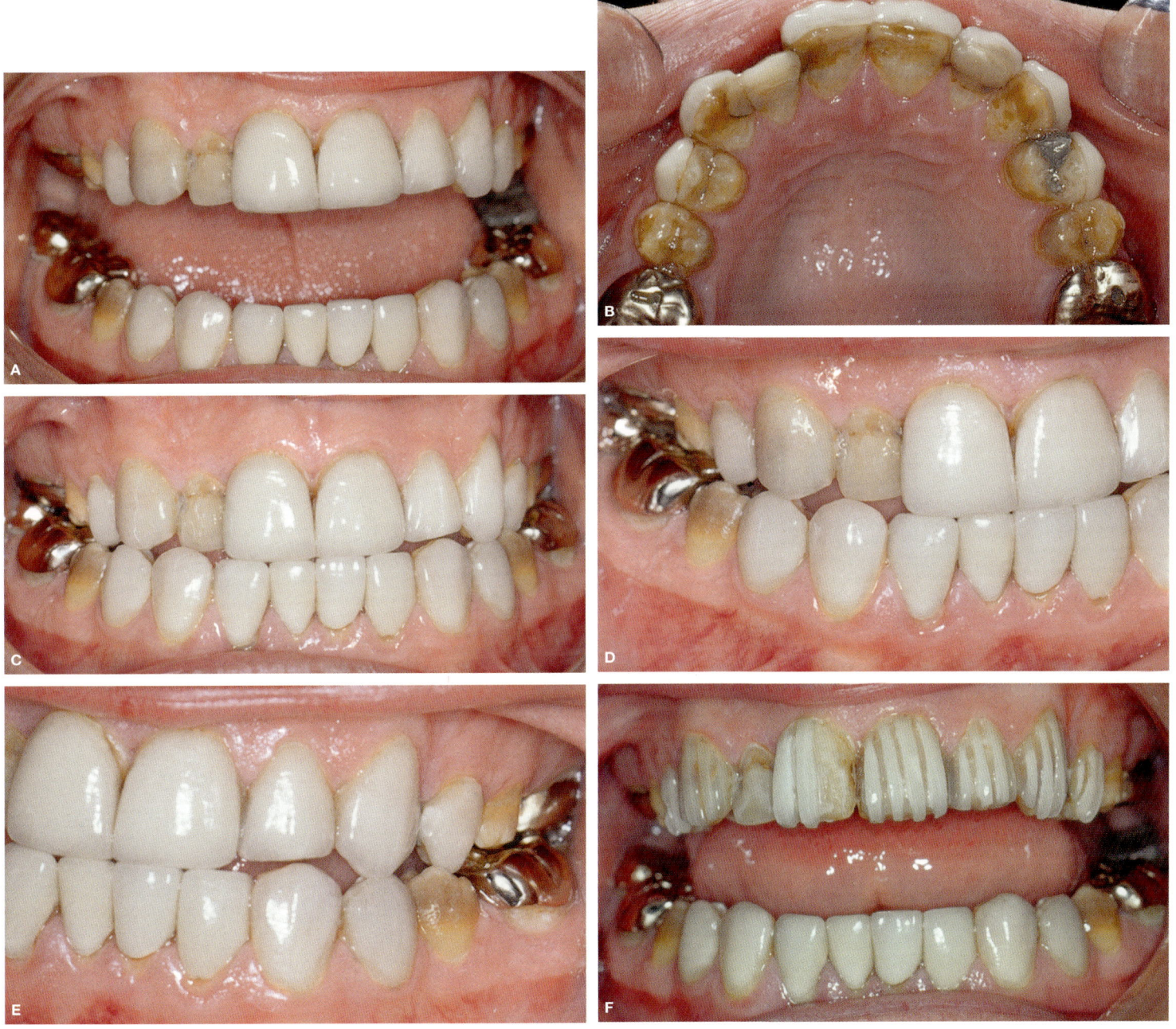

169

Figure 5.21 A-F - Male patient with amelogenesis imperfecta (severe enamel hypoplasia) that was submitted to a restorative treatment using ceramic veneers (**A**, **B**). The patient chief complaint was the missing veneer on the upper lateral incisor (12), probably due to traumatic edge-to-edge occlusion between teeth 43 and 12 and microleakage (**C**, **D**, **E**). As microleakage was present in several sites of all upper ceramic veneers, all upper restorations were replaced. During the removal of the veneers, many ceramic pieces spontaneously debonded from tooth surface (**F**), which is evidence of poor bonding.

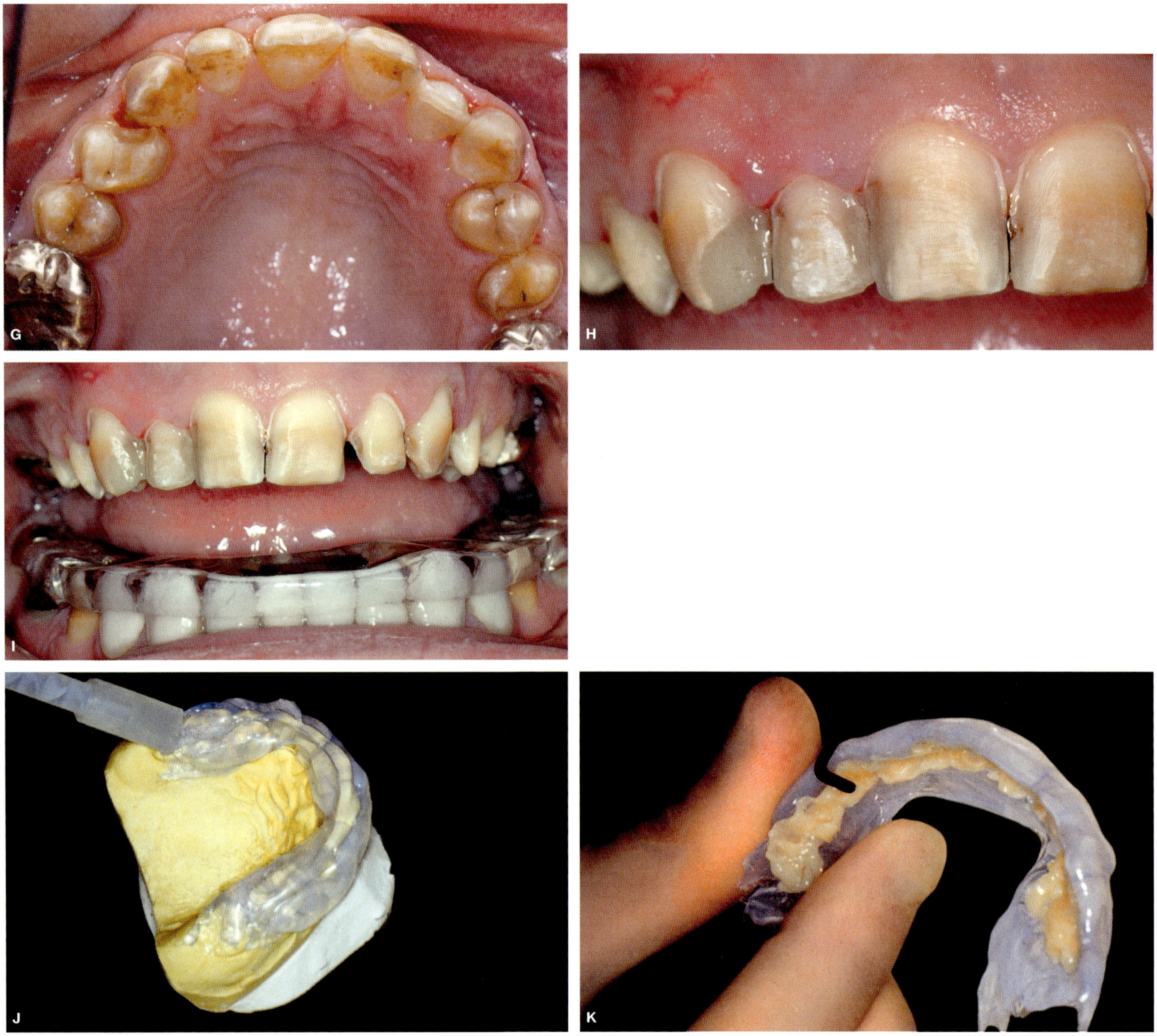

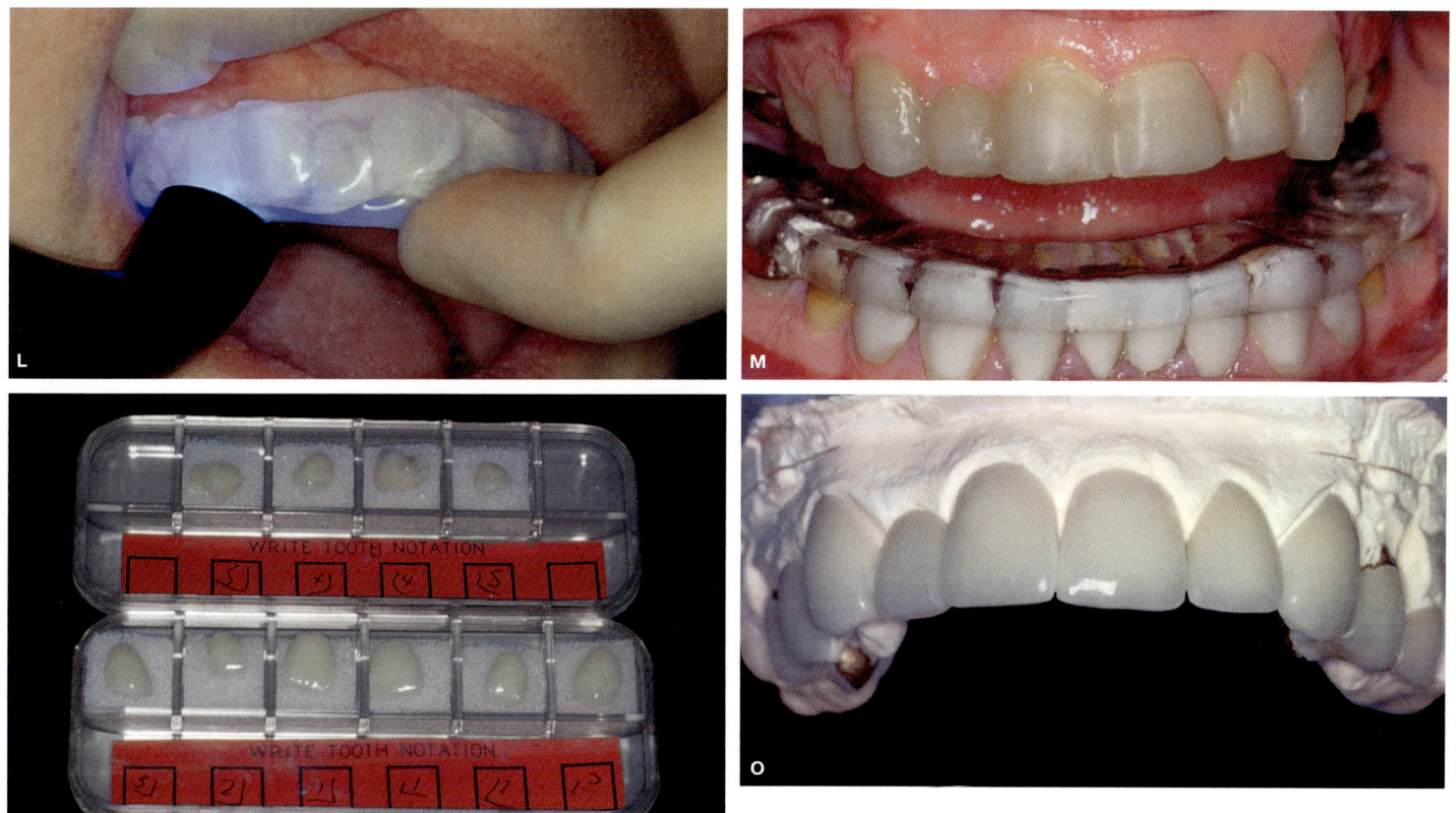

Figure 5.21 G-O - Old leaked resin-based composite restorations were substituted and teeth were re-prepared for ceramic veneers (**G**, **H**, **I**). A bite splint was fabricated during the treatment (**I**). A light-activated silicone material was used to fabricate a transparent matrix (**J**) that was used to accommodate the light-cured resin-based composite (**K**) for the provisional restorations (**L**, **M**). Ceramic veneers were made (IPS Empress, Ivoclar) and tried on the master cast (**N**, **O**).

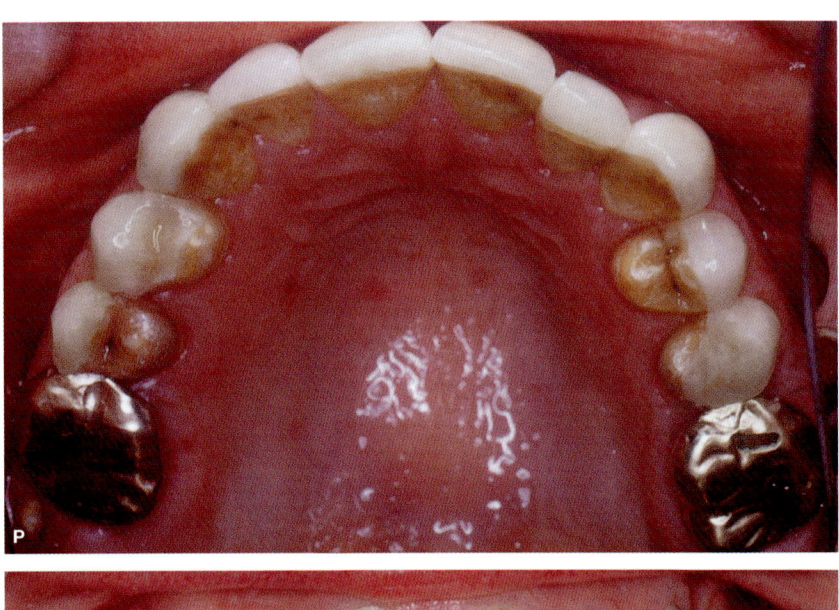

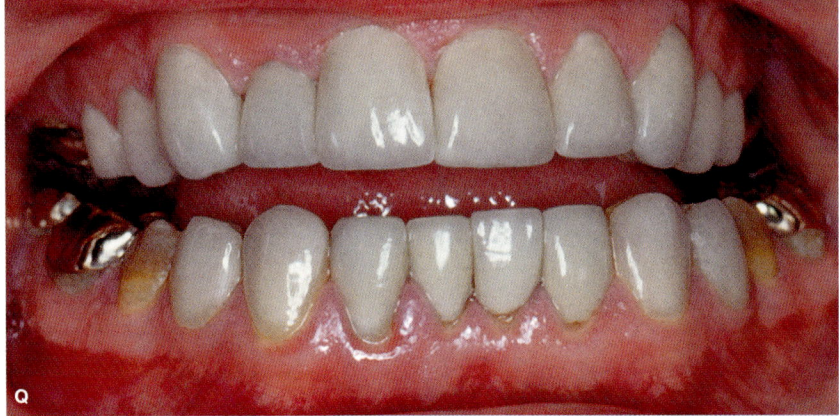

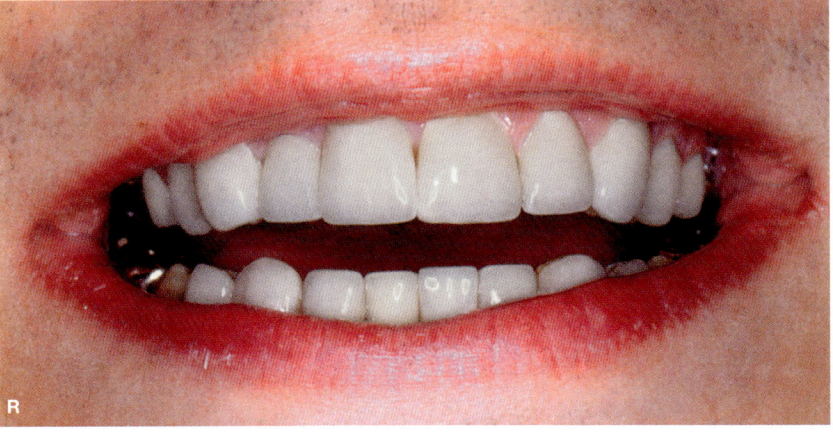

Figure 5.21 P-R - The restorations were cemented in place using an adhesive system (Scotchbond multipurpose plus, 3M) and a resin-based composite cement (RelyX ARC, 3M ESPE) (**P**, **Q**, **R**).

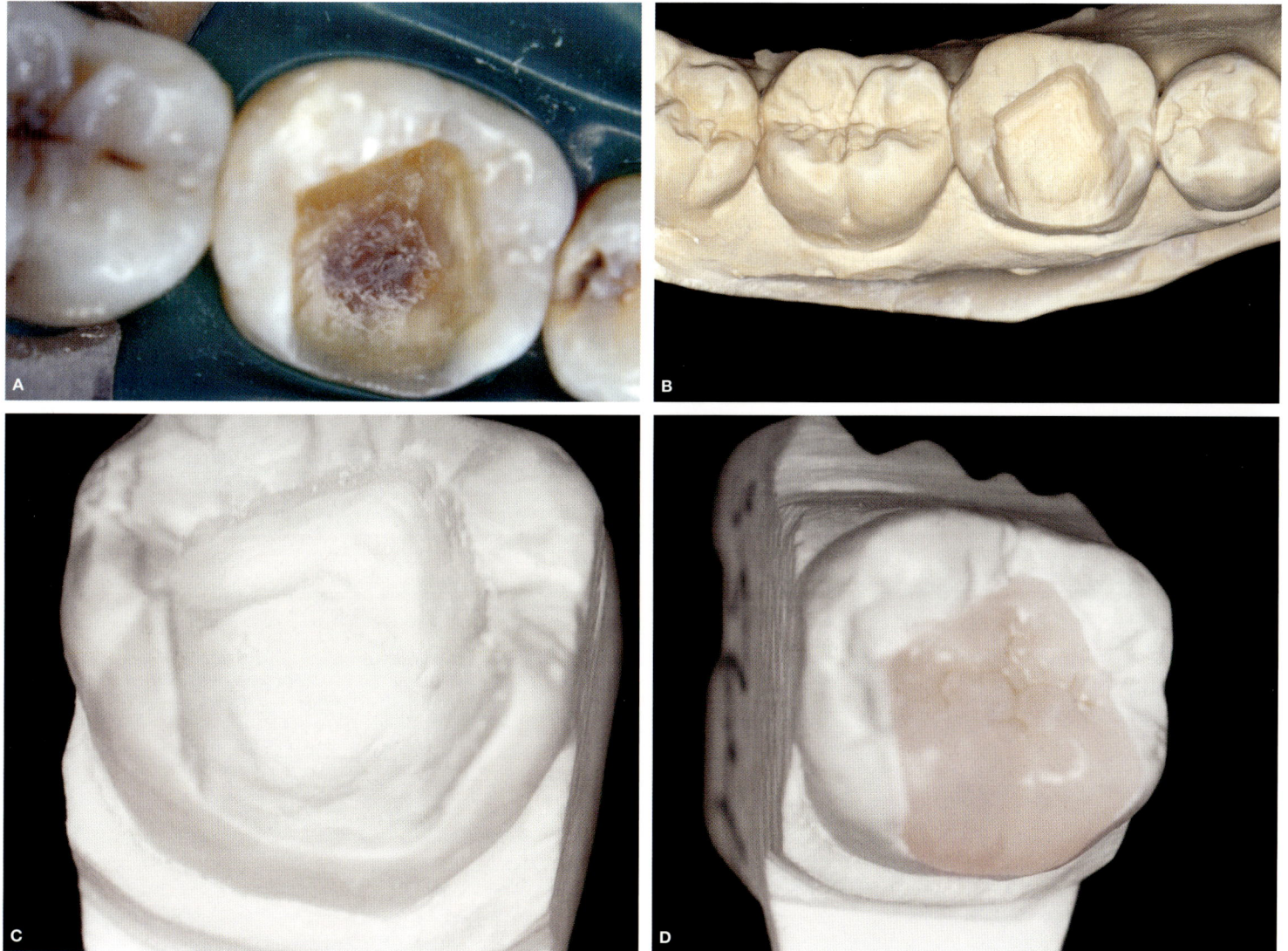

Figure 5.23 A-D - Patient had a fractured buccal surface due to a carious process in the lower first molar (46). Tooth was prepared for all-ceramic restoration (**A**), silicone impressions were taken and stone master casts were made (**B**). An investment die was obtained (**C**) and a ceramic restoration (Vitadur Alpha, Vita) was fabricated (**D**).

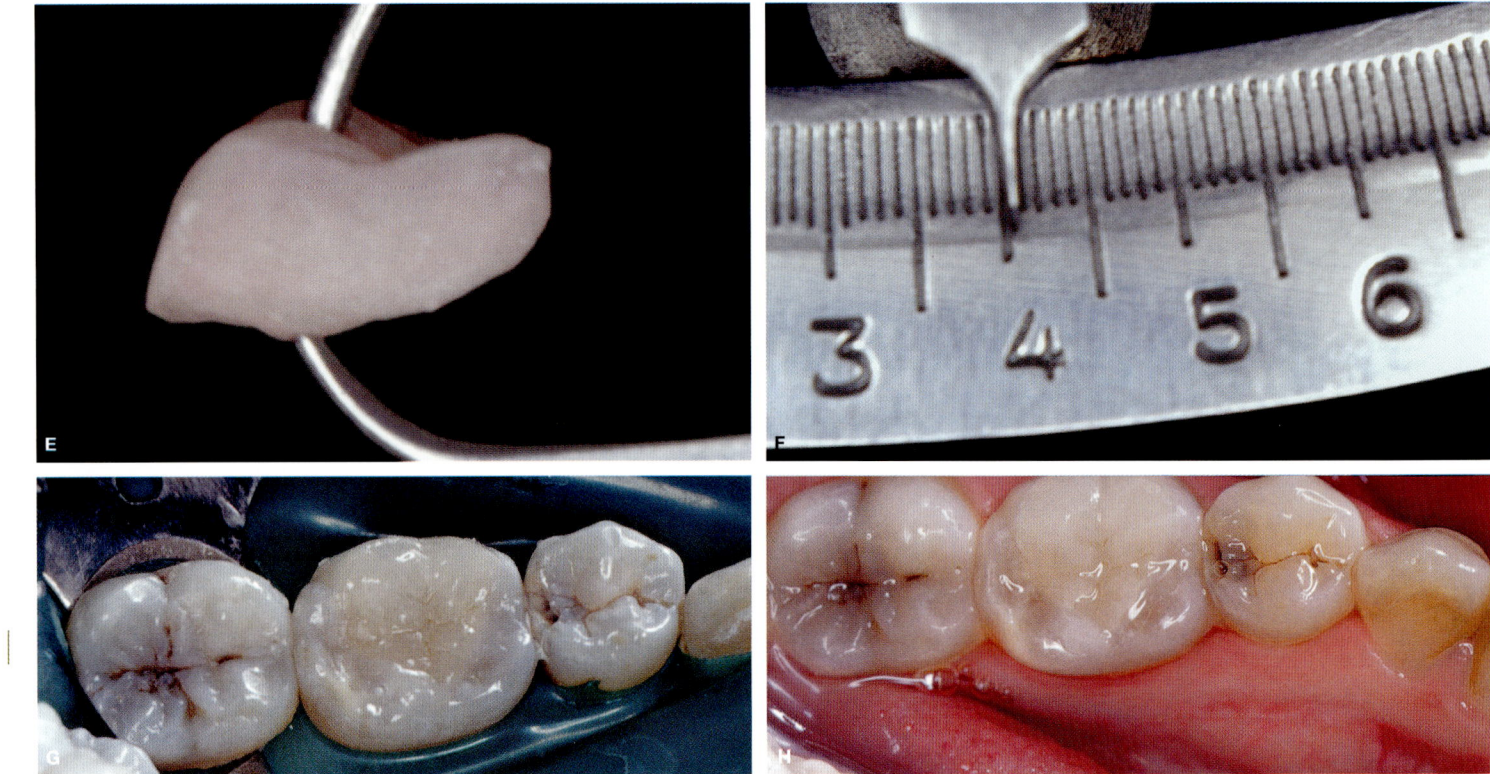

Figure 5.23 E-H - Note that the restoration is 4 mm-thick (**E**, **F**) and should be, preferably, cemented with a chemically-cured resin composite cement using rubber dam isolation (**G**), following the adhesive mechanisms appropriated for resin bonding to dentin, enamel and ceramic (Fig. 4.1) and clinically described in Table 5.2. A good esthetic blend between the tooth and the ceramic restoration was achieved on the occlusal surface (**H**). Direct resin-based composite restorations were lately done on teeth 45 and 47.

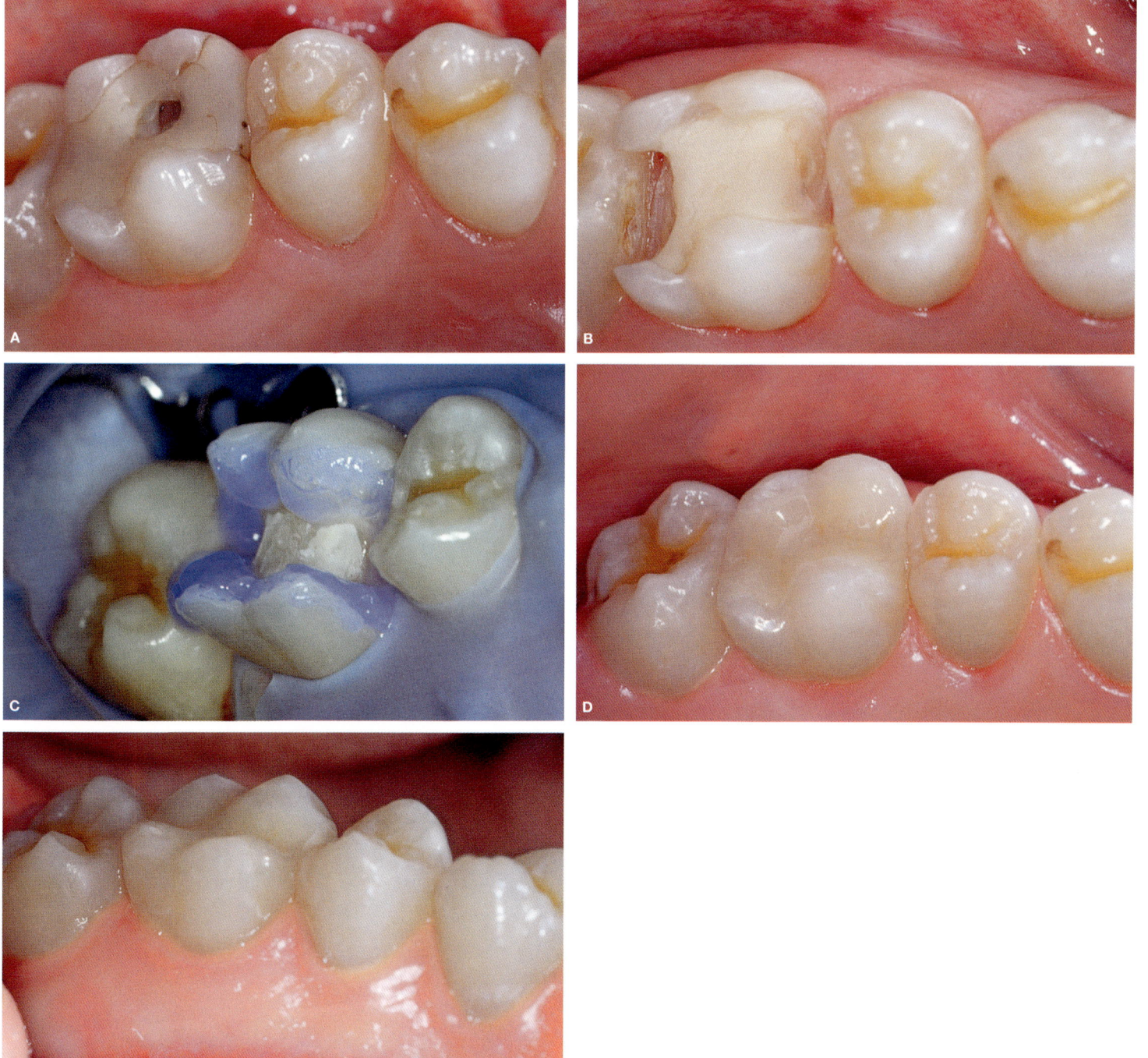

181

Figure 5.24 A-E - Occlusal fracture on class 2 resin-based composite restoration (tooth 26) probably caused by inadequate preparation depth (shallow preparation) combined with an excess occlusal load (**A**). A glass-ionomer cement was used to block-out the preparation undercuts (**B**). Tooth was isolated with rubber dam and acid etched with phosphoric acid (**C**). A ceramic restoration (IPS Empress 2, Ivoclar) was resin bonded to the tooth using HF-etching, silane coupling agent, an adhesive system and a resin-based composite cement (Fig. 4.1; Table 5.2) (**D**, **E**).

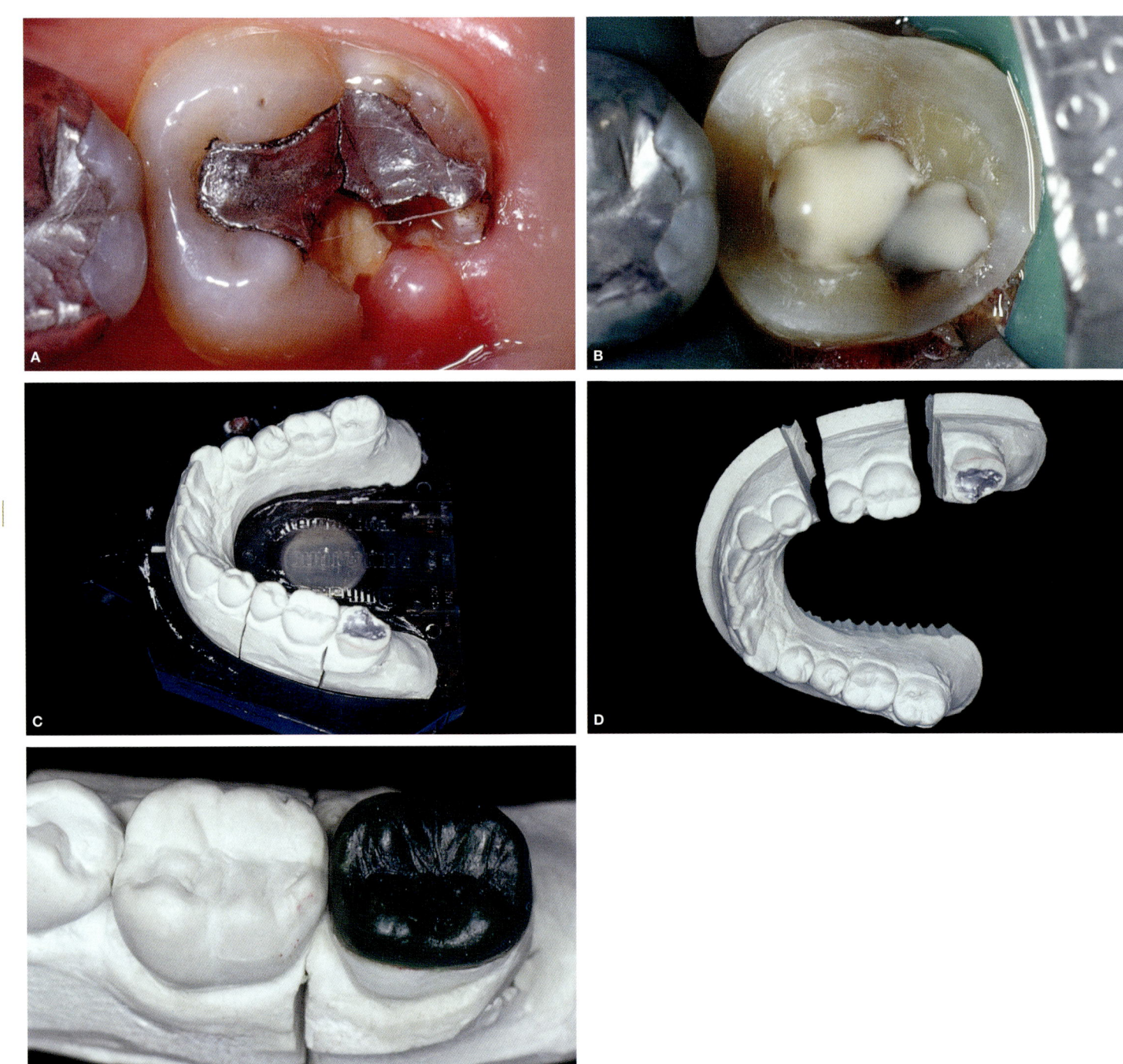

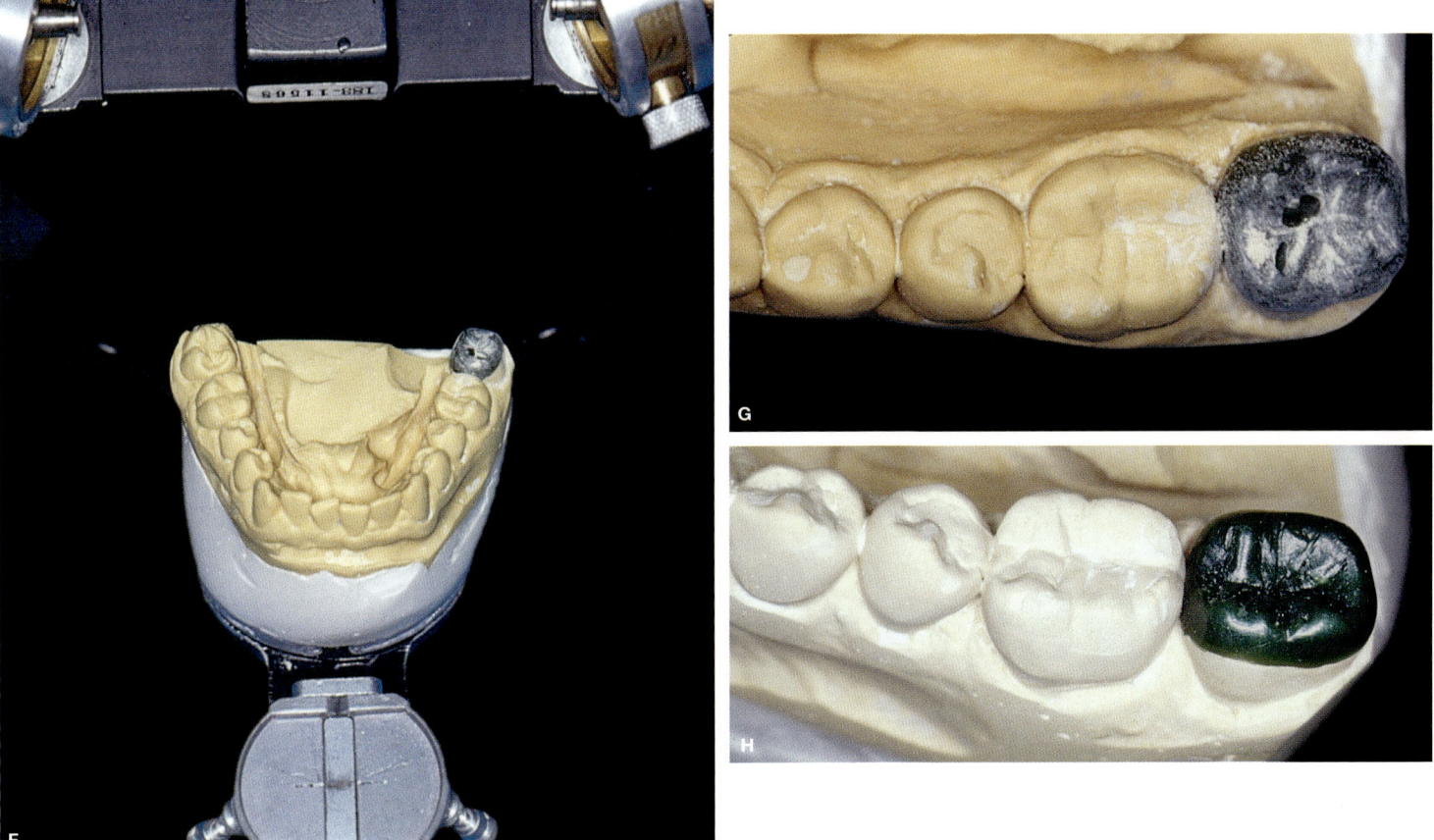

Figure 5.25 A-H - Patient fractured the distal-lingual surface of the lower second molar (37) due to a carious process (**A**). After the removal of all carious tissues, the deepest area of the onlay preparation was protected with a glass-ionomer-based liner (**B**). Silicone impressions were taken, stone casts were made and mounted in articulator to wax-up the pattern (**C-H**).

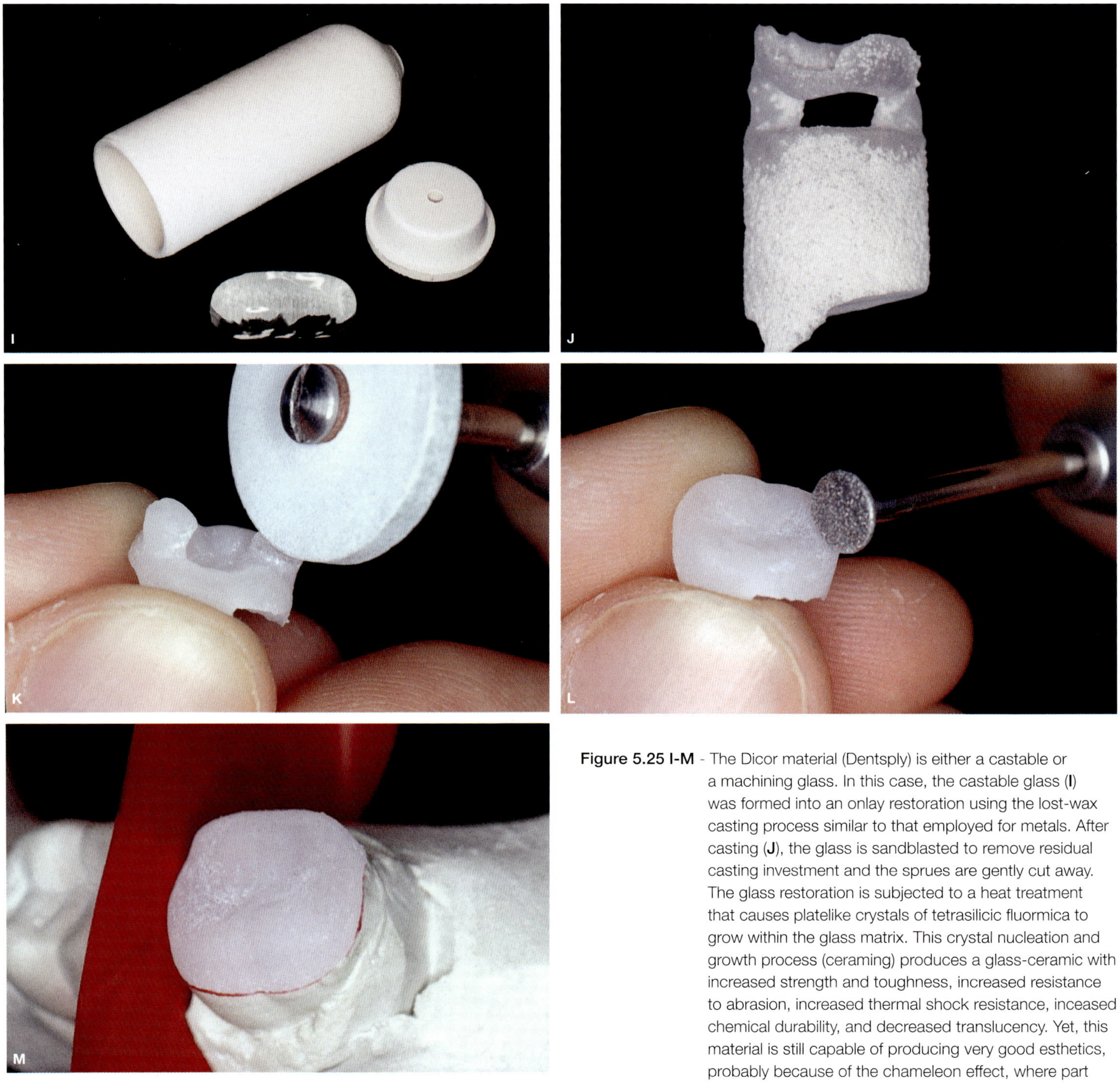

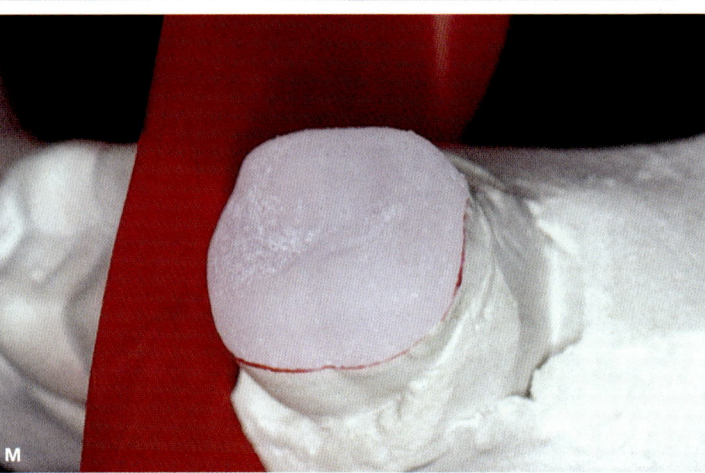

Figure 5.25 I-M - The Dicor material (Dentsply) is either a castable or a machining glass. In this case, the castable glass (**I**) was formed into an onlay restoration using the lost-wax casting process similar to that employed for metals. After casting (**J**), the glass is sandblasted to remove residual casting investment and the sprues are gently cut away. The glass restoration is subjected to a heat treatment that causes platelike crystals of tetrasilicic fluormica to grow within the glass matrix. This crystal nucleation and growth process (ceraming) produces a glass-ceramic with increased strength and toughness, increased resistance to abrasion, increased thermal shock resistance, inceased chemical durability, and decreased translucency. Yet, this material is still capable of producing very good esthetics, probably because of the chameleon effect, where part of the color of the restoration is picked up from the remaining tooth structure and adjacent teeth. Finally, the remaining portion of the sprues were gently removed from the glass-ceramic restoration (**K**, **L**) that was fit to the master cast (**M**).

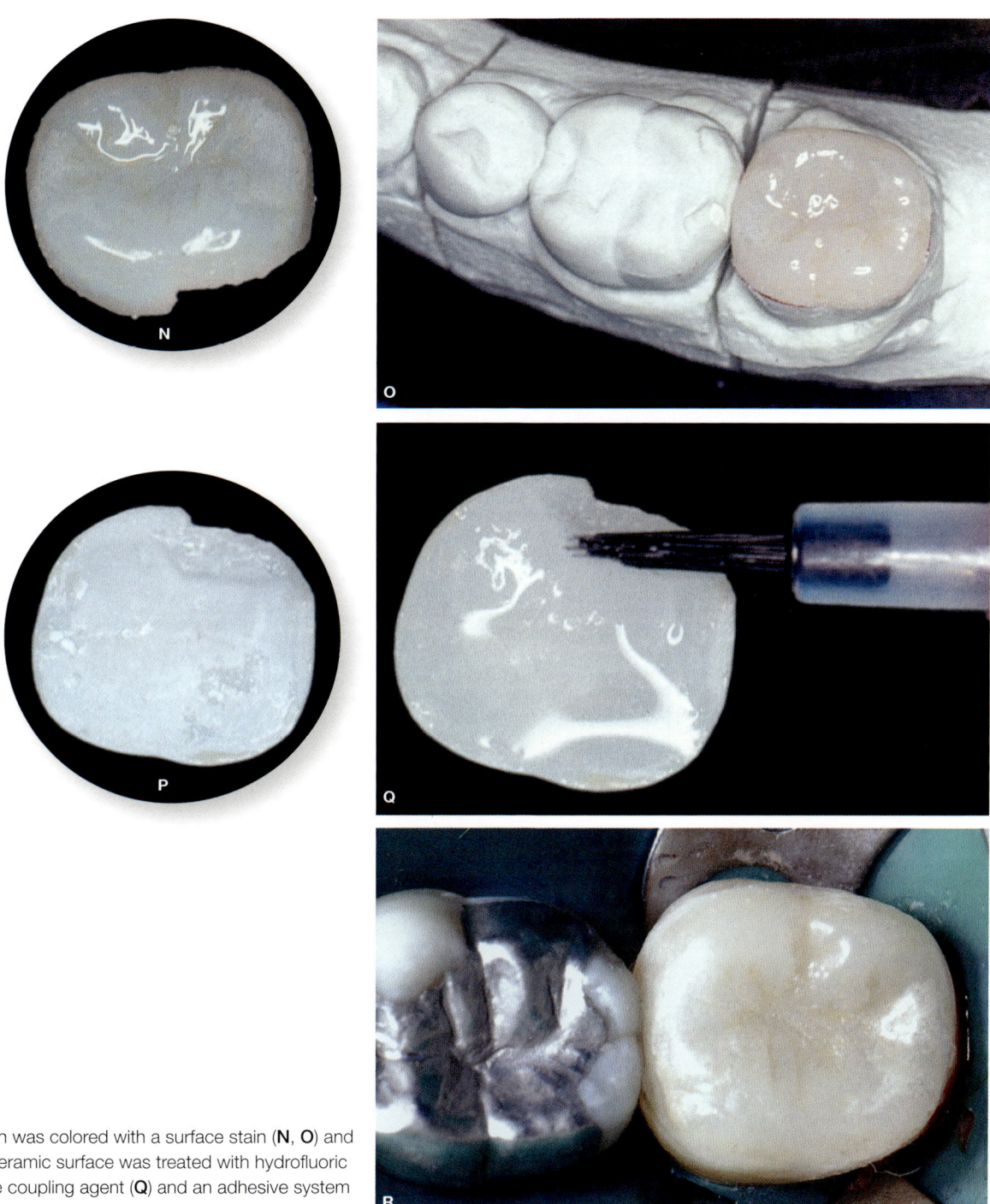

Figure 5.25 N-R - The restoration was colored with a surface stain (**N**, **O**) and the bonding ceramic surface was treated with hydrofluoric acid (**P**), silane coupling agent (**Q**) and an adhesive system before resin cement to tooth (**R**).

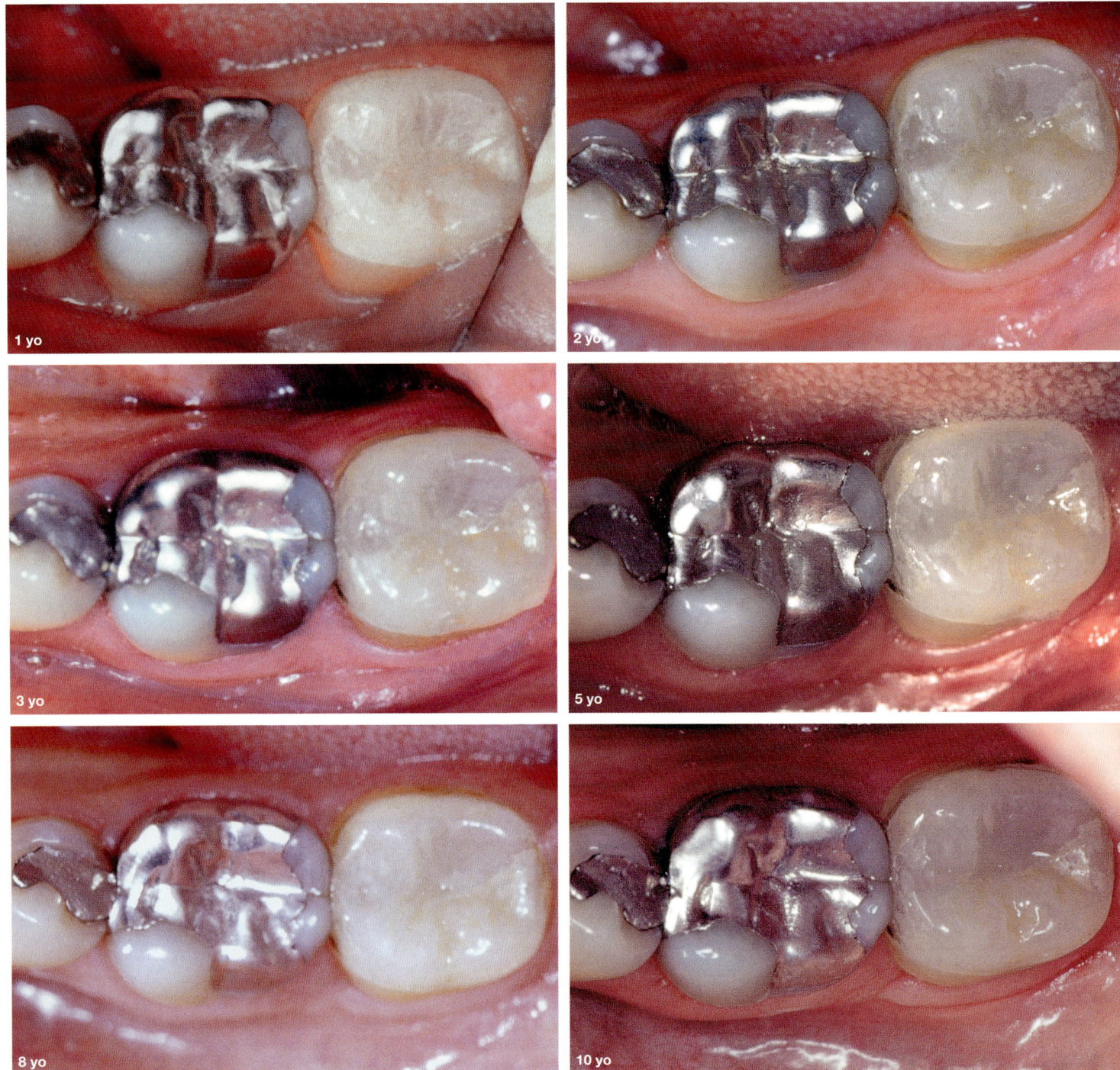

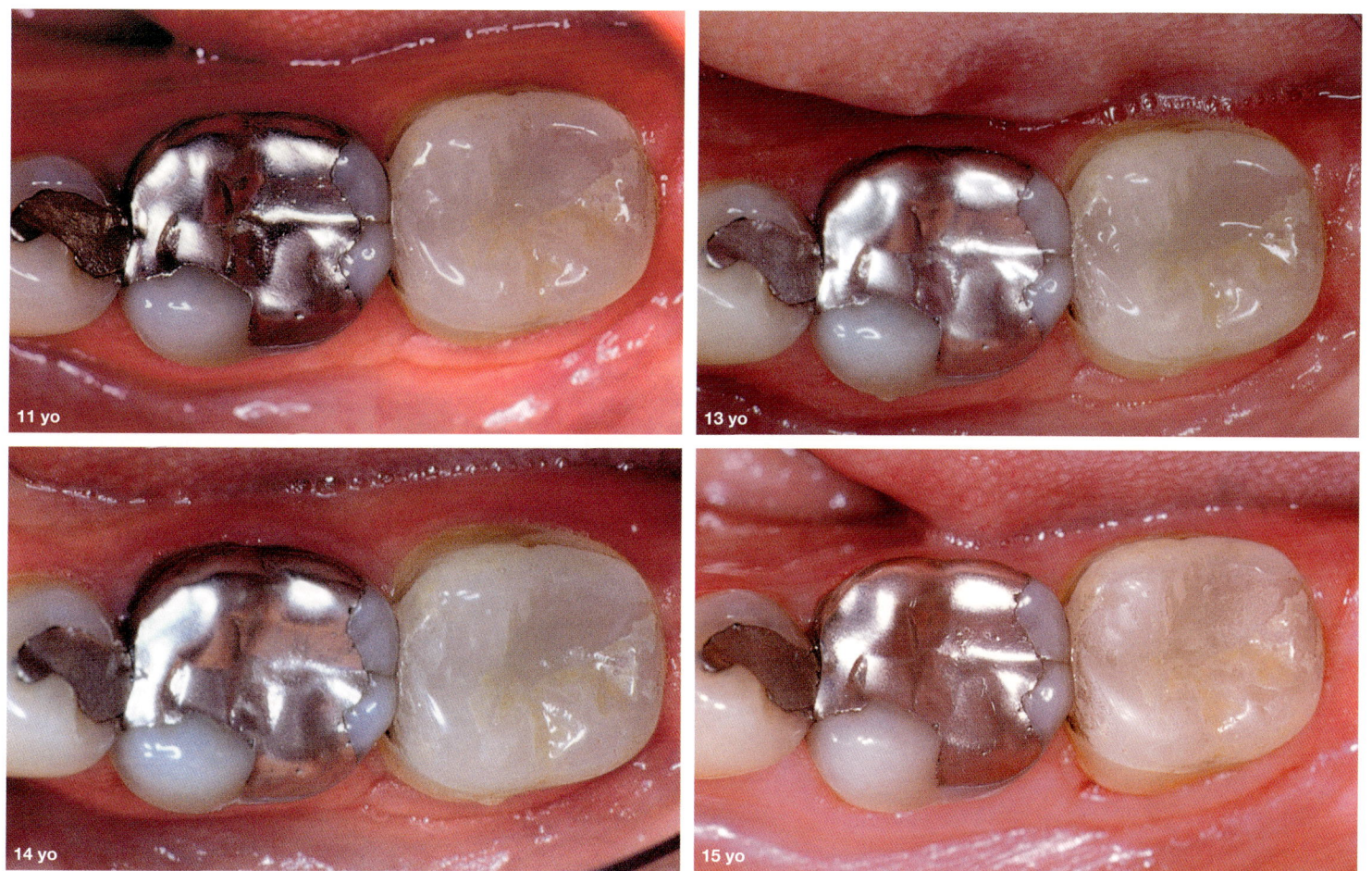

Figure 5.25 - Note that the large amalgam restoration on tooth 36 was also made at the same time. In addition, there was a 10-year old amalgam restoration on tooth 35. The remaining images are follow-up pictures after 1, 2, 3, 5, 8, 10, 11, 13, 14, and 15 years (yo) from the restorative procedure.

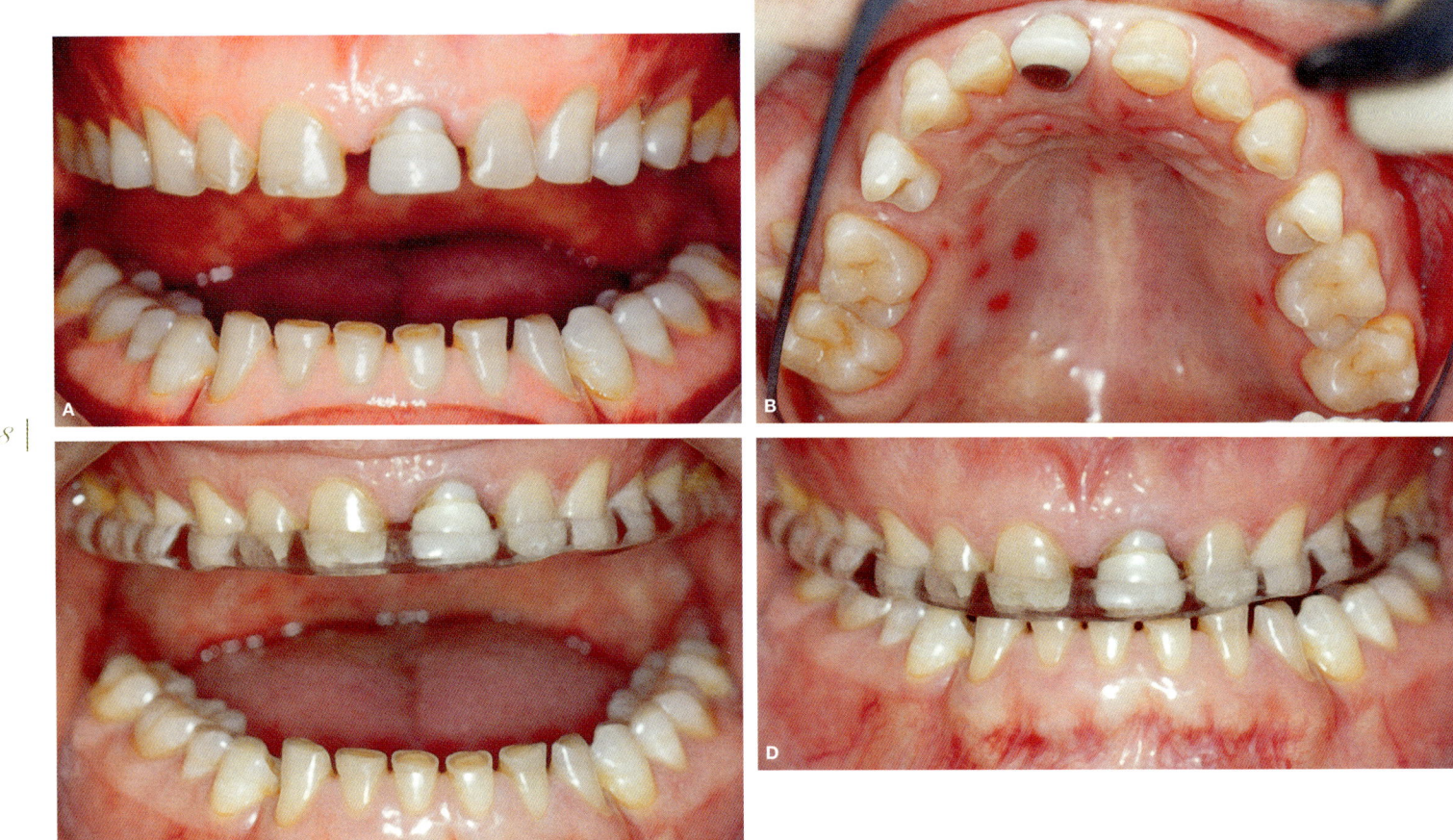

Figure 5.26 A-H - Patient with bruxism, small teeth and diastema (**A**, **B**). The treatment plan started with alginate impressions to produce stone casts used to fabricate an acrylic bite splint for the upper teeth (**C**, **D**). Study casts were mounted in articulator and diagnostic wax-up exercises were performed (**E**, **F**). The restorative treatment initiated with the preparation of the lower teeth for ceramic veneers. Provisional restorations were done with a resin-based composite (**G**, **H**) using a clear plastic matrix, as presented in Figs. 5.15 and 5.22.

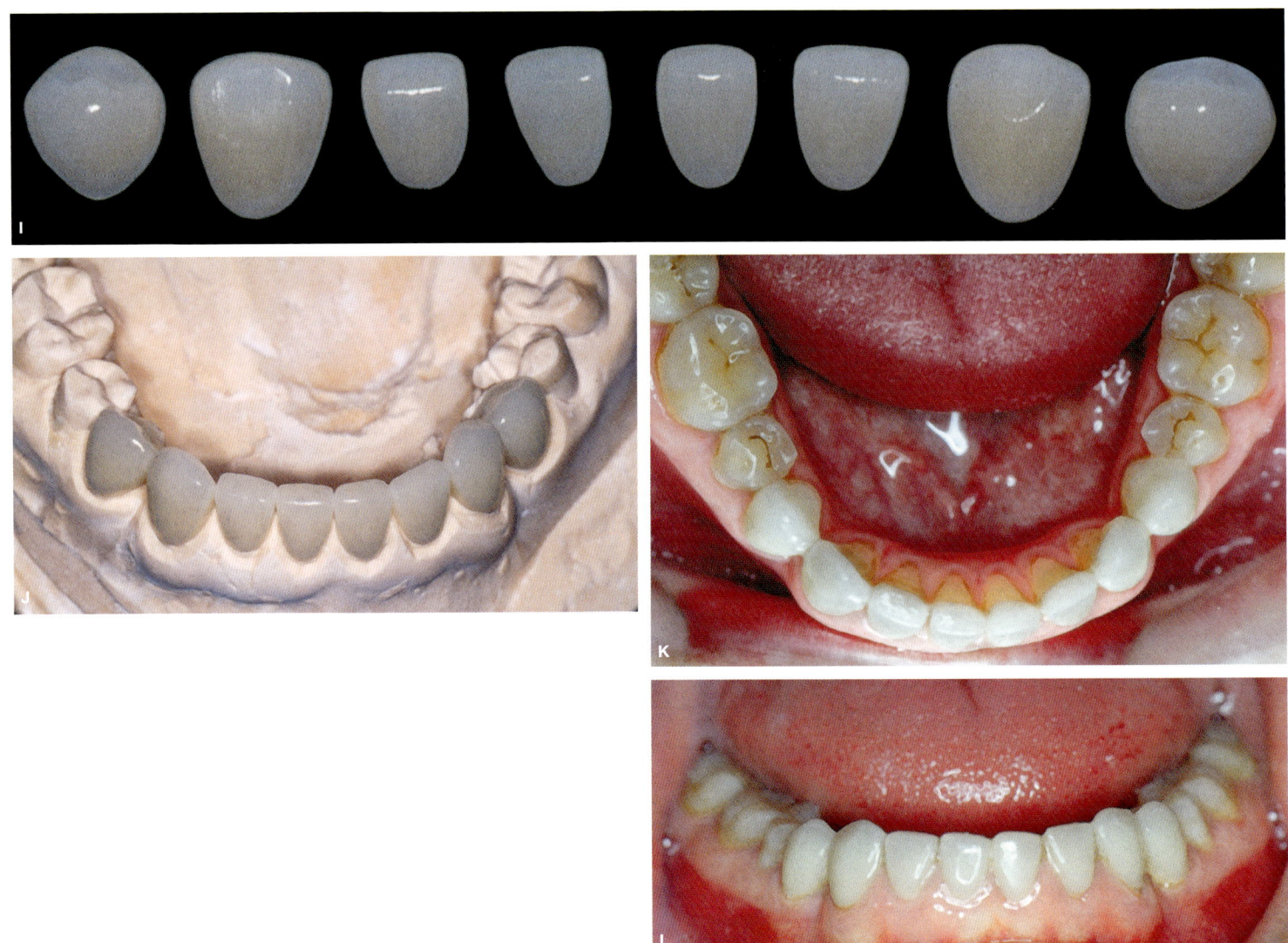

Figure 5.26 I-L - The ceramic veneers were made (Vita VM7) and tried for fit on the master cast (**I**, **J**). A resin-based composite cement system (RelyX ARC, 3M ESPE) was used to bond the restorations (**K**, **L**) considering the appropriate adhesive mechanisms for resin bonding to dentin, enamel and ceramic (Fig. 4.1) and clinically described in Table 5.2.

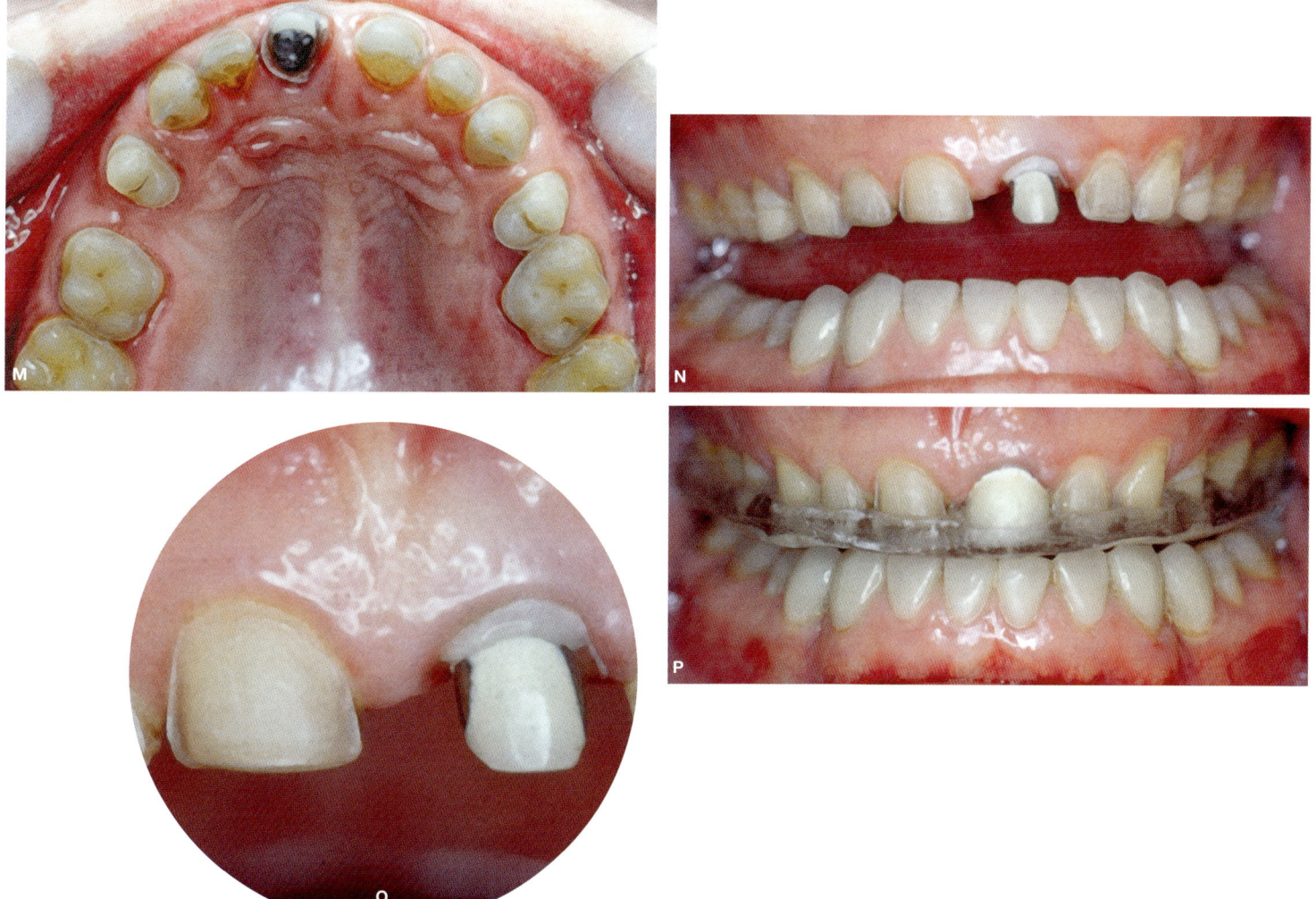

Figure 5.26 M-P - According to the diagnostic wax-up, all the upper teeth were prepared for ceramic restorations (veneers, onlays, and a crown), restoring the vertical dimension, function and esthetics. Tooth 21 (upper left central incisor) had an adequate endodontic treatment and a large cast metal post-and-core attached to a metal-ceramic crown. To prevent root fracture, the metal post was not replaced and the metal-ceramic crown was prepared for a ceramic crown. The remaining upper anterior teeth were prepared for ceramic veneers, and the upper posterior teeth were prepared for ceramic onlays (**M**, **N**, **O**). Provisional restorations were fabricated using resin-based material to fit onto the bite splint (**P**).

Figure 5.26 Q-V - Maxillary restorations were made with a feldspathic ceramic (Vita VM7), except for the crown (21) that used a substructure of In-Ceram Alumina veneered with VM7 (Vita). The restorations were examined for fit on the master cast (**Q-T**). Provisional restorations were removed and preparations were cleaned with oil-free pumice paste. The appropriate surface treatments were used to maximize the adhesive mechanisms for resin bonding to dentin, enamel, metal and ceramic (Fig. 4.1). Therefore, the crown preparation on tooth 21 (**U**) was sandblasted (airborne-particle abraded) with alumina particles (Fig. 5.15 R), etched with phosphoric acid (**V**), silane coupling agent was used on the treated ceramic surface, and the resin adhesive system (Scotchbond multi-purpose plus, 3M) was applied on the preparation according to manufacturer's instructions (Fig. 5.20). The clinical procedures for cementing the ceramic restorations are described in Table 5.2.

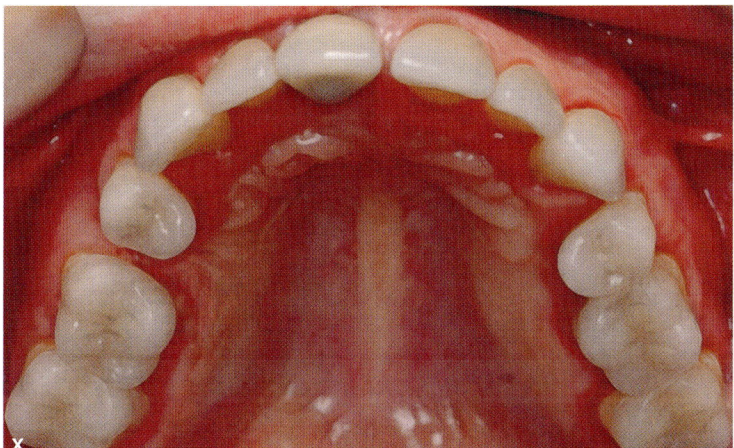
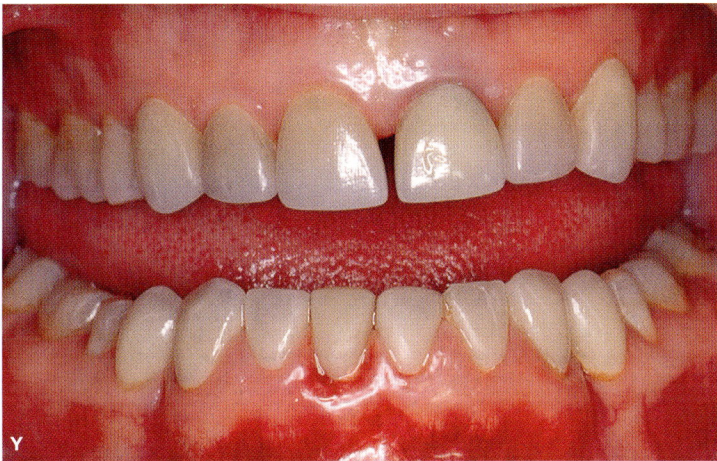
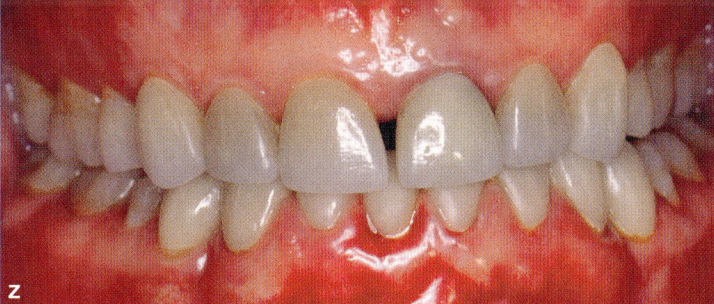

Figure 5.26 X-Z - A resin-based composite cement system (RelyX ARC, 3M ESPE) was used to cement all ceramic restorations (**X**, **Y**, **Z**). It was impossible to overcome all the gray effect from the metal post through the gingiva of tooth 21 (**O**, **Z**). A small trauma damaged the gingival area of tooth 41.

The first all-ceramic systems for single-unit crowns to appear on the market have received the most attention in peer-reviewed literature. These systems being the leucite-reinforced glass-ceramic (IPS Empress, Ivoclar), the glass-infiltrated ceramics (In-Ceram Alumina and In-Ceram Spinell, Vita), and polycrystalline alumina (Procera, Nobel Biocare). Despite the differences in their microstructure, composition, processing methods and intra-oral area of service (anterior or posterior), all clinical trials have showed survival rates greater than 90% irrespective of the time in service, except for Dicor (Dentsply Int.), a glass-ceramic no longer on the market (Table 5.3). In general, fracture rates appear to be lower for anterior crowns than for molar crowns and the two alumina-based systems are proving to be comparable (*i.e.*, In-Ceram and Procera). Higher success for anterior teeth is also the trend for IPS Empress. A study reported an overall survival rate of 95% at 11 years for 125 IPS Empress crowns, which really represents 99% in the anterior segment and 84% in the posterior segment (Fradeani and Redemagni, 2002).

The main causes of failure reported in all studies were catastrophic fractures (*i.e.*, the crown broke into two pieces; *e.g.* Fig. 5.1), chipping of the veneer ceramic (Figs. 5.2; 5.33; 5.34) and secondary caries. Again, it should be pointed out that secondary caries is a host response very likely unrelated to the materials used in fixed prostheses. Considering this rationale, a four-year study on In-Ceram alumina (n = 80; 58 anterior and 22 posterior crowns) reported that only one molar crown had fractured and the marginal ridge of one premolar crown had chipped (Haselton *et al.*, 2000). Yet, no bulk fracture was reported for 28 anterior and 68 posterior In-Ceram Alumina crowns at another four-year study (Probster, 1996).

Table 5.3 - Peer-reviewed studies of survival rate of all-ceramic single-unit crowns.

All-ceramic material	Study	No. of crowns		Fabrication method	Observation period in months (mean)	Survival rate (period)
		Anterior	Posterior			
In-Ceram Alumina*	Probster, 1993	21	40	Slip cast	4-35 (20.8)	100% (2 years)††
	Pang, 1995	35	— #	Slip cast	2.5-21 (NI)	91.5%
	Probster, 1996	28	68	Slip cast	1.3-55.9 (24.4)	100% (4 years)††
	Scotti et al., 1995	25	38	Slip cast	24-44 (37.6)	98%
	McLaren and White, 2000	223		Slip cast	36 (36)	96%
	Scherrer et al., 2001	45	23	Slip cast	NI-60 (NI)	92% (5 years)††
	Segal, 2001	177	369	Slip cast	12-72 (33.4)	99%
	Bindl and Mörmann, 2002	—	24	CAD/CAM	14-58 (40.6)	92% (5 years)††
In-Ceram Spinell*	Bindl and Mörmann, 2002	—	19	CAD/CAM	28-56 (36.3)	100% (5 years)††
	Fradeani et al., 2002	40	—	Slip cast	22-60 (50)	97.5% (5 years)††
	Bindl and Mörmann, 2004	18	—	CAD/CAM	33-57 (44.7)	92% (5 years)††
Procera†	Oden et al., 1998	17	83	CAD/CAM	60 (60)	94% (5 years)††
	Odman and Andersson, 2001	23	64	CAD/CAM	1-120 (NI)	93% (10 years)††
	Fradeani et al., 2005	50	155	CAD/CAM	6-60 (23.5)	97% (5 years)††
	Walter et al., 2006	61	46	CAD/CAM	72 (72)	94% (6 years)††
	Zitzmann et al., 2007	32	103	CAD/CAM	1-92 (55)	99% (5 years)††
IPS Empress‡	Lehner et al., 1997	41	37	Hot pressed	1-24 (20)	95% (2 years)††
	Fradeani and Aquilano, 1997	101	43	Hot pressed	6-68 (37)	95% (3 years)††
	Sorensen et al., 1998	47	28	Hot pressed	14-42 (NI)	99% (3 years)††
	Sjögren et al., 1999	43	67	Hot pressed	1-42 (3.6)	92% (3.5 years)††
	Fradeani and Redemagni, 2002	93	32	Hot pressed	48-132 (NI)	95% (11 years)††
IPS Empress 2‡	Toksavul and Toman, 2007	56	23	Hot pressed	12-60 (58)	95% (5 years)††
	Marquardt and Strub, 2006	—	27	Hot pressed	6-60 (NI)	100% (5 years)††
	Taskonak and Sertgöz, 2006	12	8	Hot pressed	24 (24)	100% (2 years)††
	Suputtamongkol et al., 2008	—	30	Hot pressed	12 (12)	100% (1 year)††
Dicor §	Sjögren et al., 1999	98		Lost wax	15-130 (74)	82%
	Scherrer et al., 2001	30		Lost wax	84 (84)	86% (7 years)††

* In-Ceram Alumina and In-Ceram Spinell are manufactured by Vita Zahnfabrik, Bad Säckingen, Germany.

† Procera is manufactured by Nobel Biocare, Göteborg, Sweden.

‡ IPS Empress is now IPS Empress Esthetic; IPS Empress 2 is now IPS e.max Press. They are manufactured by Ivoclar Vivadent, Schaan, Liechtenstein.

§ Dicor was manufactured by Dentsply, York, Pa. It is no longer on the market.

Dash indicates none.

†† Kaplan-Meier survival rate was calculated for the endpoint listed.

NI: Not included.

Nevertheless, the performance of crowns in a crown-cement-tooth system is a complex function of variables reflecting crown design, material selection, and patient specific factors. Increased stress in the crown increases the probability of crown failure. The magnitude of the maximum principal stress in a crown is in large measure a function of the crown material selected and its thickness. However, cement modulus, load position, and supporting tooth core are important contributors to the maximum stress concentration in the crown and may not contribute equally for all crown material systems. Interactions between variables may account for otherwise not recognized differences in performance of different crown materials (Rekow *et al.*, 2006).

Tooth preparation for all-ceramic crowns and bridges (FPDs) follow similar criteria mentioned for all-ceramic onlays, which are: rounded angles to prevent stress concentration; uniform and anatomic reduction to allow for adequate ceramic thickness; shoulder finish line with a rounded internal line angle (Fig. 5.27). As retention decreases as wall **taper** increases, the clinician should aim to 7^0-12^0 as the optimum degree of tooth preparation taper.

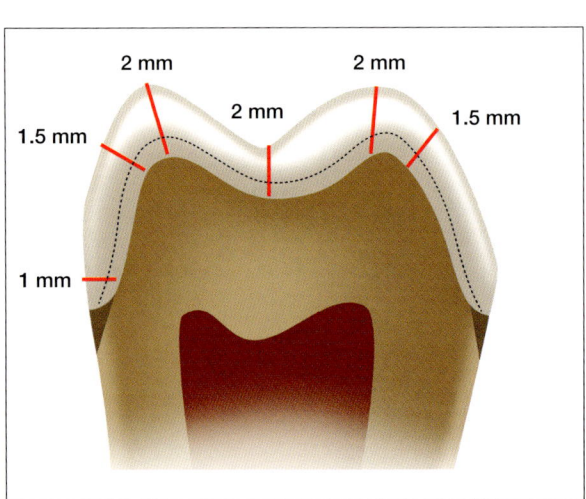

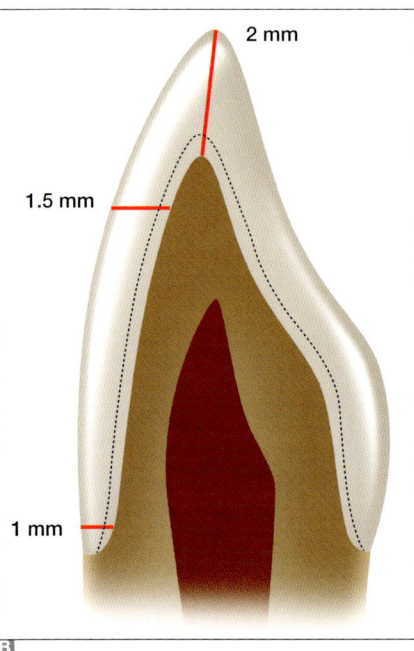

Figure 5.27 - Ceramic thickness per tooth area, including ceramic substructure thicknesses of about 0.5 mm (axial walls) and 0.7 mm (incisal/occlusal wall). These values should guide the clinician on crown preparations for posterior (**A**) and anterior (**B**) teeth. In case of all-ceramic fixed bridges, the substructure thickness of the occlusal wall of the retainers should be about 1 mm.

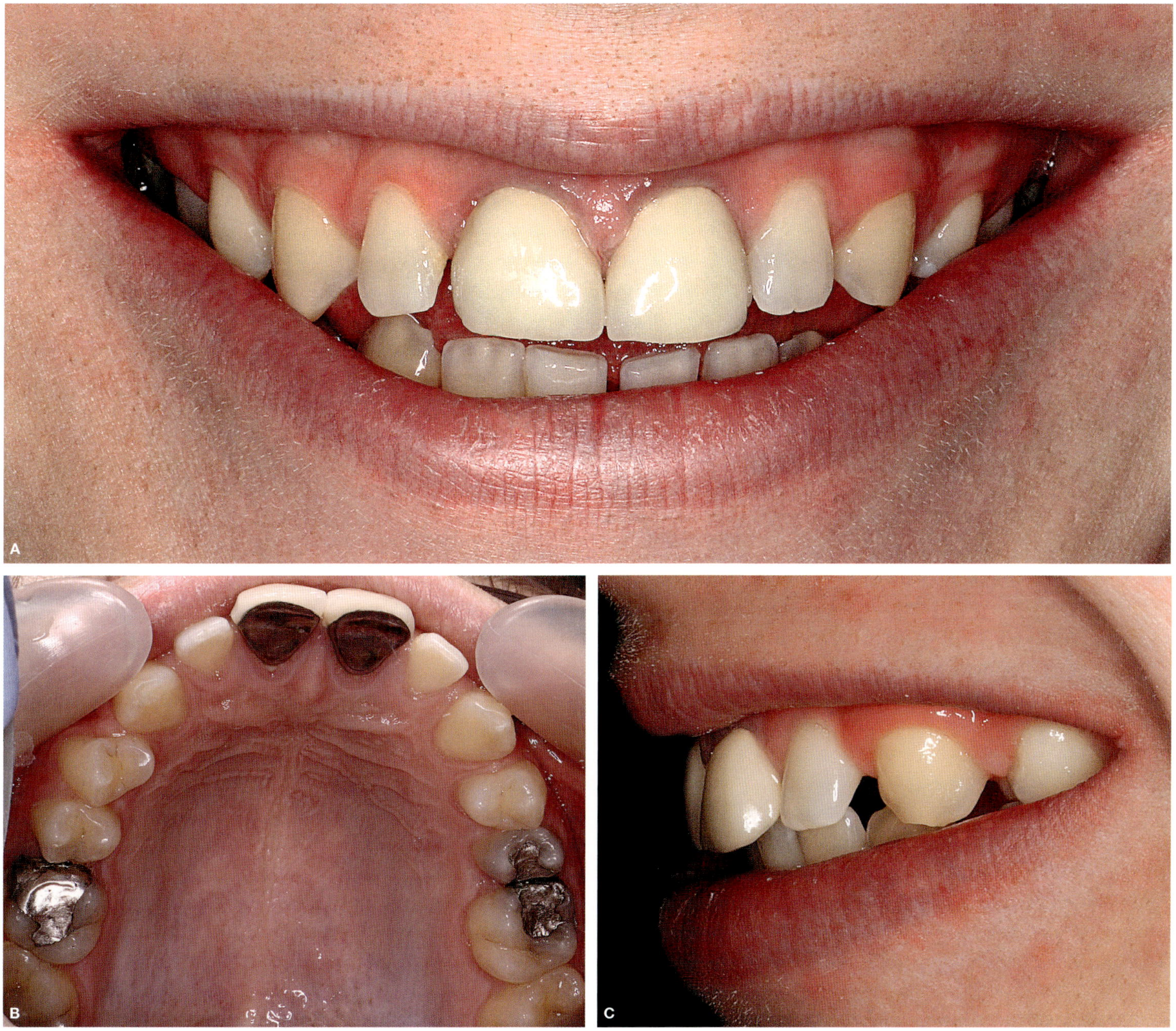

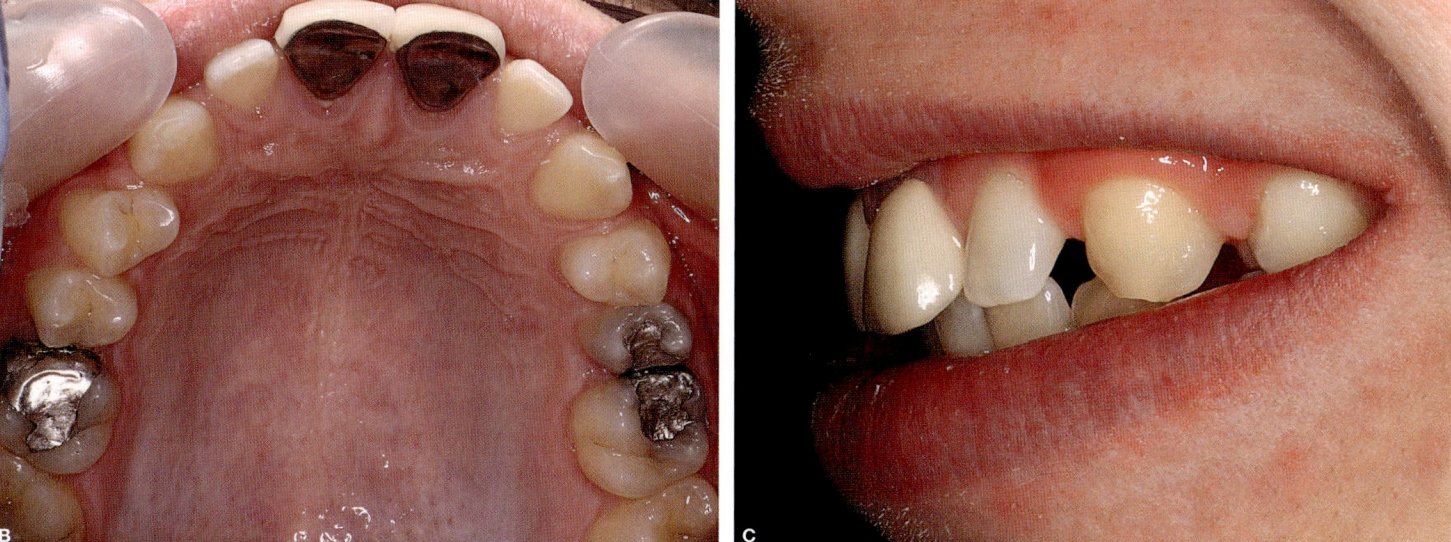

197

Figure 5.28 A-C -Young patient wishing to have lighter anterior teeth and spaces (diastema) closed (**A**, **B**, **C**). Patient was very concerned about the gray effect from the metal-ceramic crowns through the gingiva of teeth 11 and 21 (**A**).

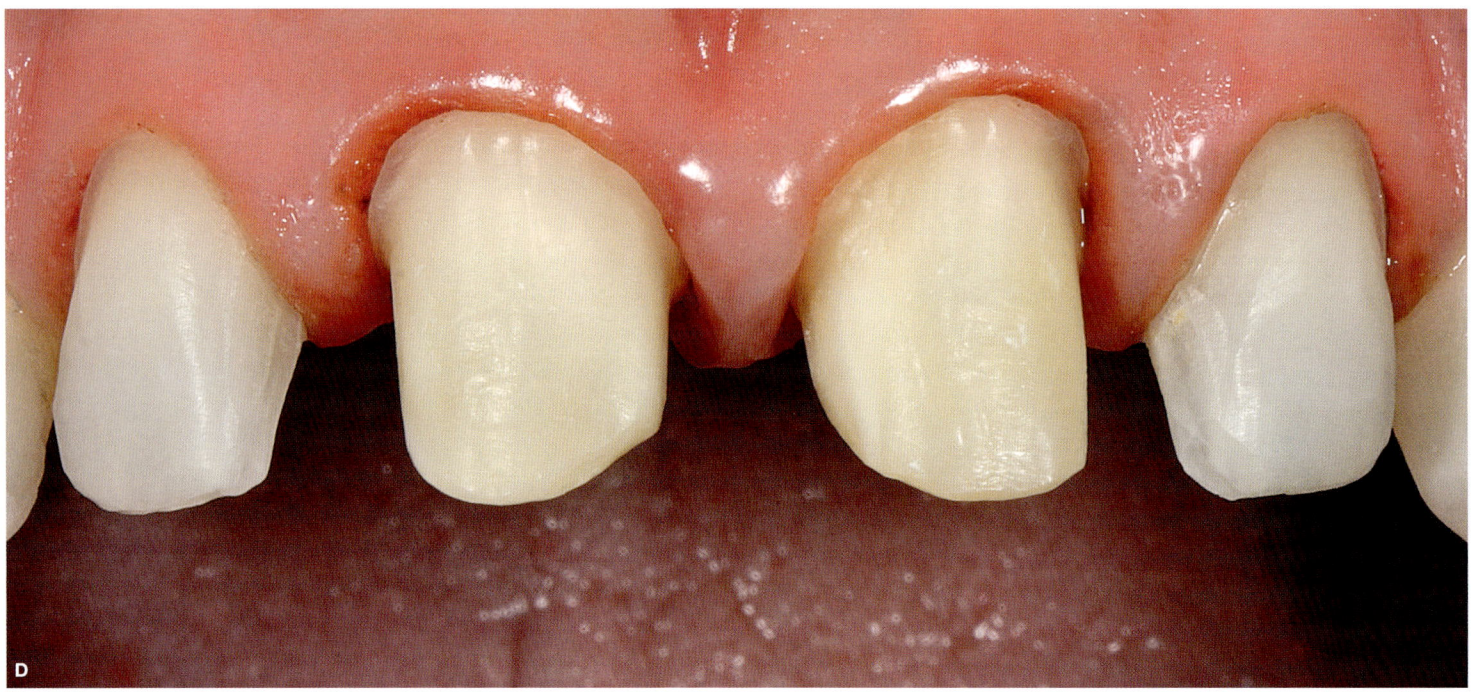

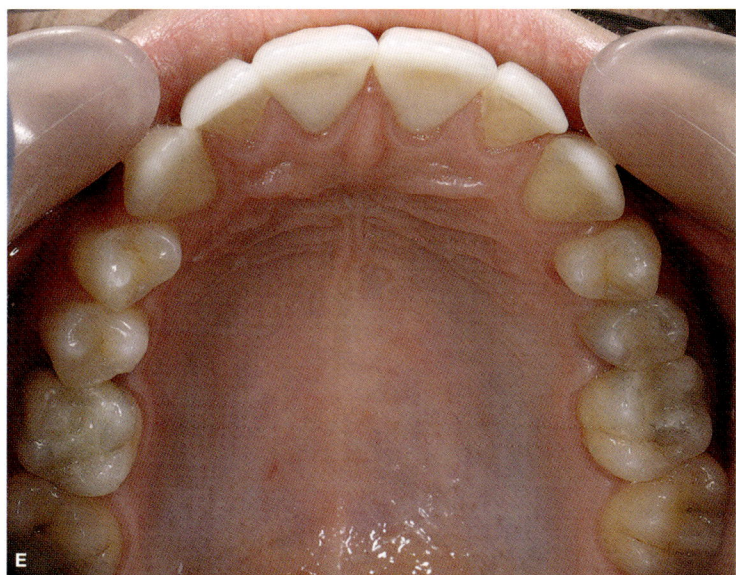

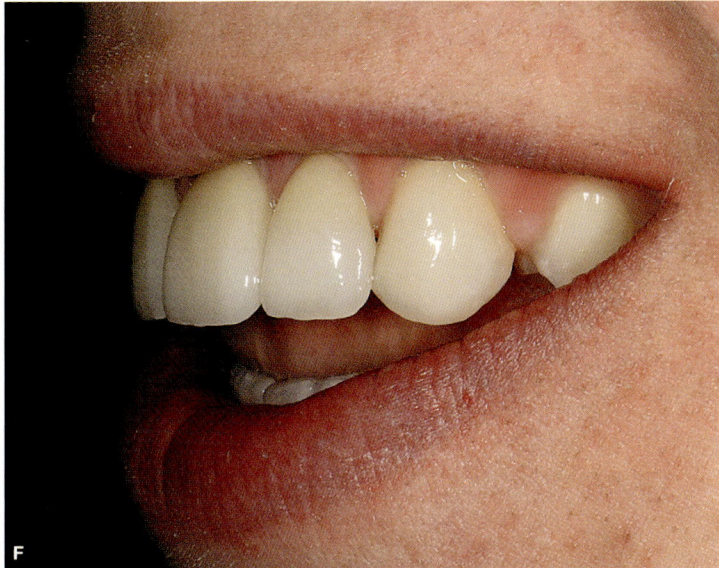

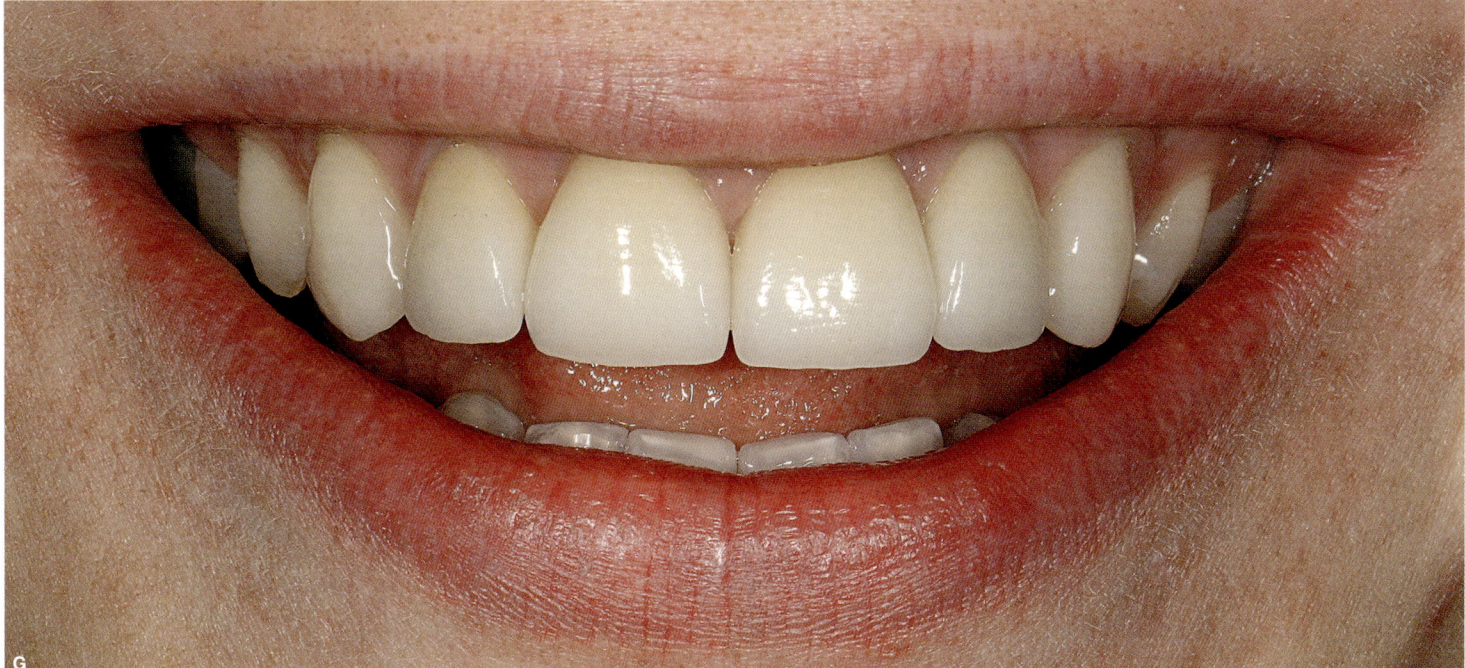

Figure 5.28 D-G - Teeth were tray bleached, the metal-ceramic crowns on the upper central incisors were removed and replaced using all-ceramic crowns (IPS e.max Press, Ivoclar). Teeth preparations show the central incisors unbleached following the removal of the metal-ceramic crowns (**D**). The upper lateral incisors were ceramic veneered (IPS e.max Press, Ivoclar) and the upper canines and lower anterior were restored, with no tooth preparation, to close the spaces using a resin-based composite (Enamel Plus HFO, Micerium). Posterior amalgam restorations were replaced with a low shrinkage resin-based composite (Filtek Silorane, 3M ESPE) (**E**, **F**, **G**). Images **A**-**G**, **B**-**E**, and **C**-**F** are, respectively, before-after pictures. This clinical case shows that similar immediate esthetic results can be achieved with three different levels of tooth preparation and restorative materials. As the lithium disilicate-based glass-ceramic (IPS e.max Press, Ivoclar) is considered an acid-sensitive ceramic, the clinical procedures for resin bonding the ceramic restorations followed Table 5.2 and are based on Fig. 4.1. This clinical case is a courtesy of Dr. Simon E Northeast.

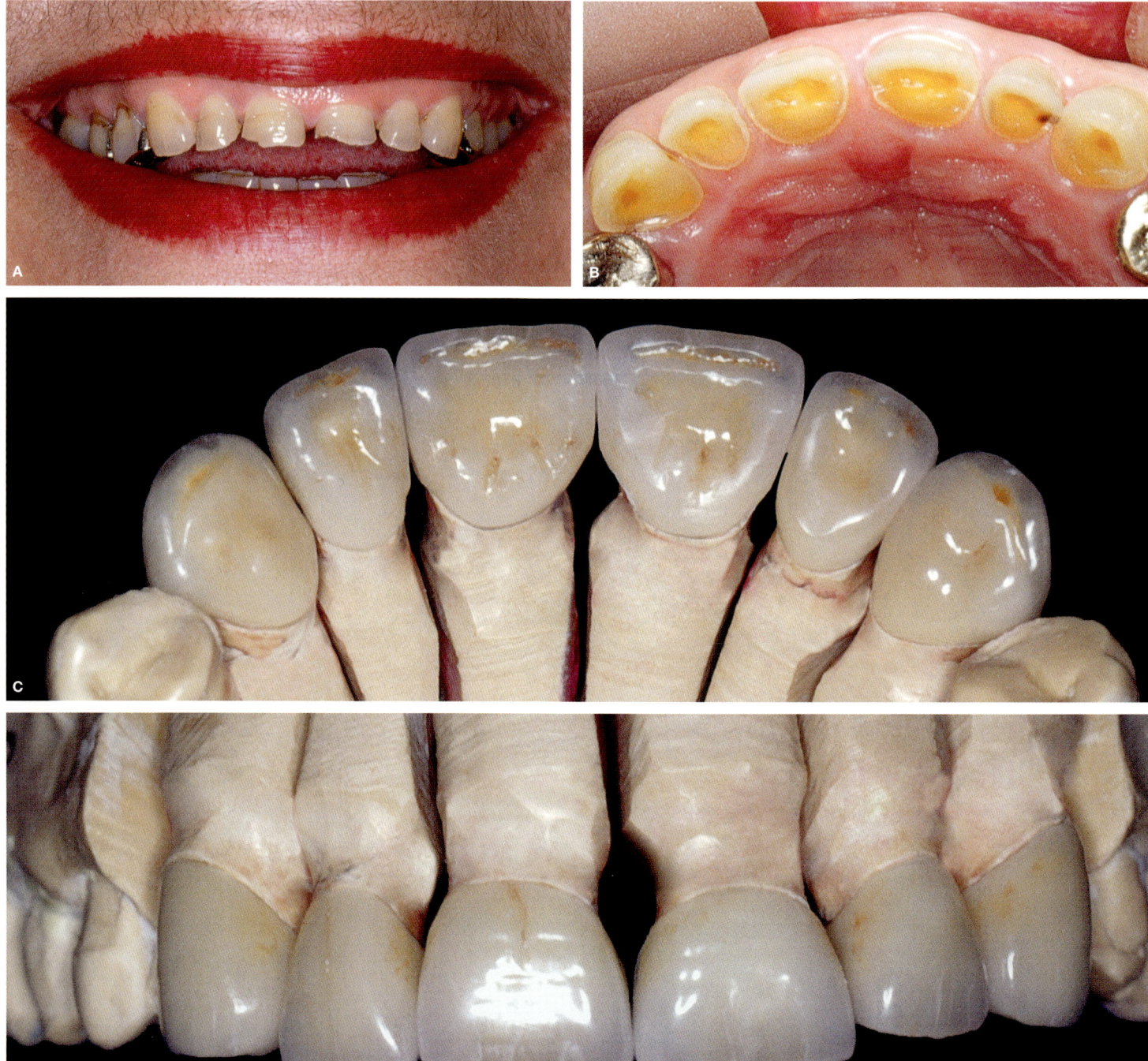

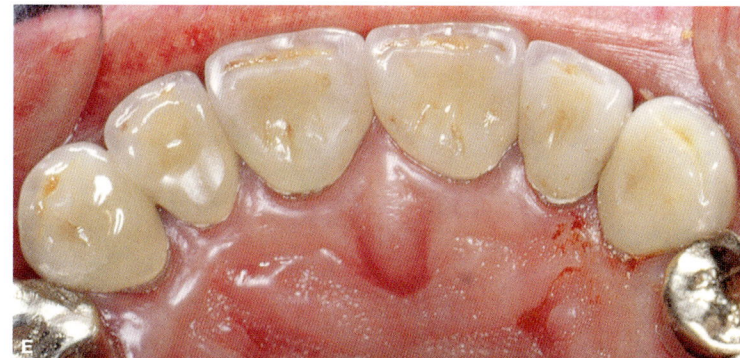
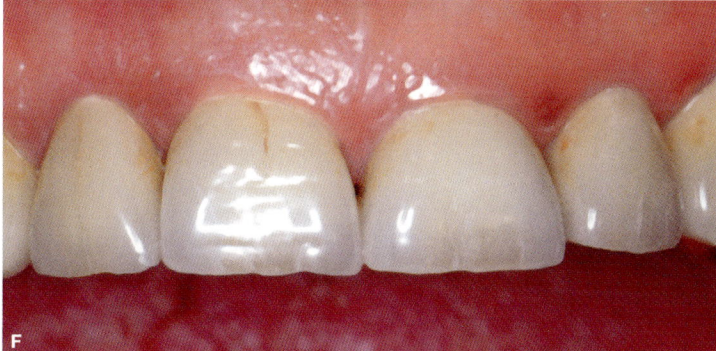

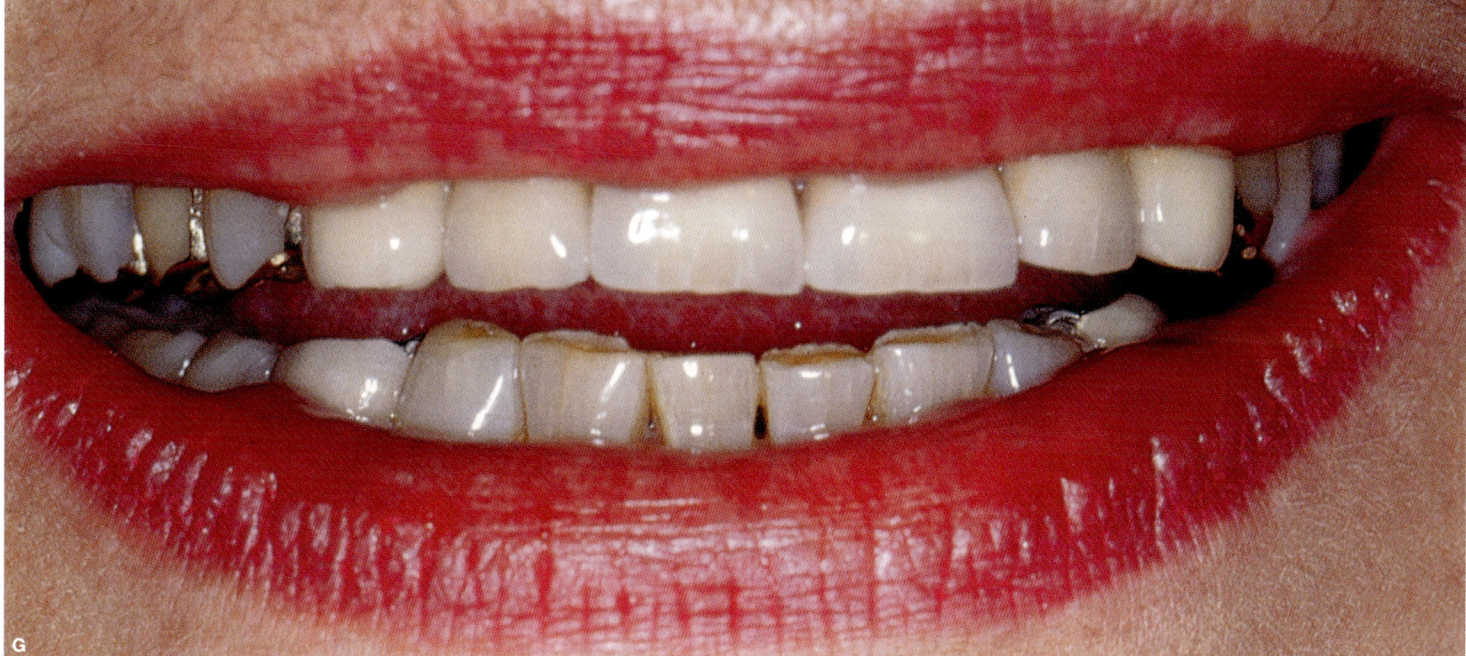

Figure 5.29 A-G - Patient with bruxism restored the posterior teeth with gold onlays but wanted esthetic restorations for the anterior teeth (**A**, **B**). Six upper anterior teeth were prepared for all-ceramic crowns made using a zirconia-reinforced, alumina-based glass infiltrated structure (In-Ceram Zirconia, Vita) that was veneered with a feldspathic ceramic (Vita VM7) (**C**, **D**). The ceramic internal surface of the restorations were silica coated (Rocatec, 3M ESPE) (Fig. 4.9), a silane coupling agent and an adhesive system were applied on the ceramic treated surface, and restorations were cemented using a resin-based composite cement (RelyX ARC, 3M ESPE) (**E**, **F**, **G**).

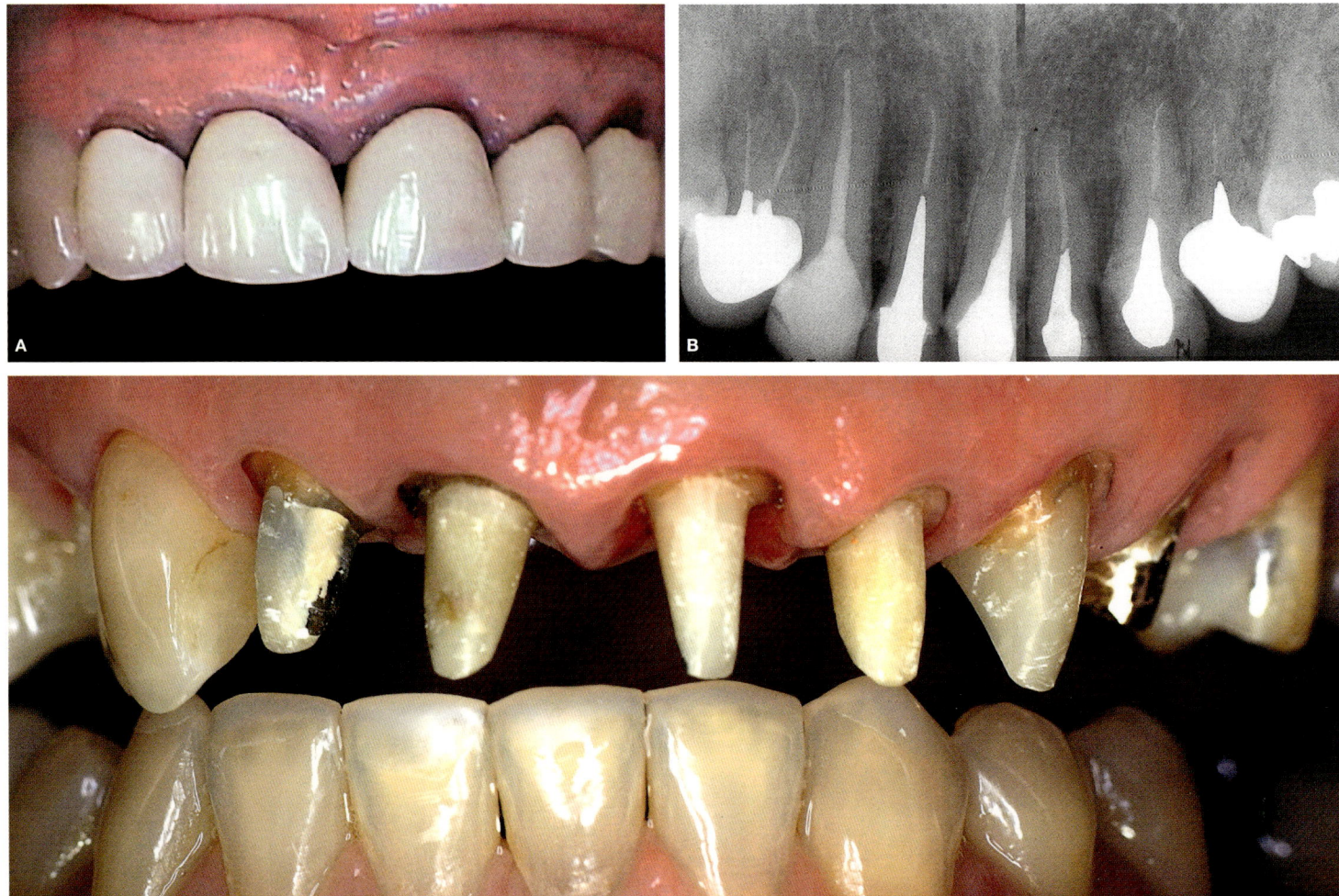

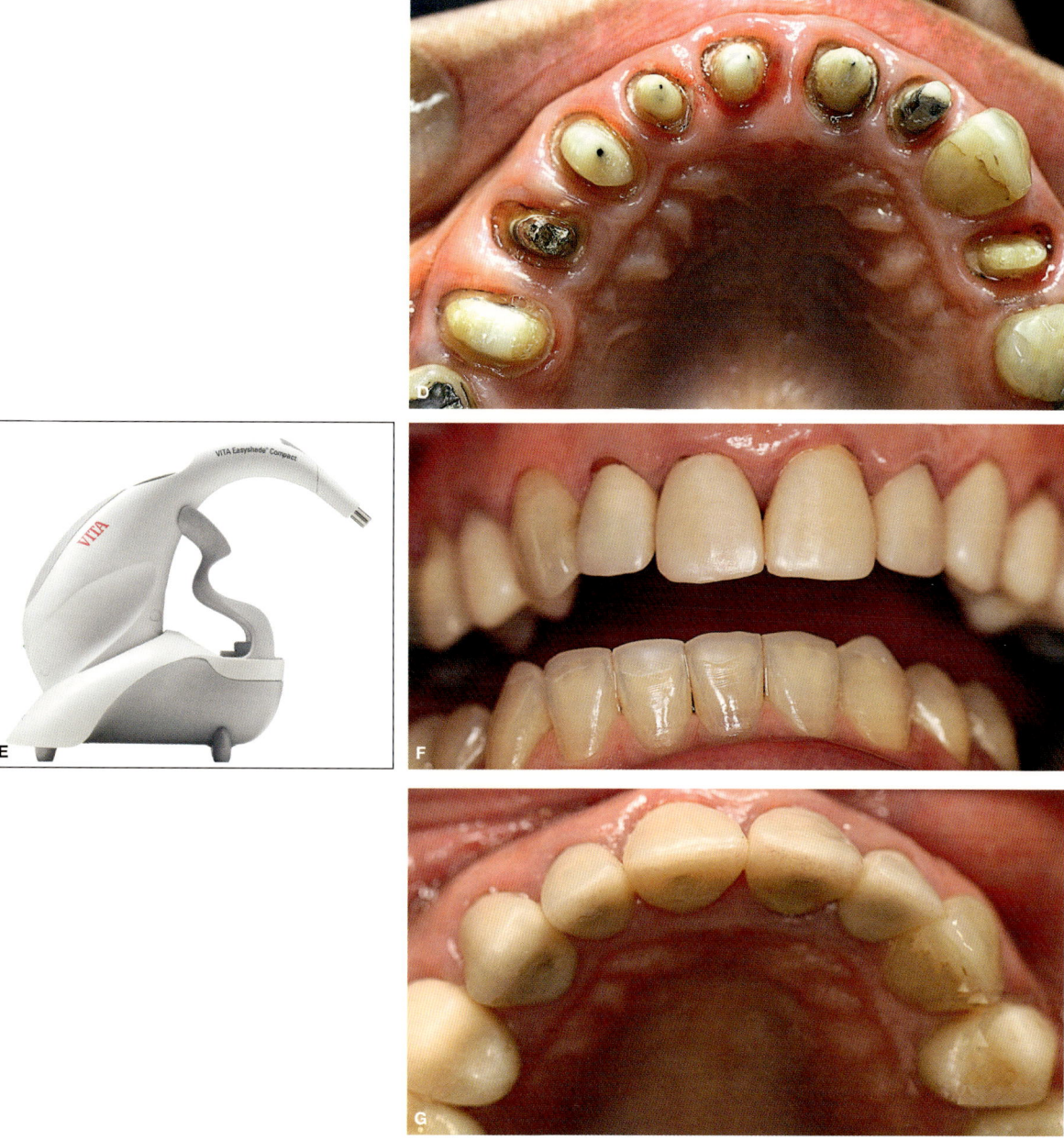

203

Figure 5.30 A-G - The patient chief complaint was poor esthetics. Note the gingivitis (redness) and the dark gray area showing through the free gingiva of the upper anterior teeth, which had been endodontically treated and restored with metal post and core and metal-ceramic (PFM) crowns (**A**, **B**). After treatment planning, the PFM crowns and most of the metal post and cores were removed, some of the endodontic treatments were redone, and carbon-reinforced glass fiber posts were placed (**C**, **D**). Tooth preparations were polished, vinyl polysiloxane impressions were taken and stone casts were made. Tooth shade was selected using the 3D-Master shade guide (Vita) and checked with an intra-oral spectrophotometer (Easyshade Compact, Vita) (**E**). Temporary restorations were done using a resin-based composite (**F**, **G**) with the assistance of a clear plastic matrix, as presented in Figs. 5.15 and 5.22.

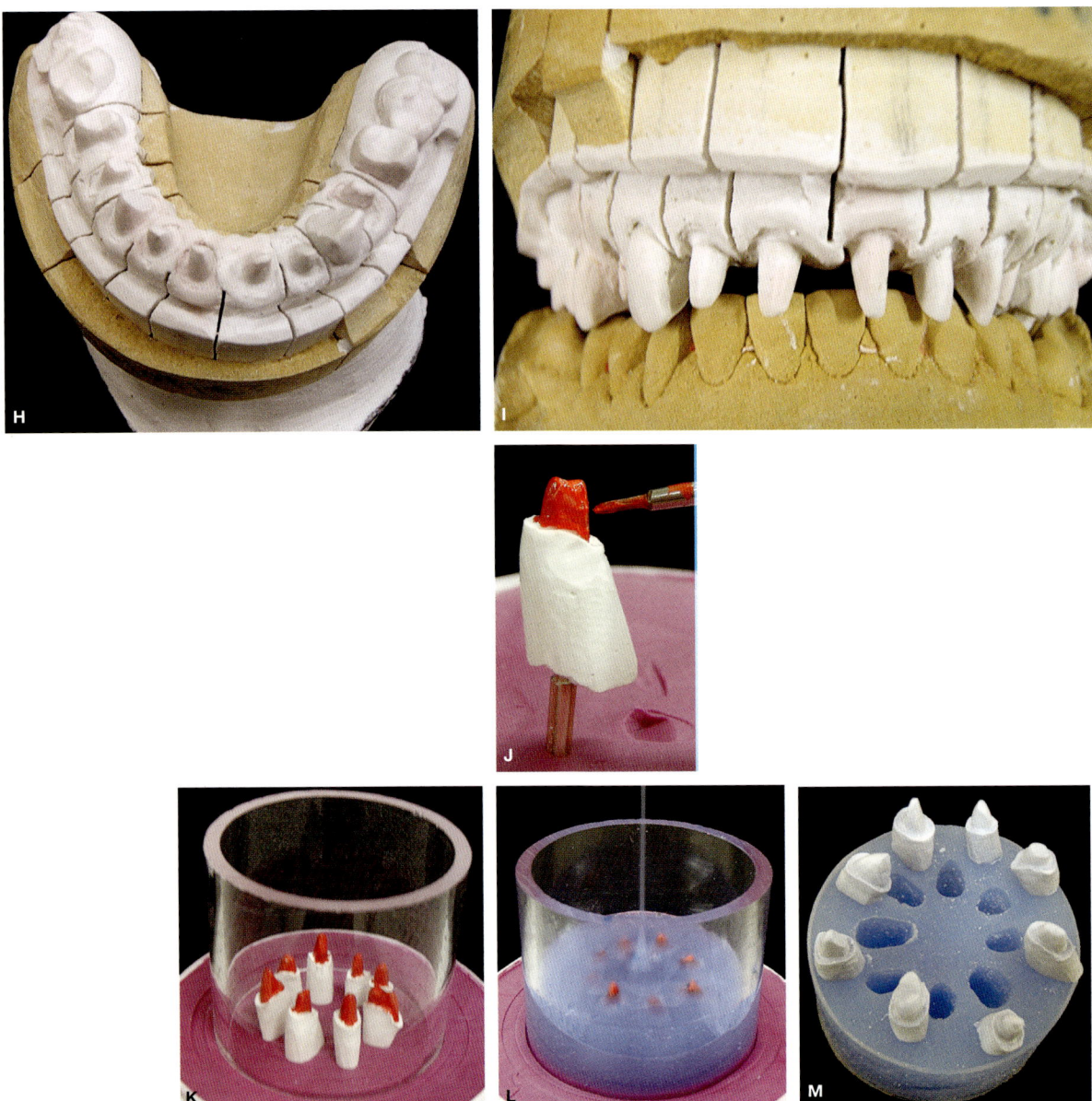

Figure 5.30 H-M - The casts were mounted in articulator and the upper cast was carefully prepared to obtain working dies (**H**, **I**). A red-colored spacer was applied on the dies (**J**). A silicone mold was fabricated and used to duplicate the dies (**K**-**M**).

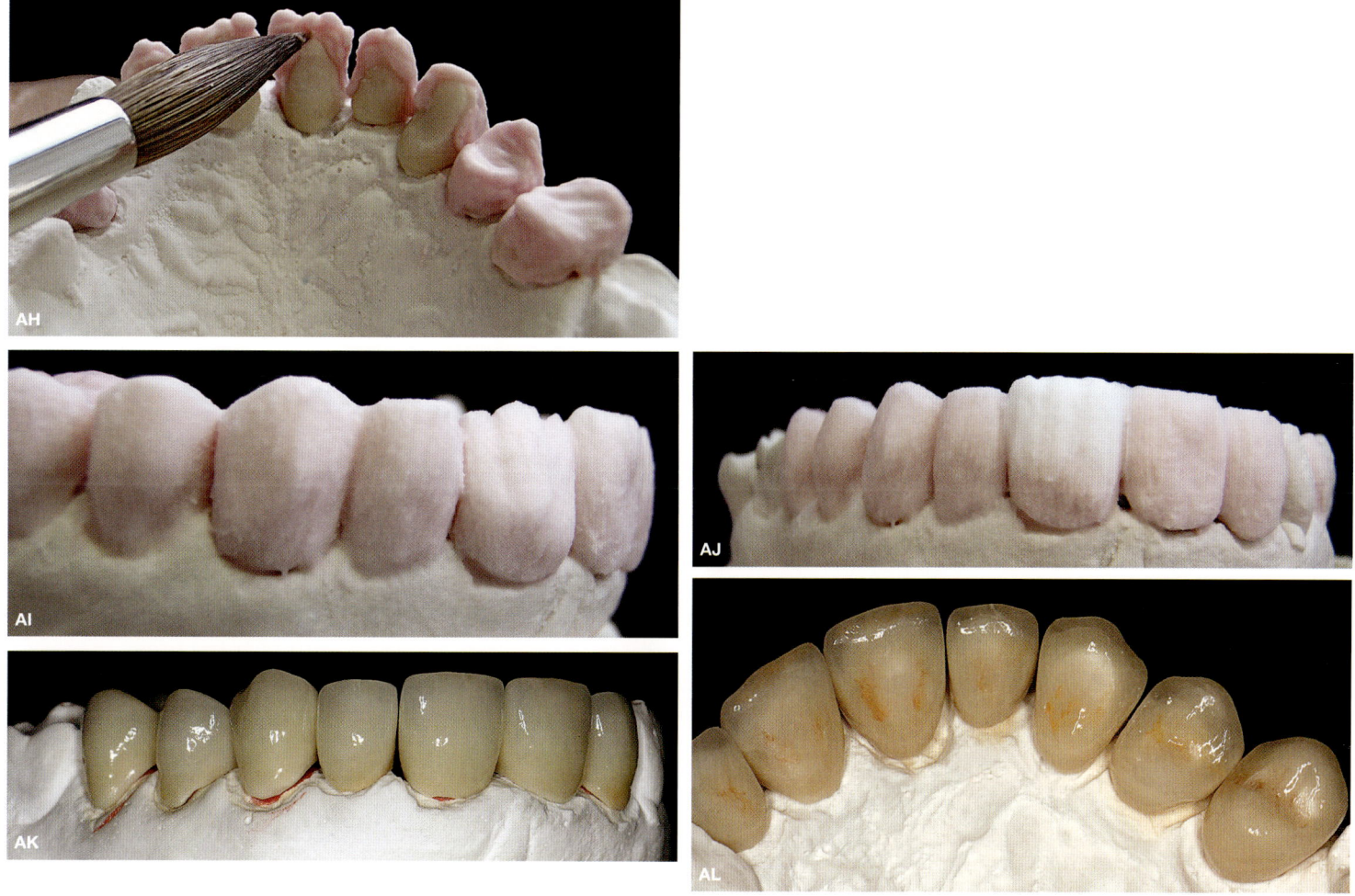

Figure 5.30 AH-AL - A feldspathic ceramic (VM7, Vita) was applied in layers for better characterization (**AH-AJ**). The veneer ceramic was sintered and the ceramic crowns were fit to the master cast (**AK**, **AL**).

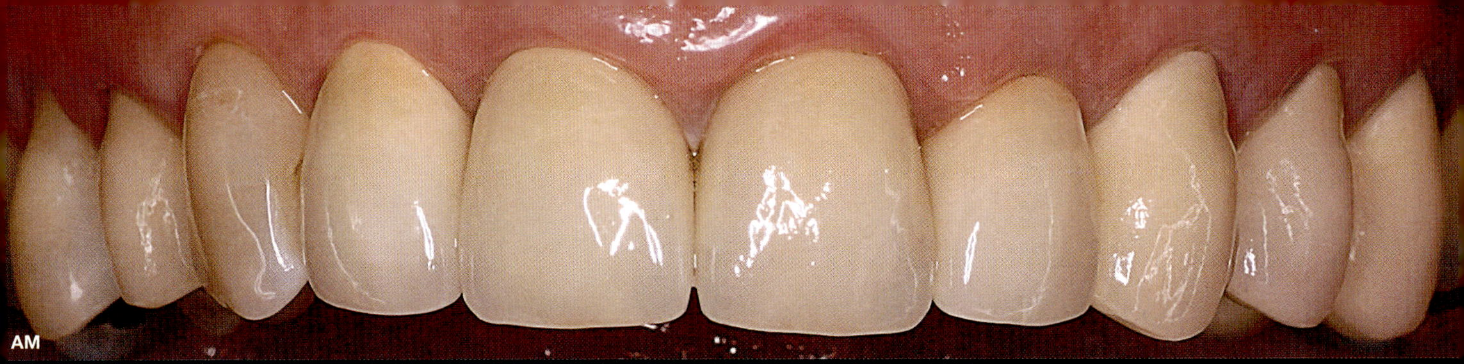

AM

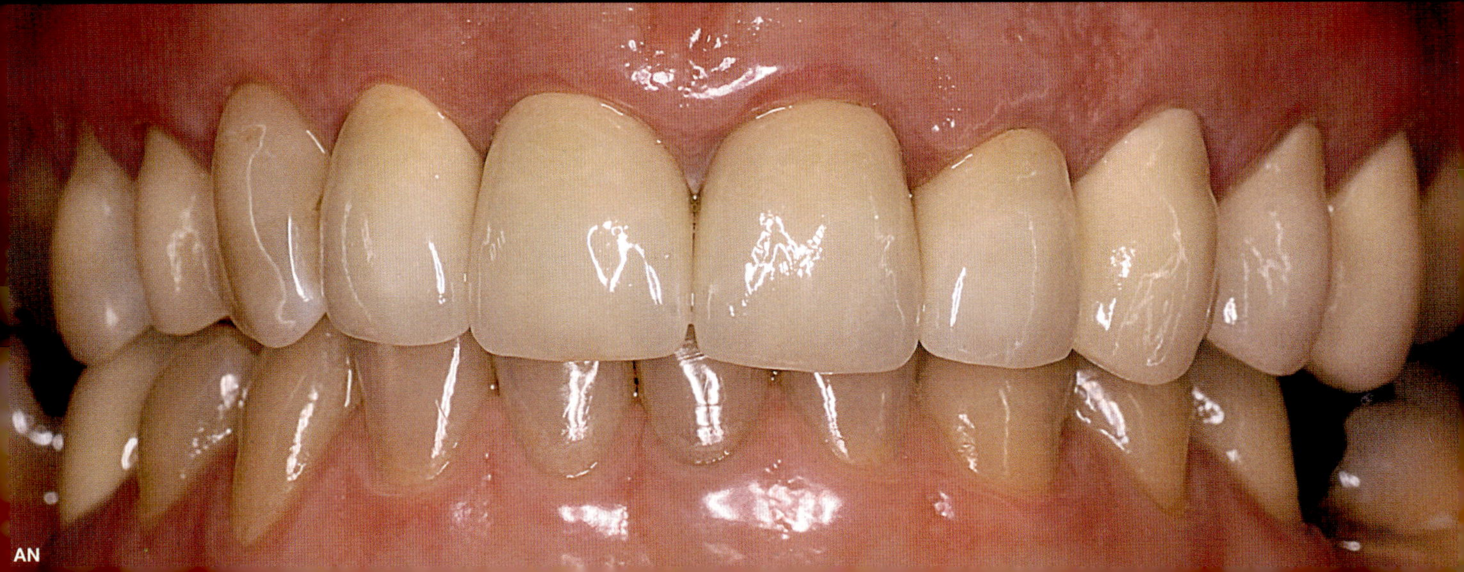

AN

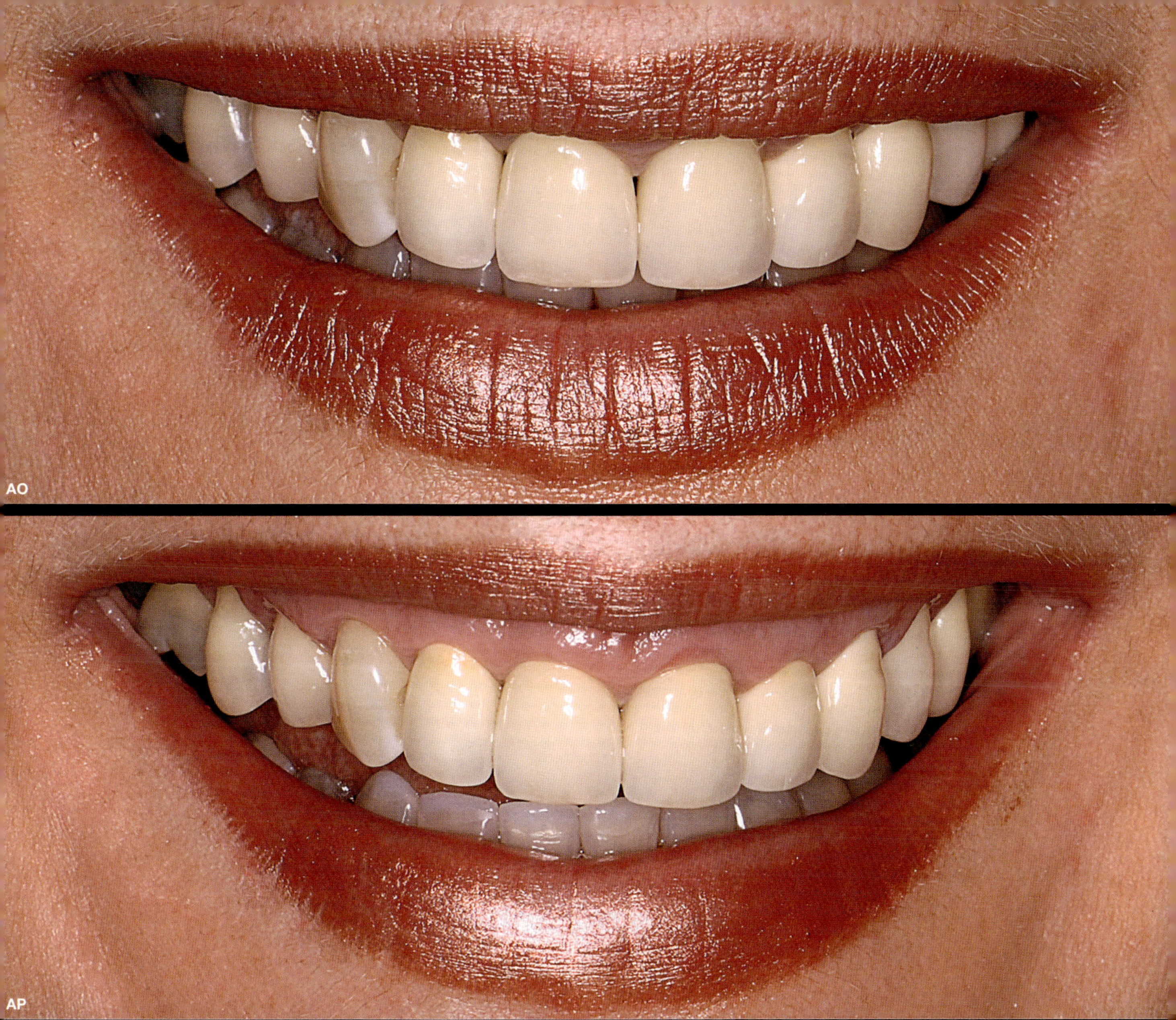

Figure 5.30 AM-AP - The ceramic restorations were cemented in place using a resin cement system with MDP (Panavia F 2.0, Kuraray) (**AM-AP**). The dark gray area that was showing through the free gingiva of the upper anterior teeth and the gingivitis (redness) (**A**) disappeared (these pictures were made immediately after cementation of the all-ceramic crowns).

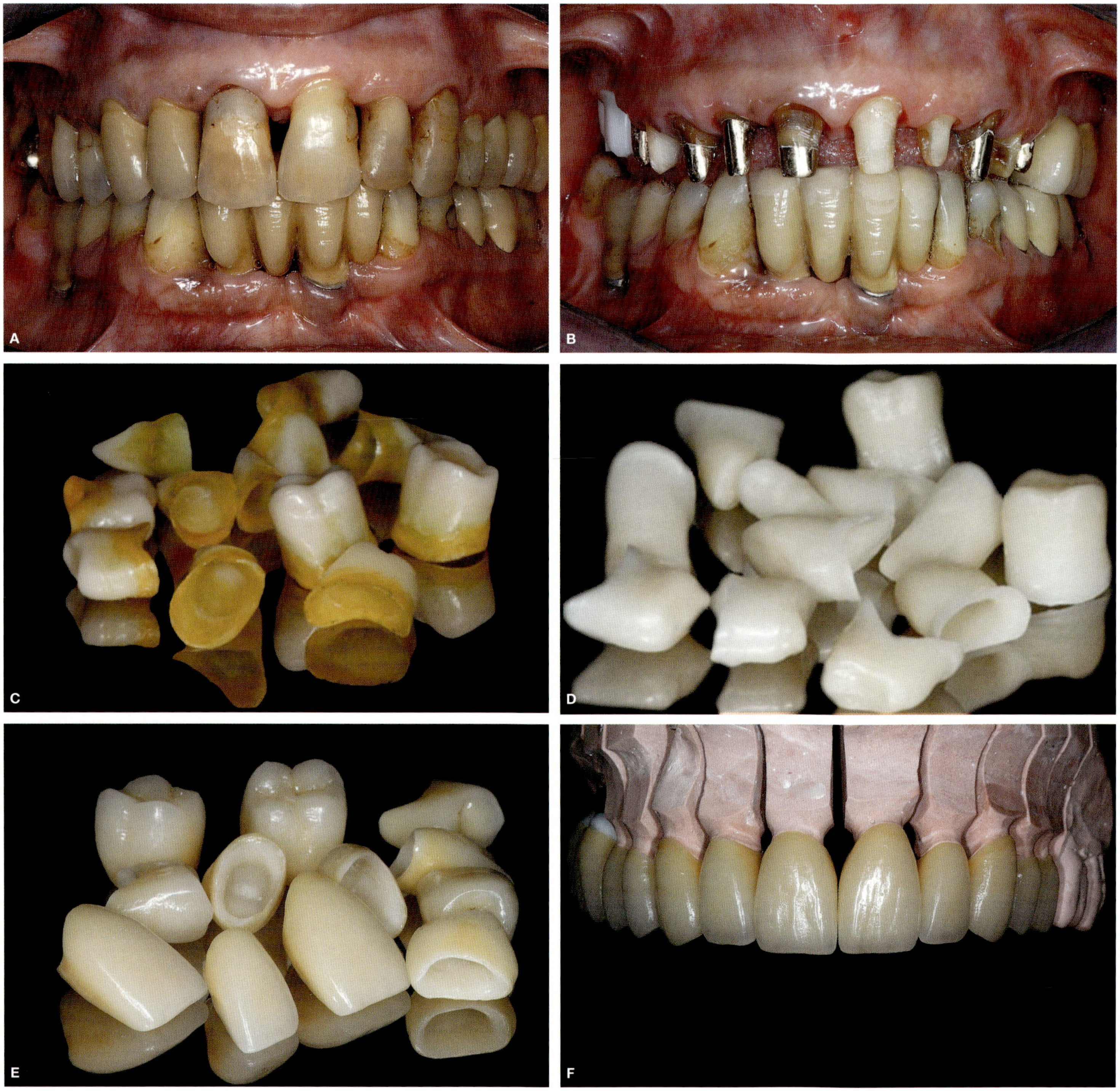

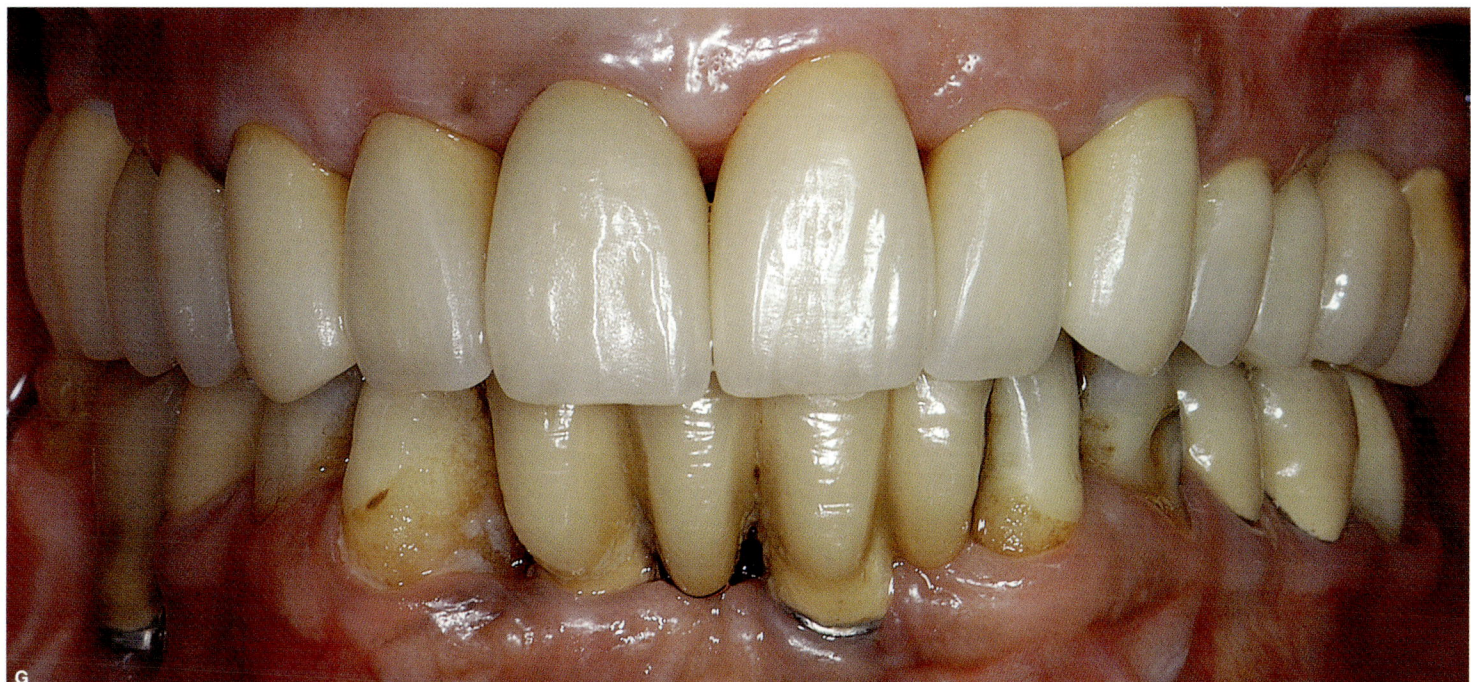

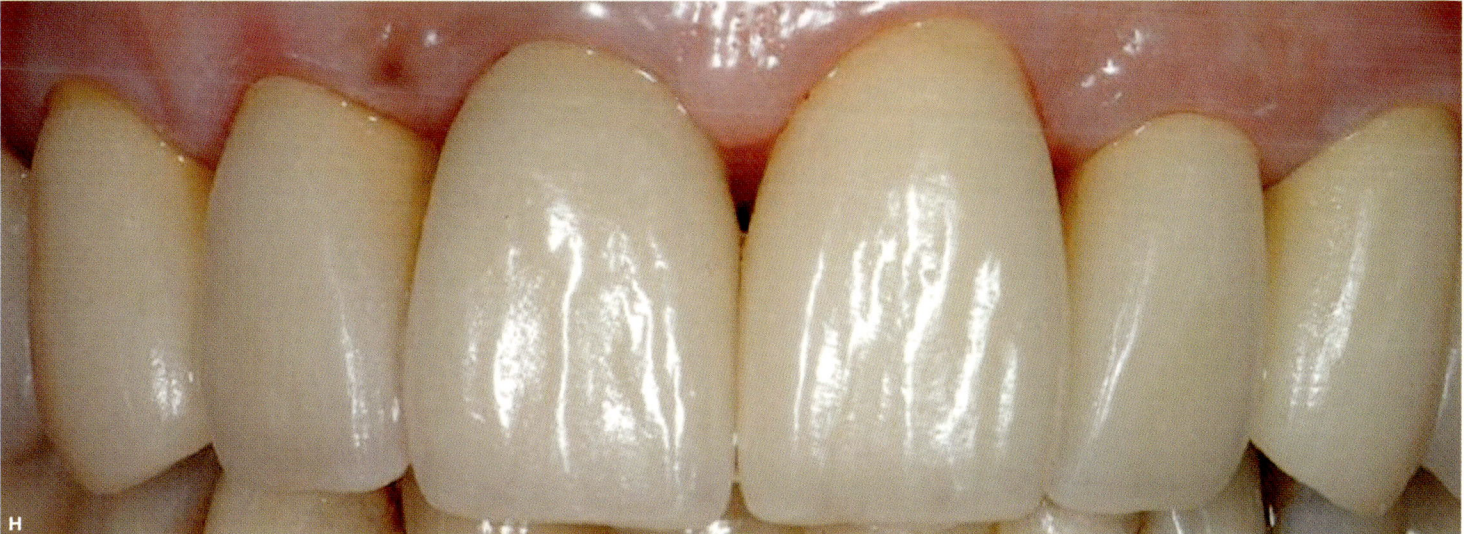

Figure 5.31 A-H - Female patient wishing to improve dental esthetics (**A**). An oral rehabilitation treatment was planned and started with the upper arch. Some teeth had to be endodontically treated and prepared for post, which were cast using a gold-based alloy. Two implants replaced the upper right molars that were lost because of periodontal disease. Temporary restorations were removed six months later (**B**), vinyl polysiloxane impressions were taken and stone casts were made. All copings were waxed-up (**C**), scanned and substructures were fabricated with alumina-based ceramic (Procera Crown Alumina, Nobel Biocare) (**D**) and veneered with porcelain (NobelRondo Alumina, Nobel Biocare) (**E**, **F**). Upper ceramic restorations were cemented (**G**, **H**) using a resin-based system (RelyX Unicem, 3M ESPE).

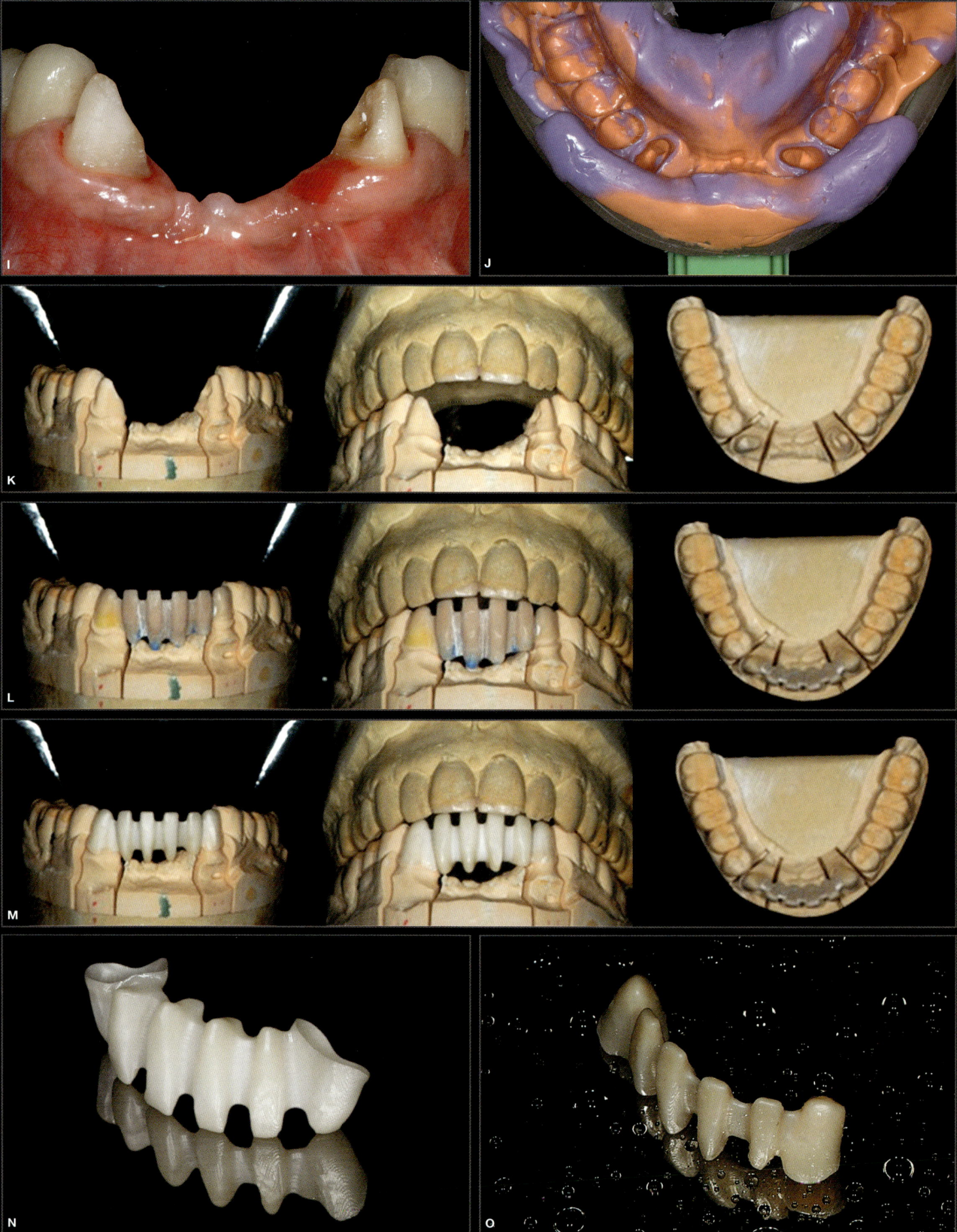

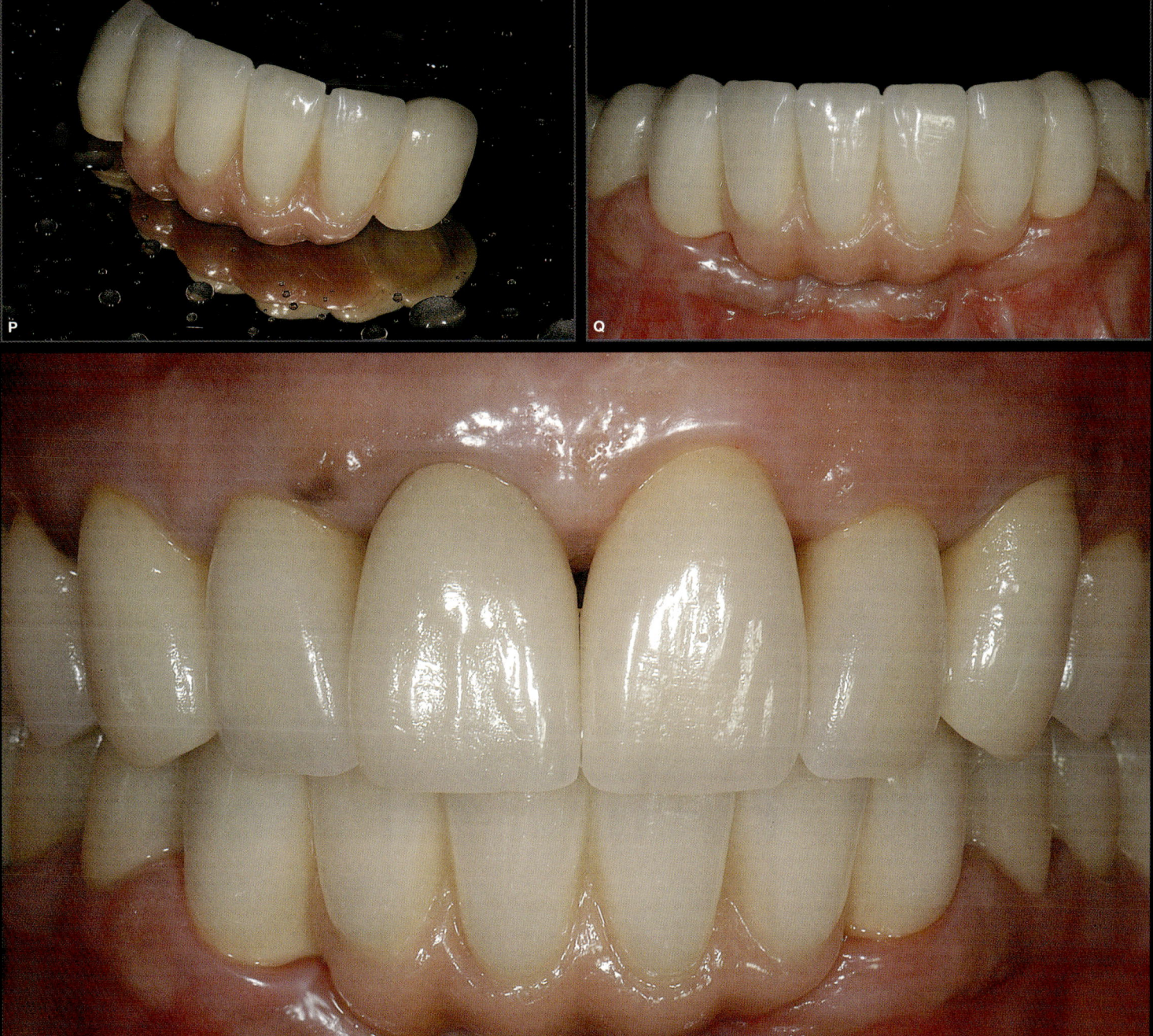

Figure 5.31 I-R - Two lower anterior implants were removed because of excessive bone loss. The patient did not want to undergo a graft procedure to replace the bone. The lower canines were prepared (**I**), vinyl polysiloxane impressions (Express, 3M ESPE) were taken and stone casts were made (**J, K**). A 6-unit FPD was waxed-up (**L**) and a zirconia-based ceramic (Lava, 3M ESPE) substructure was fabricated using the double scanning technique (**M, N, O**). The zirconia substructure was veneered using tooth-colored and pink ceramics (NobelRondo Gingiva Zirconia, Nobel Biocare) (**P**). The FPD was cemented in place using a resin-based system (RelyX Unicem, 3M ESPE) (**Q, R**). Courtesy of Dr Carlos Eduardo Sabrosa.

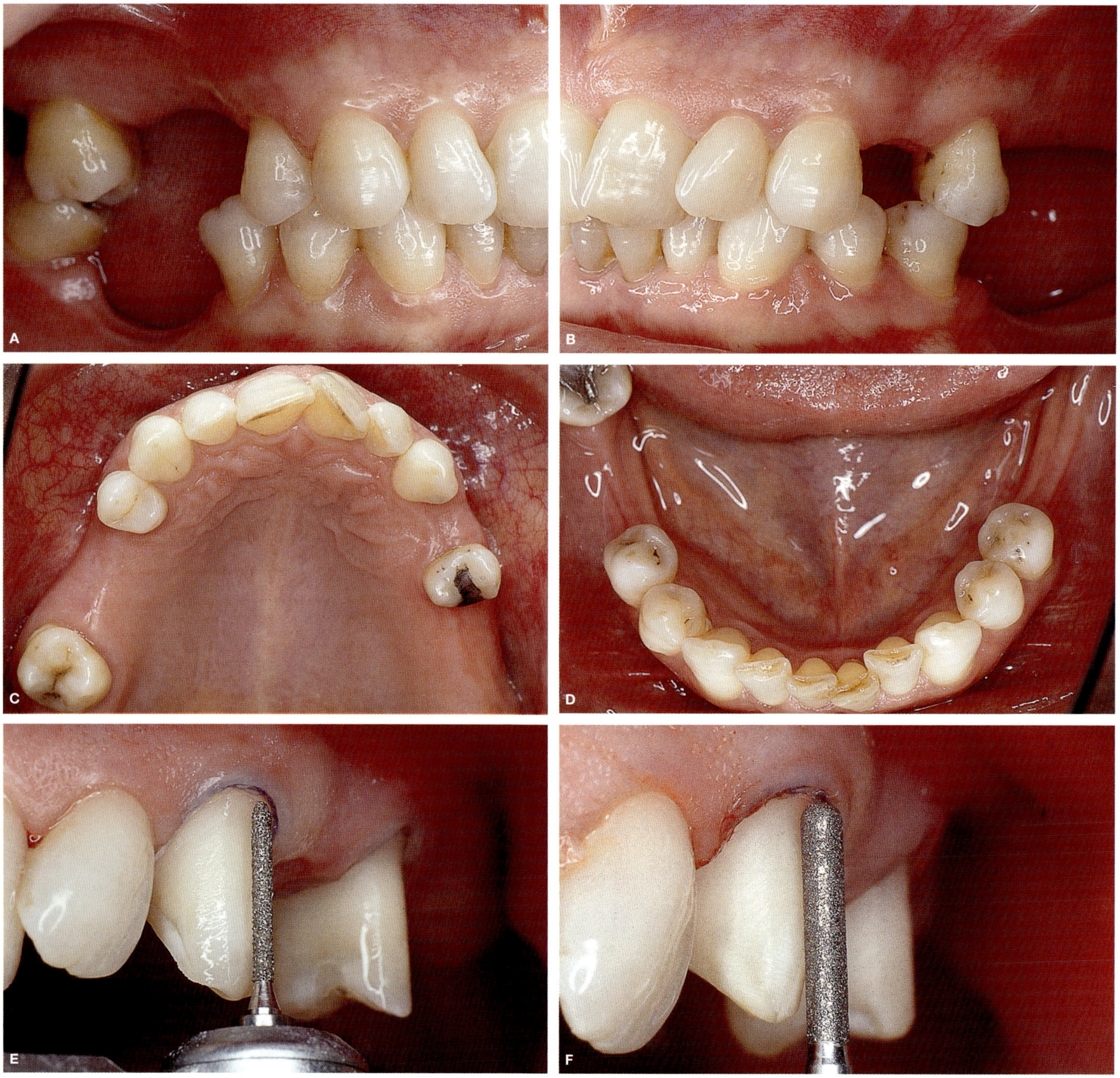

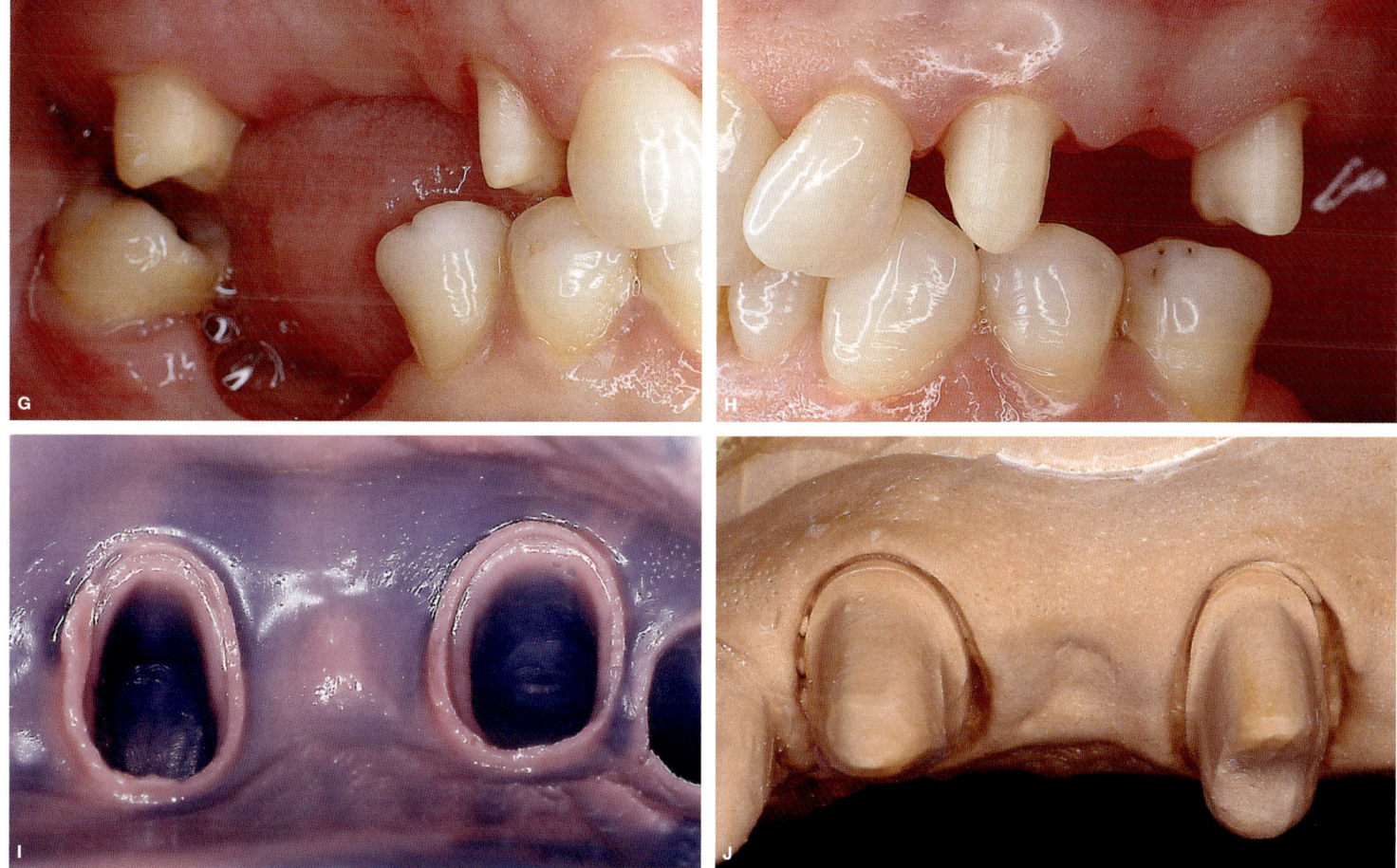

Figure 5.32 A-J - A female patient on her fifties showing some edentulous areas (**A-D**). The treatment plan involved the fabrication of three posterior all-ceramic FPD. Restorative treatment started with preparations of the upper teeth (**E-H**). Vinyl polysiloxane impressions were taken (**I**) and stone casts were made (**J**).

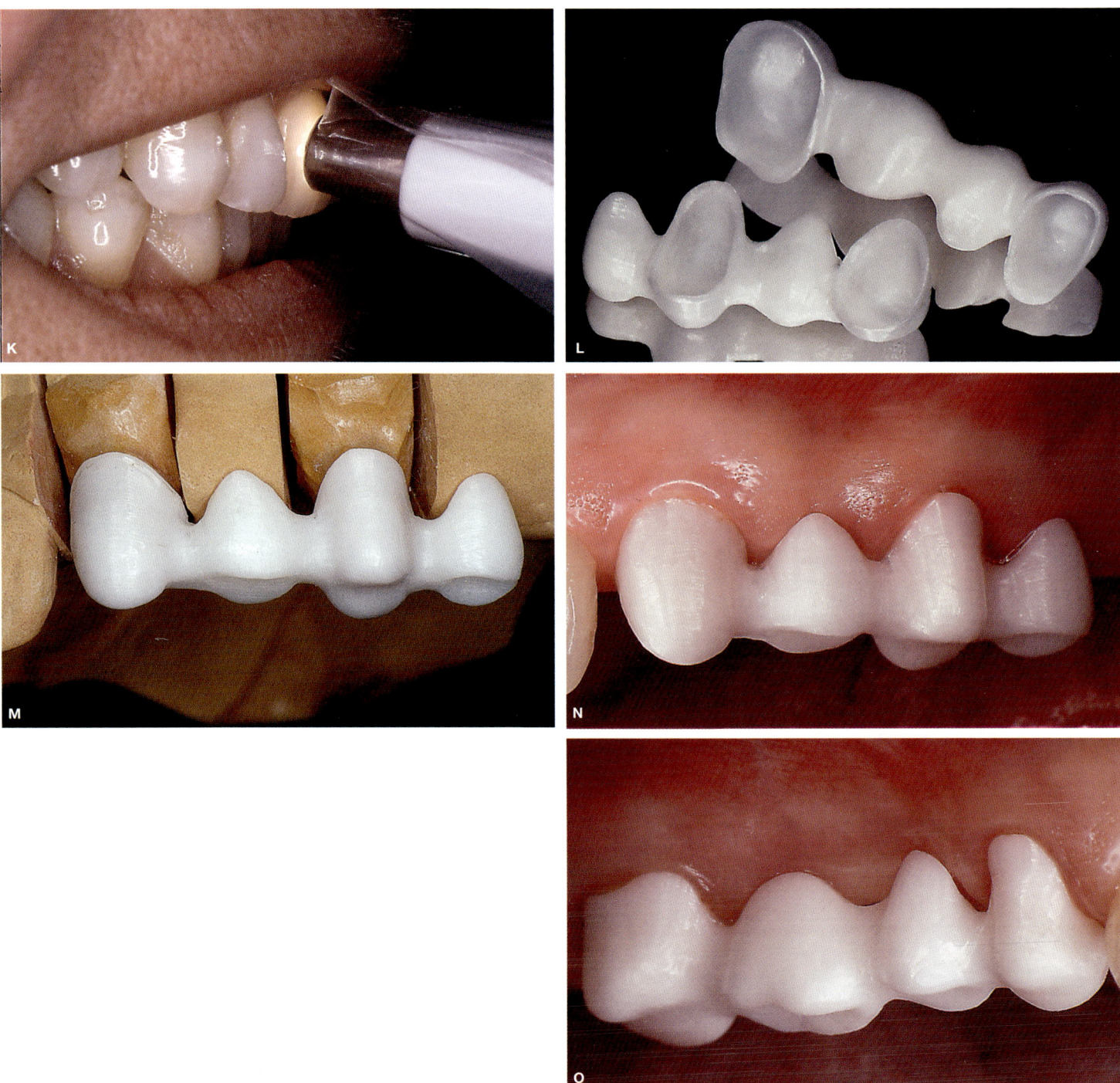

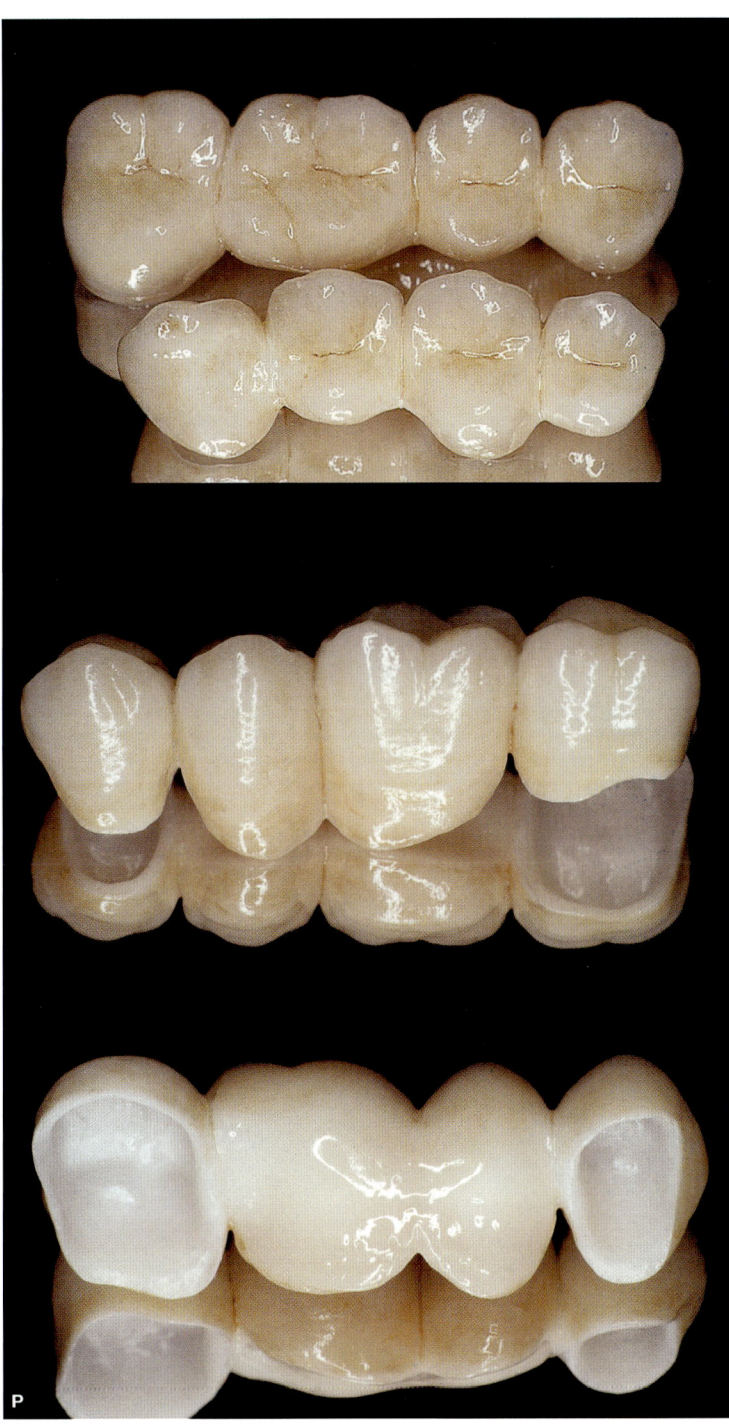

Figure 5.32 K-P - Tooth shade was selected using a shade guide (3D Master, Vita) and checked with an intra-oral spectrophotometer (Easyshade, Vita) (**K**). A CAD-CAM system (Cerec 3 InLab, Sirona) was used to scan the cast and fabricate zirconia-based ceramic substructures (In-Ceram YZ, Vita) that were tried in place (**L-O**). A feldspathic ceramic (VM9, Vita) was used to veneer the zirconia substructures (**P**).

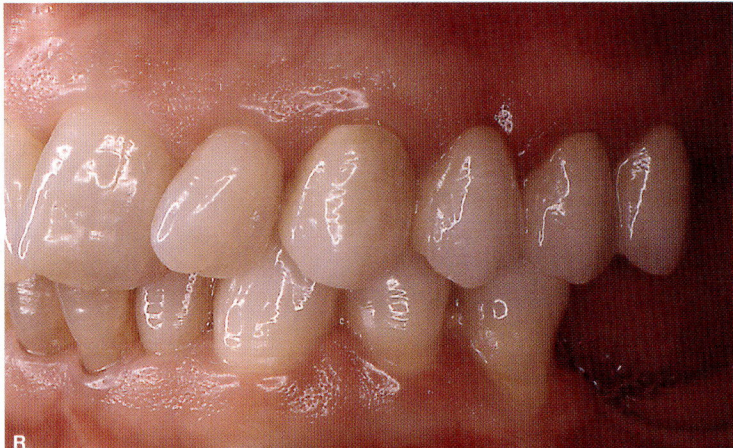

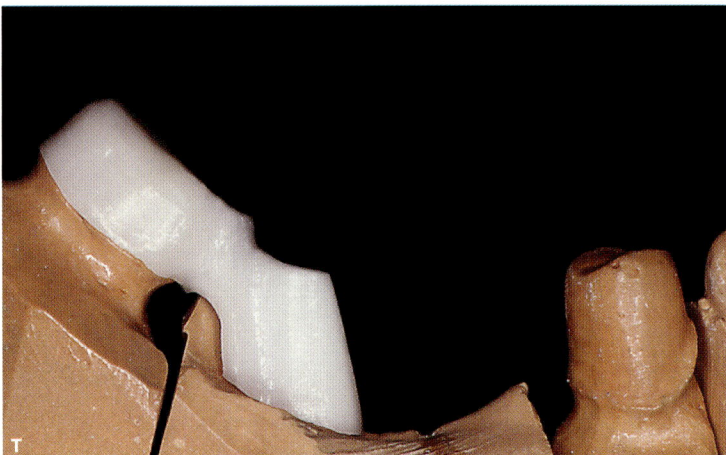

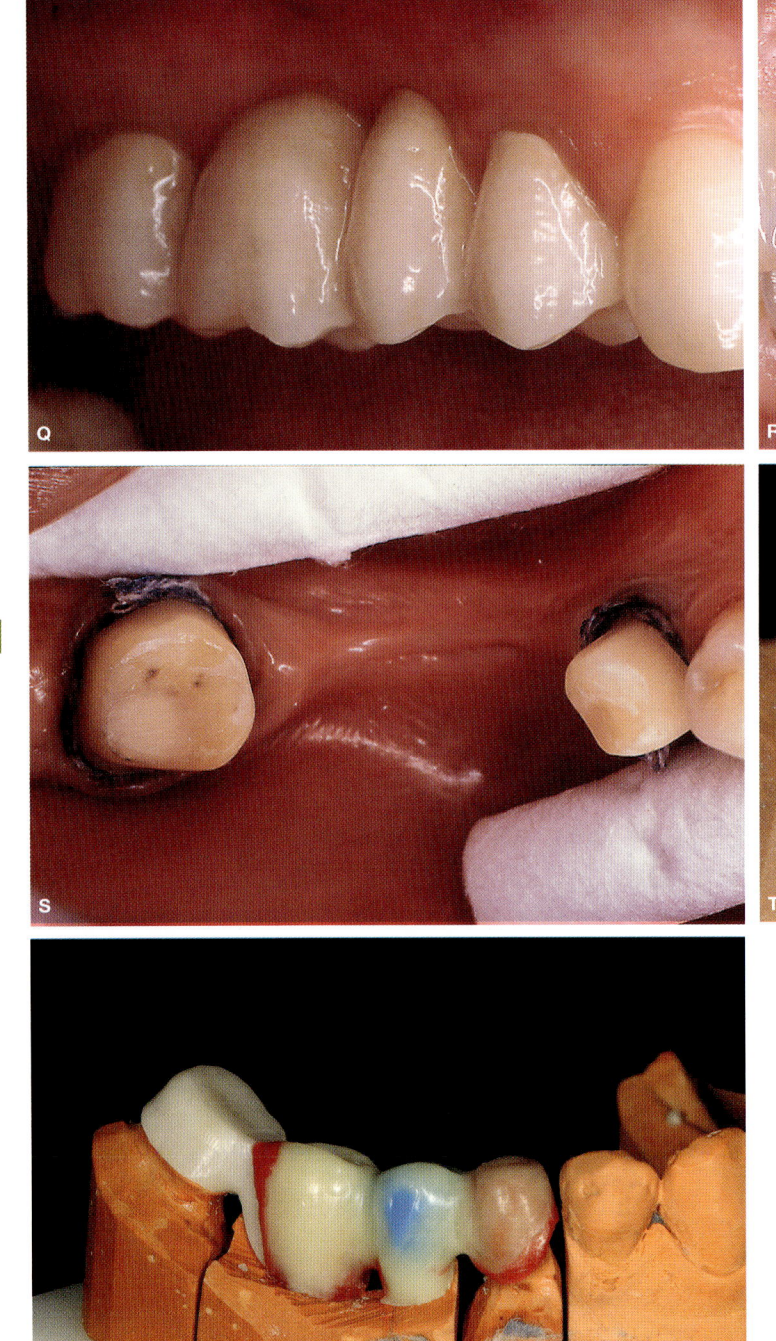

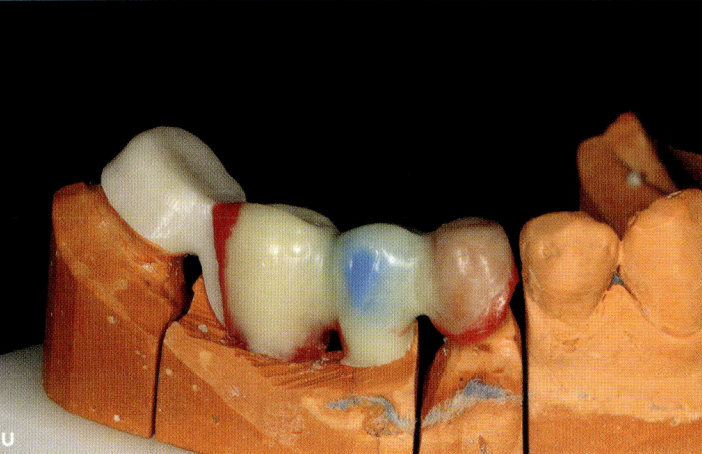

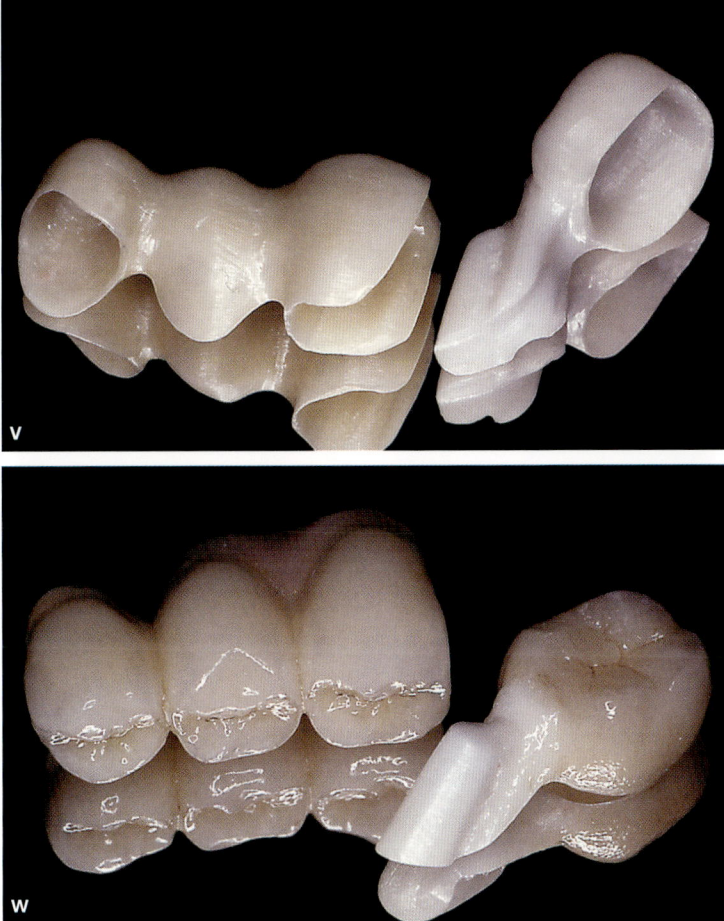

Figure 5.32 Q-W - The FPD were cemented in place using a self-etching resin-based luting system (RelyX Unicem, 3M ESPE) (**Q**, **R**). The right lower teeth were prepared (**S**), impressions were taken and stone casts made. An atypical all-ceramic FPD was designed because of the unfavorable path of insertion. A two-part bridge (In-Ceram YZ and VM9, Vita) using a precision attachment was fabricated using 3D CAD-CAM technology (Cerec 3 InLab, Sirona) (**T**-**W**).

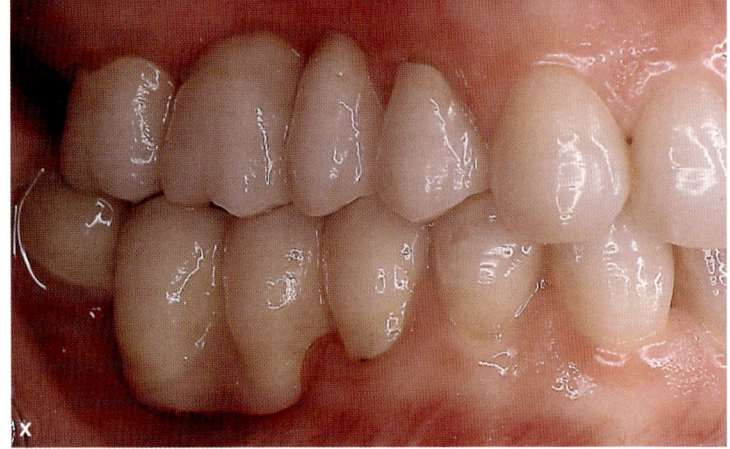

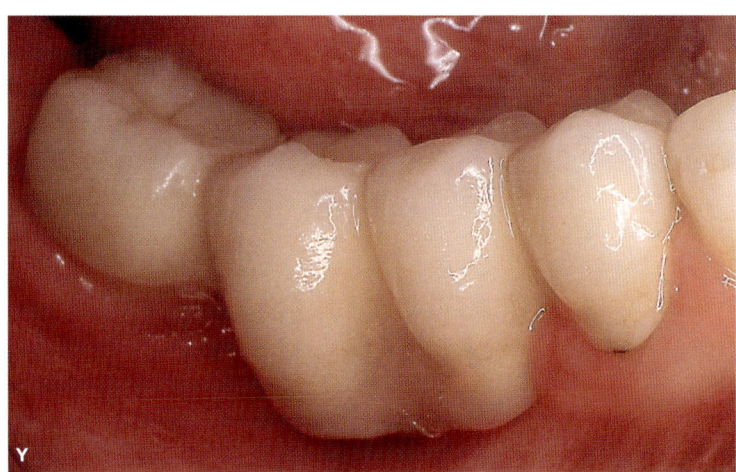

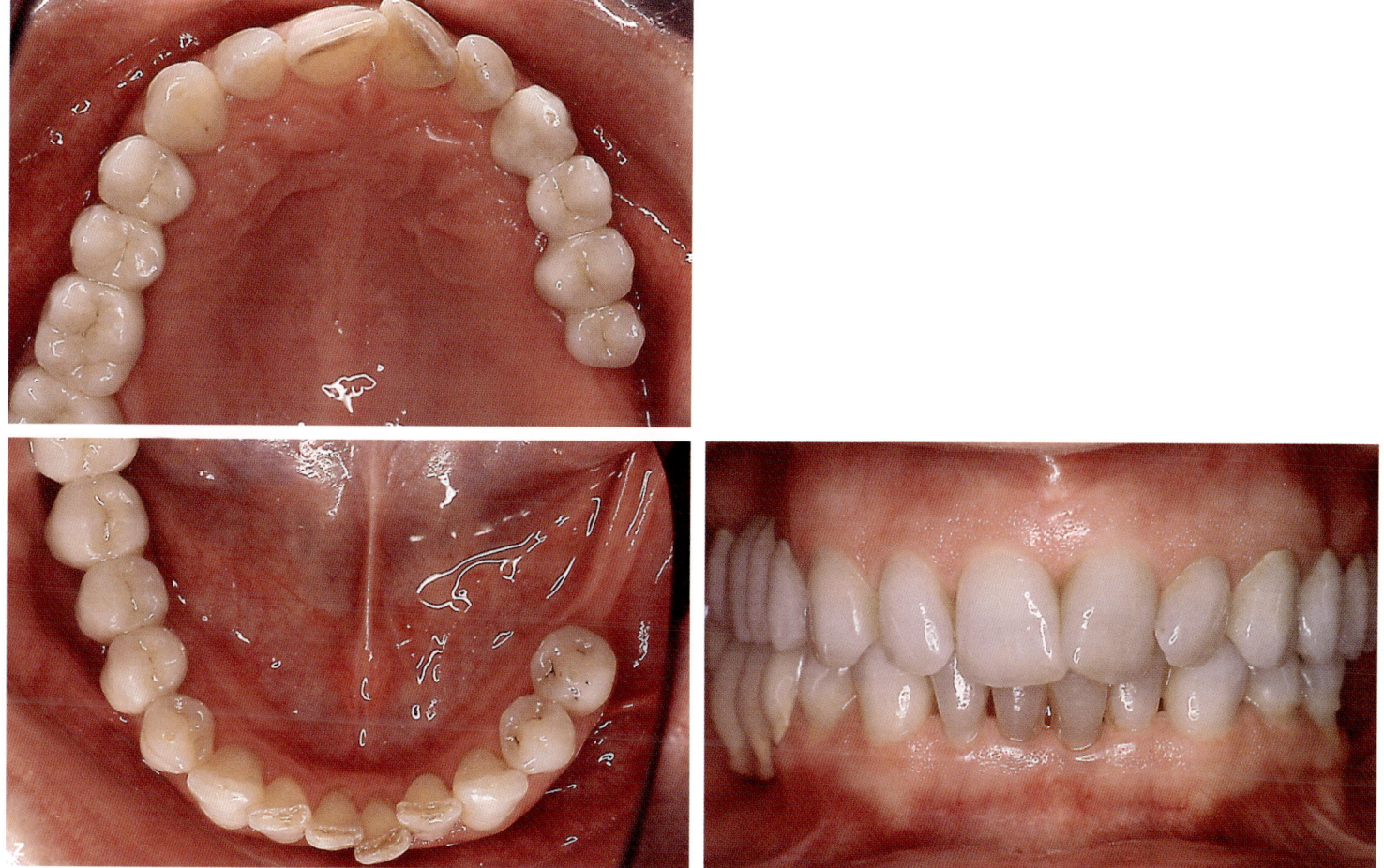

Figure 5.32 X-Z - The FPD, including the attachment, was cemented in place using a resin-based adhesive system (RelyX Unicem, 3M ESPE) (**X-Z**). Courtesy of Dr. M. Groten, University of Tübingen, Germany.

Clinical studies on FPD have reported on a variety of success rates depending on the system evaluated. Metal-ceramic restorations are well-studied and still very popular worldwide, having success rates of 72-87% at 10 years, 69-74% at 15 years, and about 55% after 30 years. However, most of the reported failures are related to secondary caries, which is often a patient-related response. Therefore, metal-ceramic restorations have become the clinical gold standard in FPD and other ceramic systems have to demonstrate similar success rate in order to replace them.

Notwithstanding, the esthetic demand and the less biocompatible non-noble alloy systems are the main reasons for the increasing interest and use of all-ceramic systems. In this context, the zirconia-based core ceramics, *e.g.* Y-TZP, have been considered the best candidate to substitute the metal frameworks (Lawn *et al.*, 2001; Raigrodski, 2004). This can be explained comparing the mechanical properties of the zirconia-based ceramics with other dental ceramics (Table 3.3 and Fig. 3.22).

The competition for high strength ceramics has led the manufacturers to launch many high crystalline content ceramics with few of them claiming strength values above 1,000 MPa (Table 3.3 and Fig. 3.22). Yet, the fracture toughness values are still well below the ones for metals. In addition, the mechanical properties of the veneering ceramics, which are exposed to direct occlusal contact, have not been significantly improved and ceramic chipping is still a clinical problem. Nevertheless, the first clinical studies on all-ceramic three-unit FPD were only reported in the 1990s.

Some of the all-ceramic systems used for single-unit crowns are also recommended by their manufacturers for anterior 3-unit FPD: a glass-infiltrated alumina (In-Ceram alumina, Vita) and a lithium disilicate-based glass-ceramic (IPS Empress 2, Ivoclar – now IPS e.max Press). Although, some clinical studies also used the In-Ceram alumina for FPDs involving the posterior teeth (Table 5.4). A 3-year study on 61 three-unit In-Ceram alumina FPDs cemented with glass ionomer cement reported survival rates of 100% for anteriors and 83% for posterior teeth, with fractures occurring through the connector area (Sorensen *et al.*, 1998). In another study of 42 FPDs (27 cantilevered 2-unit FPDs and 15 3-unit FPDs; 62% of all FPDs involving a posterior tooth), the overall survival rate was 93% at 5 years and 83% after 10 years, but 88% after 10 years for the 3-unit FPDs (Olsson *et al.*, 2003). Cantilevered 2-unit (n=21) and conventional 3-unit (n=16) anterior In-Ceram alumina FPDs were examined in another study that reported a 5-year survival rate of 74% for the 3-unit FPDs and 92% for the 2-unit FPDs (Kern, 2005). The results of this study also showed that when one connector fractured, the other was quite stable when left as a cantilevered unit. The survival rates for IPS Empress 2 FPDs range from 50% to 93% at 2 years (Table 5.4).

The indication of all-ceramic FPD to restore the posterior region (molars) was only possible with the introduction of tougher core materials such as the zirconia reinforced glass-infiltrated alumina (In-Ceram Zirconia, Vita), and the yttrium oxide partially-stabilized tetragonal zirconia polycrystal material (Y-TZP) such as: Cercon Zirconia (Dentsply Ceramco), Lava (3M ESPE) (Fig. 5.31), and In-Ceram YZ (Vita) (Fig. 5.32). A study evaluated the clinical performance of In-Ceram Zirconia posterior FPDs (n=18) after 3 years of service and reported just 1 failure due to root fracture, resulting in a survival rate of 94.5% (Suárez *et al.*, 2004). In another study, the success rate of 33 posterior zirconia-based FPDs (Cercon) was 98%. However, the overall survival rate was 74% due to other complications, such as secondary caries (22%) and chipping of the veneering ceramic (15%) (Sailer *et al.*, 2007). In these two clinical studies (n=51) only one fracture of the zirconia-based framework was reported, which shows a very promising trend for all-ceramic FPDs (Table 5.4).

It is important to remind clinicians and researchers that the Consolidated Standards of Reporting Trials (CONSORT) is an evidence-based, minimum set of recommendations for planning and reporting randomized controlled trials.

Table 5.4 - Peer-reviewed studies of survival rate of all-ceramic three-unit fixed partial dentures (two conventional retainers).

All-ceramic material	Study	No. of FPD		Fabrication method	Observation period in months (mean)	Survival rate (period)
		Anterior	Posterior			
In-Ceram Alumina*	Pröbster, 1993	7	8	Slip cast	2-35 (16.3)	93% (1 year)††
	Pang, 1995	7	— #	Slip cast	4.5-21 (NI)	100%
	Sorensen *et al.*, 1998	21	40	Slip cast	36 (36)	88.5%
	Steyern *et al.*, 2001	—	20	Slip cast	60 (60)	90%
	Olsson *et al.*, 2003	8	7	Slip cast	2-110 (76)	88% (10 years)††
	Kern, 2005	16	—	Slip cast	3-146 (76)	67% (5 years)††
In-Ceram Zirconia*	Suárez *et al.*, 2004	—	18	Slip cast	32-36 (NI)	94.5% (3 years)††
IPS Empress 2‡	Marquardt and Strub, 2006	31	—	Hot pressed	6-60 (NI)	70% (5 years)††
	Taskonak and Sertgöz, 2006	12	8	Hot pressed	24 (24)	50% (2 years)††
	Esquivel-Upshaw *et al.*, 2004	—	30	Hot pressed	24 (24)	93%
Cercon Zirconia†	Sailer *et al.*, 2007	—	33	CAD/CAM	1-60 (53.4)	74% (5 years)††

* In-Ceram Alumina and In-Ceram Zirconia are manufactured by Vita Zahnfabrik, Bad Sackingen, Germany.

‡ IPS Empress 2 is now IPS e.max Press. It is manufactured by Ivoclar Vivadent, Schann, Liechtenstein.

† Cercon Zirconia is manufactured by Dentsply Ceramco, York, Pa.

Dash indicates none.

†† Kaplan-Meier survival rate was calculated for the endpoint listed.

NI: Not included.

In the clinical studies presented above, the most common causes of all-ceramic structural failures were (1) fracture initiated in the connector area of FPDs, either at the core-veneer interface or at the gingival embrasure; and (2) chipping of the veneering material. Few well designed in vitro studies using elaborated FEA models (Fig. 3.18 C-F) have showed that the connector area is the point of higher stress concentration, mainly depending on the cross-sectional area of the connector (Fig. 3.17) and the design of the embrasures. Two in vitro studies suggested that the connector of an all-ceramic 3-unit FPD should not be veneered in the gingival area, which is under tension during mastication, to avoid delamination of the veneer ceramic (Guazzato et al., 2004; White et al., 2005). Yet, this subject should also be examined considering the deleterious LTD effect on zirconia-base substructures exposed to the oral environment.

A stress concentration at the core-veneer interface is resulted from great differences in the elastic modulus of the two ceramics. The causes of veneer chipping may be related to: (1) residual stresses at the core-veneer interface, (2) differences in thermal conductivity (thermal incompatibility) between core and veneer materials (Table 1.1), (3) thick veneer layer, (4) sliding Hertzian-type contact (Fig. 5.33), and (4) poor bonding between core and veneer ceramics. Clinically, sliding occlusal contacts cause more damage than uniaxial contacts (Fig. 5.33). It is worth mentioning that bite force, and consequently the occlusal contact area, may change among patients but the contact pressure is basically around 38 MPa (Hidaka et al., 1999). Nevertheless, chipping should be classified as a fracture failure, since a permanent and esthetically long-term intra-oral repair is often not possible.

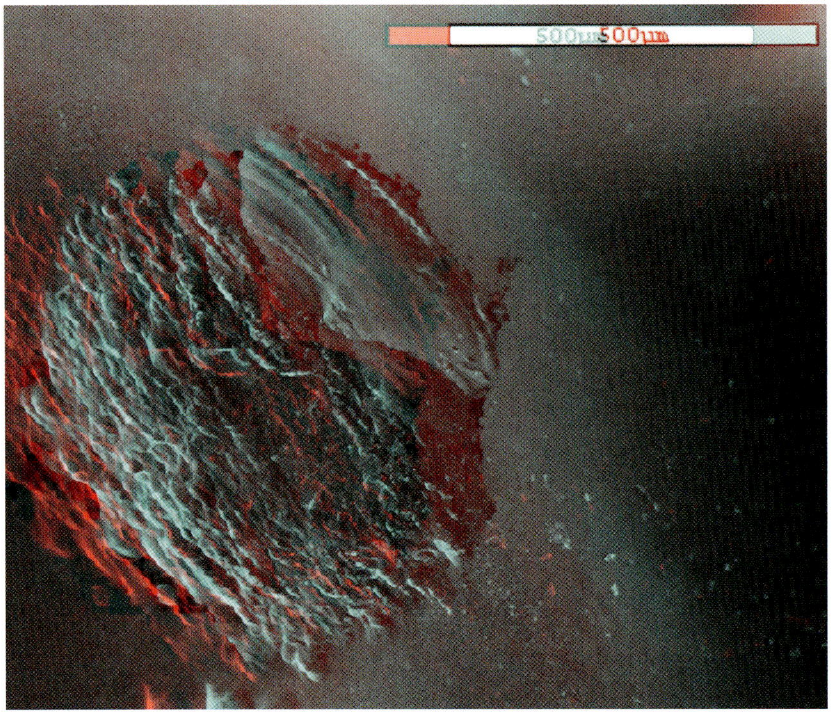

Figure 5.33 - Sliding occlusal contact causing surface roughness and chipping of the veneering ceramic.

The presented clinical data is related to the increase of crystalline content (alumina and zirconia particles) in dental ceramics, resulting in a significant improvement in the mechanical properties of these materials and allowing for all-ceramic FPDs. However, these polycrystalline ceramics are hard to machine and resistant to acid etching. Therefore, the creation of mechanically retentive ceramic surfaces for resin bonding is a challenge for the clinician.

The adhesive principles and mechanisms for bonding to all types of ceramics were presented in the previous chapters and clinically illustrated in this chapter. It has been explained that the use of silica coating (silicatization) systems (*e.g.* Rocatec and Cojet, 3M ESPE) create a silica layer on acid-resistant ceramic surfaces (Fig. 4.9 and Table 4.1) because of the high-speed surface impact of the silica-modified alumina particles on the ceramic surface, producing a tribochemical effect that promotes the resin bonding via two mechanisms: (1) the creation of a rough and retentive ceramic surface allowing for micromechanical bonding to resin; and (2) the promotion of a chemical bond between the silanated silica coated ceramic surface and the resin-based material. Another way of improving adhesion to acid-resistant ceramics is using an adhesive resin system containing the phosphate (MDP) monomers.

Therefore, there are two clinical strategies to resin bond acid-resistant ceramic restorations:

1. Improving mechanical retention and introducing an irregular silica layer onto the high crystalline content or polycrystalline ceramic surface

using a silica coating system (*e.g.* Rocatec or Cojet systems, 3M ESPE) followed by a silane coupling agent, which promotes a chemical bond to any resin-based adhesive/cement system.

2. Improving the chemical bond using an adhesive/cement system containing a ceramic primer such as MDP monomer (*e.g.* Panavia F2.0, Kuraray).

Airborne particle abrasion using alumina particles (sand blasting) is a controversial ceramic surface treatment. Some studies suggested the use of this treatment to create a rough ceramic surface, which is activated for resin bonding. Other reports showed that sand blasting the ceramic significantly decreased the failure load of cemented ceramic samples. As not many clinical trials are reported on the resin adhesion to acid-resistant ceramics, clinicians should avoid using non evidence-based bonding procedures. Future studies should examine processes to deposit a regular silica layer on the bonding surface of acid-resistant ceramics, which could be traditionally treated as for acid-sensitive ceramics, that is, HF-etched, silanated and resin bonded. Another alternative is to investigate other "metal" primers with monomers such as thiophosphoric methacrylate (MEPS), vinylbenzyl-n-propyl amino-triazine-dithiol (VBATDT), and thiouracil (MTU-6), which may also promote resin bond to metal oxide-based ceramics. Nevertheless, resin bonded ceramic restorations are complex function multi-layered systems where structural and bonding properties are crucial.

As mentioned, dental ceramic restorations may fracture and a critical interpretation of the fracture surfaces should be used to understand and explain the failure process and to improve materials, design and techniques. However, it has been shown (Fig 3.19) that interpreting fractured surfaces from glassy materials is fairly straightforward, but recognizing clear surface markings on some of the coarse-grained or polycrystalline ceramics, may become an intricate procedure.

Clinically, a small veneer chipped restoration may often be salvaged via resin-based composite repair (Figs. 5.2, 5.17), but larger factures generally result in the complete removal of the failed restorations (Fig. 5.1). Therefore, the fractured surface should be left undisturbed after failure occurred, that is, no subsequent grinding, scratching, rubbing or smearing should occurred, which in effect "erases" the surface features left during the fracture process. Often direct examination of fracture surface under the microscope is not possible because one part of the restoration is still strongly cemented onto its abutment while the other was lost. In these instances a replica of the remaining fracture surface must be obtained. To this end an intra-oral impression of the exposed fractured surface using a low viscosity impression material is taken. The impression is poured with cold mounting epoxy resin and gold coated for SEM analysis (Fig 5.34).

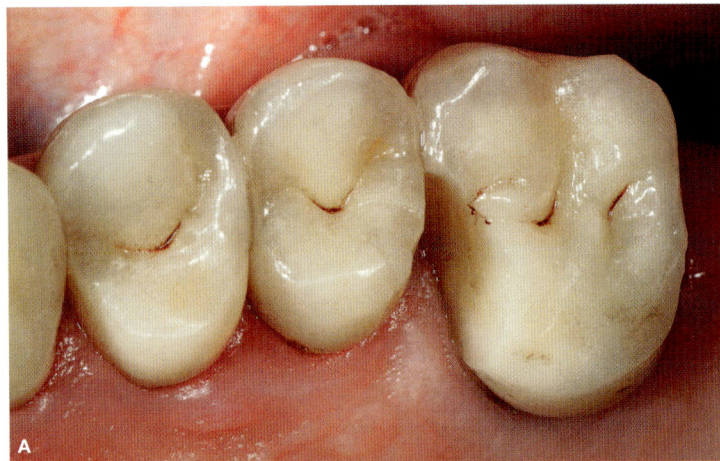

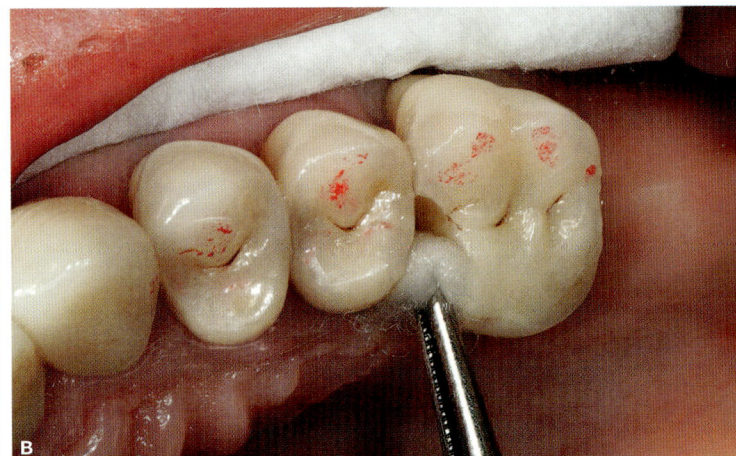

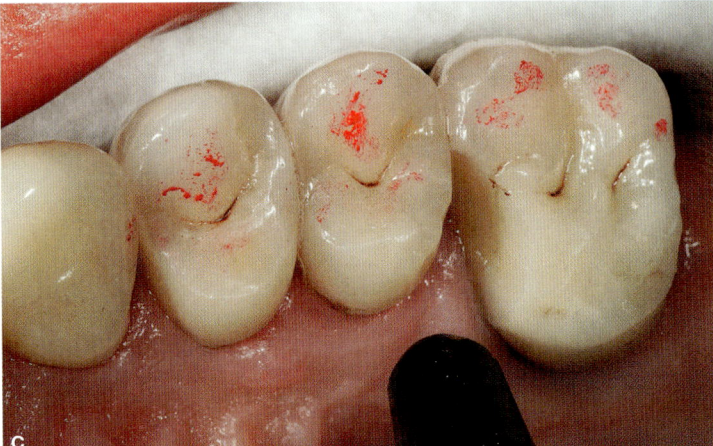

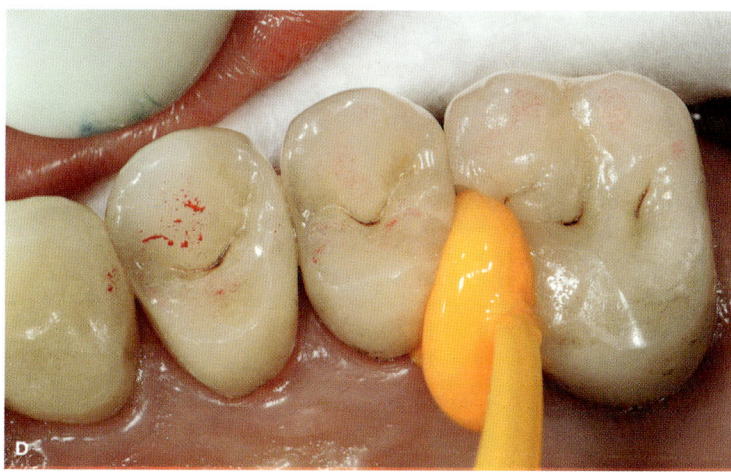

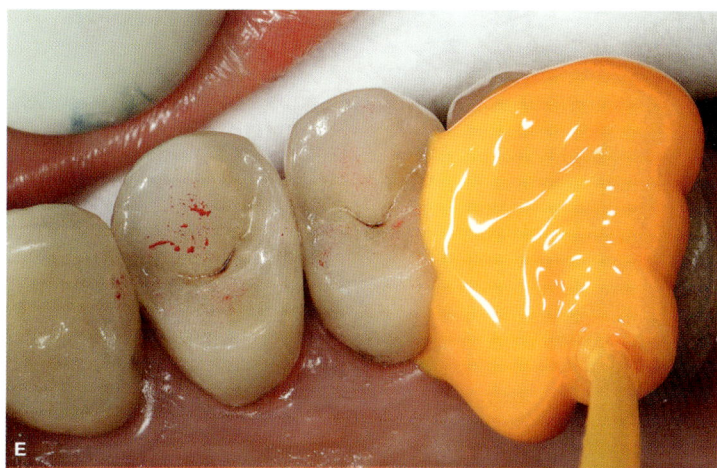

Figure 5.34 A-F - A- Fracture of the veneering ceramic (Procera AllCeram on Procera Alumina substructure, Nobel Biocare) of an upper left molar after 4.2 years of service. After having cleaned the fractured surface with an alcohol cotton pellet (**B**) and air-dried (**C**), an ultralight vinyl polysiloxane impression material (Express (USA) or Imprint (Europe), 3M ESPE) was injected first on the fractured zone (**D**) then around the whole crown (**E**). After set, the impression mold was removed (**F**) and a replica was cast with epoxy resin reproducing the fractured crown.

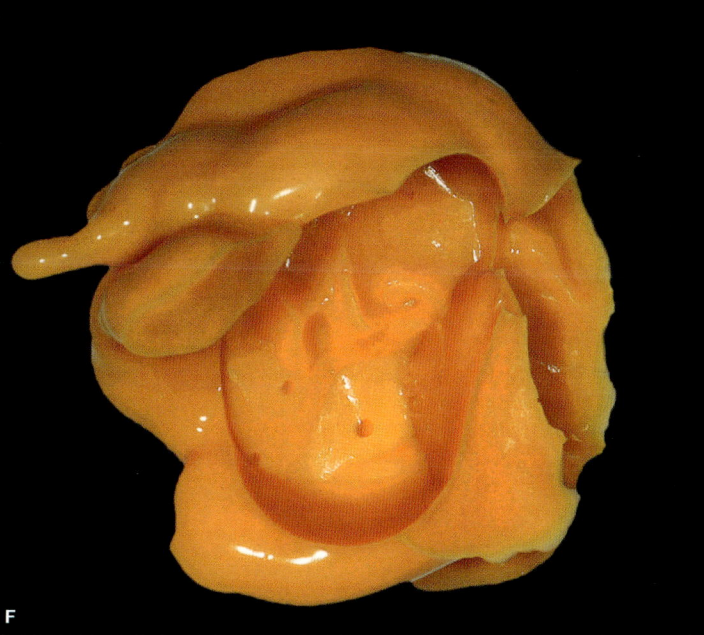

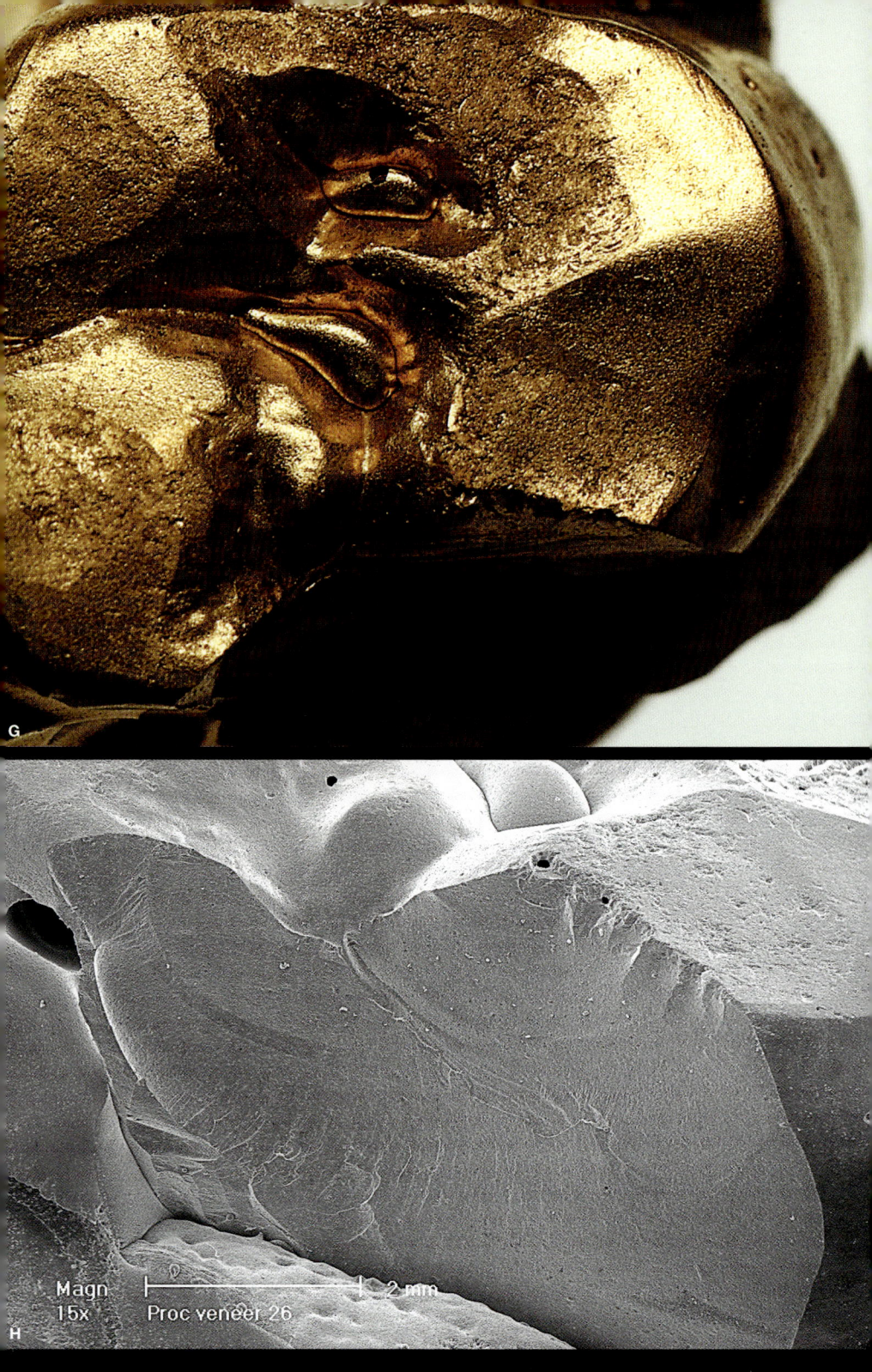

Magn
15x   Proc veneer 26   2 mm

Figure 5.34 G-H - The replica is gold coated (**G**) for SEM examination (**H**).

Final considerations

It is universally true that the stronger (and tougher) ceramics are more opaque (less translucent) than esthetic ceramics (porcelains, glasses). Therefore, where tooth restoration involves esthetic demands without much structural need, single layers of tooth-colored ceramics can be used (*i.e.* monolithic veneers). When structural demands require higher strength materials, the substructure of less esthetic ceramics has to be veneered with tooth-colored porcelains. Layered ceramics are also used to mask discolored preparations. These information along with evidence from many clinical studies suggest that clinicians may chose from any all-ceramic system based on esthetic needs for veneers, intra-coronal, and full-coverage restoration of single-rooted anterior teeth. Only a few all-ceramic systems have been successful for the restoration of molars, and additional clinical factors such as adequate preparation depth and cementation can overwhelm materials considerations.

Although no equivalent long-term data exists as for metal-ceramics (74% at 15 years), many all-ceramic systems have greater than 90% success after 5 years. Reasonable evidence is available for anterior three-unit FPDs in lithium disilicate-based ceramic, In-Ceram Alumina and In-Ceram Zirconia. For 3-unit FPDs involving a molar, expert consensus from the ISO working group responsible for dental ceramic standards suggest that only zirconia-based systems are indicated.

In the future, transformation-toughened zirconia may stand out as the most successful all-ceramic system, irrespective of the clinical indication.

Nevertheless, chipping of the veneering ceramic on zirconia restoration remains a problem to be solved. The evidence provided in this book should enable clinicians to enter into informed-consent decisions with their patients who desire all-ceramic restorations.

Clinical data strongly suggests that higher success rates are achieved when ceramics can be bonded to teeth using resin-based cements, instead of glass ionomer or zinc phosphate cements. On the ceramic side, bonding requires a heterogeneous material that can be selectively etched to create micromechanical adherence features (acid-sensitive ceramics), or the acid-resistant ceramic surface has to be activated by a primer (Fig. 4.1). Manufacturers routinely provide cementation recommendations that should be given serious consideration.

This chapter presented current evidence suggesting an acceptable clinical longevity of resin bonded all-ceramic restorations to go along with their long lasting esthetics.

Selected readings

- Albert FE, El-Mowafy OM. Marginal adaptation and microleakage of Procera AllCeram crowns with four cements. *Int J Prosthodont*, 17:529-535, 2004.
- Banks RG. Conservative posterior ceramic restorations: a literature review. *J Prosthet Dent*, 63:619-626, 1990.
- Berman MA. The clinical performance of ceramic inlays: a review. *Aust Dent J*, 44:157-168, 1999.
- Bindl A, Mörmann WH. An up to 5-year clinical evaluation of posterior In-Ceram CAD/CAM core crowns. *Int J Prosthodont*, 15:451-456, 2002.
- Bindl A, Mörmann WH. Survival rate of mono-ceramic and ceramic-core CAD/CAM-generated anterior crowns over 2-5 years. *Eur J Oral Sci*, 112:197-204, 2004.
- Bogacki RE, Hunt RJ, del Aguila M, Smith WR. Survival analysis of posterior restorations using an insurance claims database. *Oper Dent*, 27:488-492, 2002.
- Boscato N, Della Bona A, Cury AADB. Influence of ceramic pre-treatments on tensile bond strength and mode of failure of resin bonded to ceramics. *Am J Dent*, 20:103-108, 2007.
- Della Bona A, Barghi N. Removal of partially or fully polymerized resin from porcelain veneers. *J Prosthet Dent*, 69:443-444, 1993.
- Della Bona A, Kelly JR. The clinical success of all-ceramic restorations. *J Am Dent Assoc*, 139 (9 suppl):8S-13S, 2008.
- Della Bona A, Barrett AA, Rosa V, Pinzetta C. Visual and instrumental agreement in dental shade selection: Three distinct observer populations and shade matching protocols. *Dent Mater*, in press.
- Denry I, Kelly JR. State of the art of zirconia for dental applications. *Dent Mater*, 24:299-307, 2008.
- El-Mowafy O, Brochu JF. Longevity and clinical performance of IPS-Empress ceramic restorations: a literature review. *J Can Dent Assoc*, 68:233-237, 2002.
- Esquivel-Upshaw JF, Anusavice KJ, Young H, Jones J, Gibbs C. Clinical performance of a lithia disilicate-based core ceramic for three-unit posterior FPDs. *Int J Prosthodont*, 17:469-475, 2004.
- Fasbinder DJ. Clinical performance of chairside CAD/CAM restorations. *J Am Dent Assoc*, 137(Suppl):22S-31S, 2006.
- Fradeani M, Aquilano A. Clinical experience with Empress crowns. *Int J Prosthodont*, 10:241-247, 1997.
- Fradeani M. Six-year follow-up with Empress veneers. *Int J Periodontics Restorative Dent*, 18:216-225, 1998.
- Fradeani M, Aquilano A, Corrado M. Clinical experience with In-Ceram Spinell crowns: 5-year follow-up. *Int J Periodontics Restorative Dent*, 22:525-533, 2002.
- Fradeani M, Redemagni M. An 11-year clinical evaluation of leucite-reinforced glass-ceramic crowns: a retrospective study. *Quintessence Int*, 33:503-510, 2002.
- Fradeani M, Redemagni M, Corrado M. Porcelain laminate veneers: 6- to 12-year clinical evaluation--a retrospective study. *Int J Periodontics Restorative Dent*, 25:9-17, 2005.

- Fradeani M, D'Amelio M, Redemagni M, Corrado M. Five-year follow-up with Procera all-ceramic crowns. *Quintessence Int*, 36:105-113, 2005.
- Guazzato M, Proos K, Sara G, Swain MV. Strength, reliability, and mode of fracture of bilayered porcelain/core ceramics. *Int J Prosthodont*, 17:142-149, 2004.
- Haselton DR, Diaz-Arnold AM, Hillis SL. Clinical assessment of high-strength all-ceramic crowns. *J Prosthet Dent*, 83:396-401, 2000.
- Heffernan MJ, Aquilino SA, Diaz-Arnold AM, Haselton DR, Stanford CM, Vargas MA. Relative translucency of six all-ceramic systems. Part II: core and veneer materials. *J Prosthet Dent*, 88:10-15, 2002.
- Hidaka O, Iwasaki M, Saito M, Morimoto T. Influence of clenching intensity on bite force balance, occlusal contact area, and average bite pressure. *J Dent Res*, 78:1336-1344, 1999.
- Kelly JR. Dental ceramics: current thinking and trends. *Dent Clin North Am*, 48:513-530, 2004.
- Kelly JR. Machinable Ceramics. In: Mörmann WH (ed.) State of the Art of CAD/CAM Restorations. 20 Years of CEREC. Berlin: *Quintessenz Verlags-GmbH*, 2006.
- Kelly JR, Denry I. Stabilized zirconia as a structural ceramic: An overview. *Dent Mater*, 24:289-298, 2008.
- Kern M. Clinical long-term survival of two-retainer and single-retainer all-ceramic resin-bonded fixed partial dentures. *Quintessence Int*, 36:141-7, 2005.
- Krämer N, Frankenberger R. Clinical performance of bonded leucite-reinforced glass ceramic inlays and onlays after eight years. *Dent Mater*, 21:262-271, 2005.
- Lawn BR, Deng Y, Thompson VP. Use of contact testing in the characterization and design of all-ceramic crown-like layer structures: a review. *J Prosthet Dent*, 86:495-510, 2001.
- Layton D, Walton T. An up to 16-year prospective study of 304 porcelain veneers. *Int J Prosthodont*, 20:389-396, 2007.
- Lehner C, Studer S, Brodbeck U, Schärer P. Short-term results of IPS-Empress full-porcelain crowns. *J Prosthodont*, 6:20-30, 1997.
- Lohbauer U, Krämer N, Petschelt A, Frankenberger R. Correlation of in vitro fatigue data and in vivo clinical performance of a glass-ceramic material. *Dent Mater*, 24:39-44, 2008.
- Magne P. Immediate dentin sealing: a fundamental procedure for indirect bonded restorations. *J Esthet Restor Dent*, 17:144-154, 2005.
- Magne P, So WS, Cascione D. Immediate dentin sealing supports delayed restoration placement. *J Prosthet Dent*, 98:166-174, 2007.
- Marquardt P, Strub JR. Survival rates of IPS empress 2 all-ceramic crowns and fixed partial dentures: results of a 5-year prospective clinical study. *Quintessence Int*, 37:253-259, 2006.
- Martin N, Jedynakiewicz NM. Clinical performance of CEREC ceramic inlays: a systematic review. *Dent Mater*, 15:54-61, 1999.
- McLaren EA, White SN. Survival of In-Ceram crowns in a private practice: a prospective clinical trial. *J Prosthet Dent*, 83:216-222, 2000.
- Nasedkin JN. Porcelain posterior resin-bonded restorations: current perspectives on esthetic restorative dentistry: Part II. *J Can Dent Assoc*, 54:499-506, 1988.

- Oden A, Andersson M, Krystek-Ondracek I, Magnusson D. Five-year clinical evaluation of Procera AllCeram crowns. *J Prosthet Dent*, 80:450-456, 1998.
- Odman P, Andersson B. Procera AllCeram crowns followed for 5 to 10.5 years: a prospective clinical study. *Int J Prosthodont*, 14:504-509, 2001.
- Olsson KG, Furst B, Andersson B, Carlsson GE. A long-term retrospective and clinical follow-up study of In-Ceram Alumina FPDs. *Int J Prosthodont*, 16:150-156, 2003.
- Otto T, De Nisco S. Computer-aided direct ceramic restorations: a 10-year prospective clinical study of Cerec CAD/CAM inlays and onlays. *Int J Prosthodont*, 15:122-128, 2002.
- Pallesen U, van Dijken JWV. An 8-year evaluation of sintered ceramic and glass ceramic inlays processed by the CEREC CAD/CAM system. *Eur J Oral Sci*, 108:239-246, 2000.
- Pang SE. A report of anterior In-Ceram restorations. *Ann Acad Med Singapore*, 24:33-37, 1995.
- Peumans M, Van Meerbeek B, Lambrechts P, Vanherle G. Porcelain veneers: a review of the literature. *J Dent*, 28:163-177, 2000.
- Probster L. Survival rate of In-Ceram restorations. *Int J Prosthodont*, 6:259-263, 1993.
- Probster L. Four-year clinical study of glass-infiltrated, sintered alumina crowns. *J Oral Rehab*, 23:147-151, 1996.
- Raigrodski AJ. Clinical and laboratory considerations for the use of CAD/CAM Y-TZP-based restorations. *Pract Proced Aesthet Dent*, 15:469-476, 2003.
- Raigrodski AJ. Contemporary materials and technologies for all-ceramic fixed partial dentures: a review of the literature. *J Prosthet Dent*, 92:557-562, 2004.
- Rekow ED, Harsono M, Janal M, Thompson VP, Zhang G. Factorial analysis of variables influencing stress in all-ceramic crowns. *Dent Mater*, 22:125-132, 2006.
- Sailer I, Fehér A, Filser F, Gauckler LJ, Lüthy H, Hämmerle CH. Five-year clinical results of zirconia frameworks for posterior fixed partial dentures. *Int J Prosthodont*, 20:383-388, 2007.
- Scherrer SS, De Rijk WG, Wiskott HW, Belser UC. Incidence of fractures and lifetime predictions of all-ceramic crown systems using censored data. *Am J Dent*, 14:72-80, 2001.
- Schwartz R, Davis R, Mayhew R. Effect of a ZOE temporary cement on the bond strength of a resin luting cement. *Am J Dent*, 3:28-30, 1990.
- Schwartz R, Davis R, Hilton TJ. Effect of temporary cements on the bond strength of a resin cement. *Am J Dent*, 5:147-150, 1992.
- Scotti R, Catapano S, D'Elia A. A clinical evaluation of In-Ceram crowns. *Int J Prosthodont*, 8:320-323, 1995.
- Segal BS. Retrospective assessment of 546 all-ceramic anterior and posterior crowns in a general practice. *J Prosthet Dent*, 85:544-550, 2001.
- Sjögren G, Lantto R, Granberg A, Sundström BO, Tillberg A. Clinical examination of leucite-reinforced glass-ceramic crowns (Empress) in general practice: a retrospective study. *Int J Prosthodont*, 12:122-128, 1999.
- Sjögren G, Lantto R, Tillberg A. Clinical evaluation of all-ceramic crowns (Dicor) in general practice. *J Prosthet Dent*, 81:277-284, 1999.
- Sjögren G, Molin M, van Dijken JW. A 10-year prospective evaluation of CAD/CAM-manufactured (Cerec) ceramic inlays cemented with a chemically cured or dual-cured resin composite. *Int J Prosthodont*, 17:241-246, 2004.

- Sorensen JA, Choi C, Fanuscu MI, Mito WT. IPS Empress crown system: three-year clinical trial results. *J Calif Dent Assoc*, 26:130-136, 1998.
- Sorensen JA, Kang SK, Torres TJ, Knode H. In-Ceram fixed partial dentures: three-year clinical trial results. *J Calif Dent Assoc*, 26:207-214, 1998.
- Steyern PV, Jönsson O, Nilner K. Five-year evaluation of posterior all-ceramic three-unit (In-Ceram) FPDs. *Int J Prosthodont*, 14:379-384, 2001.
- Stoll R, Cappel I, Jablonski-Momeni A, Pieper K, Stachniss V. Survival of inlays and partial crowns made of IPS empress after a 10-year observation period and in relation to various treatment parameters. *Oper Dent*, 32:556-563, 2007.
- Suárez MJ, Lozano JF, Paz Salido M, Martínez F. Three-year clinical evaluation of In-Ceram Zirconia posterior FPDs. *Int J Prosthodont*, 17:35-38, 2004.
- Summitt JB, Robbins JW, Hilton TJ, Schwartz RS. *Fundamentals of operative dentistry: a contemporary approach*. 3rd ed. Chicago: Quintessence Publishing Co., 2006.
- Suputtamongkol K, Anusavice KJ, Suchatlampong C, Sithiamnuai P, Tulapornchai C. Clinical performance and wear characteristics of veneered lithia-disilicate-based ceramic crowns. *Dent Mater*, 24:667-673, 2008.
- Taskonak B, Sertgöz A. Two-year clinical evaluation of lithia-disilicate-based all-ceramic crowns and fixed partial dentures. *Dent Mater*, 22:1008-1013, 2006.
- Toksavul S, Toman M. A short-term clinical evaluation of IPS Empress 2 crowns. *Int J Prosthodont*, 20:168-172, 2007.
- Walter MH, Wolf BH, Wolf AE, Boening KW. Six-year clinical performance of all-ceramic crowns with alumina cores. *Int J Prosthodont*, 19:162-163, 2006.
- White SN, Miklus VG, McLaren EA, Lang LA, Caputo AA. Flexural strength of a layered zirconia and porcelain dental all-ceramic system. *J Prosthet Dent*, 94:125-131, 2005.
- Zitzmann NU, Galindo ML, Hagmann E, Marinello CP. Clinical evaluation of Procera AllCeram crowns in the anterior and posterior regions. *Int J Prosthodont*, 20:239-241, 2007.

Index

A

B

C

D

E

F

G

H

I

K

L

M

T

V

W

"Those who stop their questioning at 75, 60, even at 30 - cut short their explorations and end up with permanently unfinished lives."

Sidney Poitier

"Our lives begin to end the day we become silent about things that matter."

Martin Luther King, Jr.

The last page does not need to be the end...

Commentary is welcome and invited at dbona@upf.br.

Please use the subject heading "Bonding to Ceramics book".

Your comments will be appreciated.